Injury & Trauma Sourcebook

Learning Disabilities Sourcebook,
2nd Edition

Leukemia Sourcebook

Liver Disorders Sourcebook

Lung Disorders Sourcebook

Medical Tests Sourcebook, 2nd Edition

Men's Health Concerns Sourcebook,
2nd Edition

Mental Health Disorders Sourcebook,
3rd Edition

Mental Retardation Sourcebook

Movement Disorders Sourcebook

Muscular Dystrophy Sourcebook

Obesity Sourcebook

Osteoporosis Sourcebook

Pain Sourcebook, 2nd Edition

Pediatric Cancer Sourcebook

Physical & Mental Issues in Aging
Sourcebook

Podiatry Sourcebook, 2nd Edition

Pregnancy & Birth Sourcebook,
2nd Edition

Prostate Cancer Sourcebook

Prostate & Urological Disorders
Sourcebook

Rehabilitation Sourcebook

Respiratory Diseases & Disorders
Sourcebook

Sexually Transmitted Diseases
Sourcebook, 3rd Edition

Sleep Disorders Sourcebook,
2nd Edition

Smoking Concerns Sourcebook

Sports Injuries Sourcebook, 3rd Edition

Stress-Related Disorders Sourcebook

Stroke Sourcebook

Substance Abuse Sourcebook

Surgery Sourcebook

Thyroid Disorders Sourcebook

Transplantation Sourcebook

Traveler's Health Sourcebook

Urinary Tract & Kidney Diseases &
Disorders Sourcebook, 2nd Edition

Vegetarian Sourcebook

Women's Health Concerns Sourcebook,
2nd Edition

Workplace Health & Safety Sourcebook

Worldwide Health Sourcebook

Teen Health Series

Abuse & Violence Information
for Teens

Alcohol Information for Teens

Allergy Information for Teens

Asthma Information for Teens

Body Information for Teens

Cancer Information for Teens

Complementary & Alternative
Medicine Information for
Teens

Diabetes Information for Teens

Diet Information for Teens,
2nd Edition

Drug Information for Teens,
2nd Edition

Eating Disorders Information
for Teens

Fitness Information for Teens

Learning Disabilities Information
for Teens

Mental Health Information for
Teens, 2nd Edition

Pegnancy Information for Teens

Sexual Health Information for
Teens

Skin Health Information for
Teens

Sports Injuries Information
for Teens

Suicide Information for Teens

Tobacco Information for Teens

Eye Care

SOURCEBOOK

Third Edition

Health Reference Series

Third Edition

Eye Care
SOURCEBOOK

Basic Consumer Health Information about Eye Care and Eye Disorders, Including Facts about the Diagnosis, Prevention, and Treatment of Refractive Disorders, Cataracts, Glaucoma, Macular Degeneration, and Problems Affecting the Cornea, Retina, and Lacrimal Glands

Along with Advice about Preventing Eye Injuries and Tips for Living with Low Vision or Blindness, a Glossary of Related Terms, and Directories of Resources for More Help and Information

Edited by
Amy L. Sutton

Omnigraphics

P.O. Box 31-1640, Detroit, MI 48231

Bibliographic Note
Because this page cannot legibly accommodate all the copyright notices, the Bibliographic
Note portion of the Preface constitutes an extension of the copyright notice.

Edited by Amy L. Sutton

Health Reference Series
Karen Bellenir, *Managing Editor*
David A. Cooke, M.D., *Medical Consultant*
Elizabeth Collins, *Research and Permissions Coordinator*
Cherry Stockdale, *Permissions Assistant*
EdIndex, Services for Publishers, *Indexers*

* * *

Omnigraphics, Inc.
Matthew P. Barbour, *Senior Vice President*
Kay Gill, *Vice President—Directories*
Kevin M. Hayes, *Operations Manager*

* * *

Peter E. Ruffner, *Publisher*

Copyright © 2008 Omnigraphics, Inc.

ISBN 978-0-7808-1000-6

Library of Congress Cataloging-in-Publication Data

Eye care sourcebook : basic consumer health information about eye care and eye
disorders, including facts about the diagnosis, prevention, and treatment of refractive
disorders, cataracts, glaucoma, macular degeneration, and problems affecting the cornea,
retina, and lacrimal glands; along with advice about preventing eye injuries and tips for
living with low vision or blindness, a glossary of related terms, and directories of
resources for more help and information / edited by Amy L. Sutton. -- 3rd ed.
    p. cm. -- (Health reference series)
  Includes bibliographical references and index.
  Summary: "Provides basic consumer health information about the prevention,
diagnosis, and treatment of eye diseases, disorders, and injuries. Includes index,
glossary of related terms, and other resources"--Provided by publisher.
  ISBN 978-0-7808-1000-6 (hardcover : alk. paper) 1. Eye--Diseases--Popular works.
2. Eye--Care and hygiene--Popular works. I. Sutton, Amy L.
  RE51.O64 2008
  617.7--dc22

                                                                    2007045230

Printed in the United States

Table of Contents

Visit www.healthreferenceseries.com to view *A Contents Guide to the Health Reference Series*, a listing of more than 13,000 topics and the volumes in which they are covered.

Part II: Refractive Problems and Procedures

Part V: Macular Degeneration

Part VI: Disorders of the Cornea, Retina, and Lacrimal Glands (Tear Ducts)

Part VII: Eye Infections, Muscular Problems, and Malignancies

Part VIII: Disorders with Eye-Related Complications

Part XI: Additional Help and Information

Preface

About This Book

The National Eye Institute estimates that nearly 14 million children and adults—about 6% of the population—are unable to see clearly due to ophthalmological disorders and diseases. According to vision care researchers, the problem is expected to worsen as the American population ages and the prevalence of low vision and blindness caused by macular degeneration, glaucoma, cataract, diabetic retinopathy, and other common eye diseases increases. Although these eye diseases can be linked to loss of independence and a reduced quality of life, there is hope. Research has shown that regular eye examinations, timely diagnoses, appropriate treatment, and lifestyle changes can correct, prevent, delay, and even cure many vision problems.

Eye Care Sourcebook, Third Edition provides information on the function and structures of the eye, and it describes the prevalence of vision impairment and blindness in the United States. The *Sourcebook* also includes information on corrective therapies and procedures for refractive errors, including contact lenses, eyeglasses, and surgeries. In addition, it details the symptoms, diagnosis, and treatment of cataracts, glaucoma, macular degeneration, corneal and retinal problems, and eye infections. Information about disorders with eye-related complications, such as allergies and diabetic retinopathy, is also included, along with tips on preventing eye injuries, suggestions for people recently diagnosed with vision impairment or blindness, a glossary of terms, and resources for additional help and information.

How to Use This Book

This book is divided into parts and chapters. Parts focus on broad areas of interest. Chapters are devoted to single topics within a part.

Part I: Facts about the Eyes and Eye Diseases and Disorders explains how the eye works, debunks common eye care myths, and provides information to patients preparing for eye examinations. It also offers insight into eye care concerns pertinent to specific populations with special risks, and it describes current initiatives in vision research.

Part II: Refractive Problems and Procedures offers detailed information about common refractive errors, including myopia (nearsightedness), hyperopia (farsightedness), presbyopia, and astigmatism. This part also discusses the correction of refractive errors with contact lenses, eyeglasses, and refractive surgery, including laser-assisted in situ keratomileusis (LASIK), wavefront-guided LASIK, and phakic intraocular lenses.

Part III: Cataracts describes the development and progression of a cataract—the clouding of the eye's lens. Information about cataract treatments, including cataract removal and intraocular lens implantation, is also provided.

Part IV: Glaucoma identifies common risk factors, signs, and symptoms of glaucoma, an eye disorder caused by damage to the optic nerve from too much pressure in the eye. This part highlights mainstream treatments for glaucoma, such as surgery and eyedrop medication, as well as more controversial therapeutic strategies, such as the use of alternative medicine and medical marijuana.

Part V: Macular Degeneration answers common questions about the juvenile and adult forms of macular degeneration, a leading cause of vision loss in the United States. Risk factors, nutritional therapies to halt the progression of the disease, and treatments for both the dry and wet forms of macular degeneration are also discussed.

Part VI: Disorders of the Cornea, Retina, and Lacrimal Glands (Tear Ducts) includes information on a variety of disorders affecting the cornea and retina, including keratoconus, retinal and vitreous detachment, and macular hole and pucker, as well as degenerative retinal disorders. In addition, people dealing with dry eye, floaters, or other problems related to lacrimal dysfunction can find treatment information in this part.

Part VII: Eye Infections, Muscular Problems, and Malignancies describes conjunctivitis (pinkeye), herpetic eye disease, histoplasmosis, blepharitis, and uveitis. It also discusses disorders caused by muscular weakness or imbalance in the eye, such as amblyopia and strabismus, and the types of cancer that can affect the eye.

Part VIII: Disorders with Eye-Related Complications notes the impact that certain health conditions—including allergies, diabetes, traumatic brain injury, and such hereditary disorders as albinism or color blindness—can have on vision and eye health.

Part IX: Protecting Vision by Avoiding Injury identifies steps to take in case of eye emergencies, such as corneal abrasion. Tips on preventing eye injuries at work, during sports, and while participating in outdoor activities are also offered.

Part X: Living with Low Vision or Blindness provides detailed information about low vision devices, low vision centers, and other aids for people with vision loss or impairment. This part also describes state vocational rehabilitation services and offers tips on contacting government service programs for those who are blind or have low vision.

Part XI: Additional Help and Information includes a glossary of important terms, answers to frequently asked questions about eye donation, and directories of libraries that provide information to people with vision-related disabilities and government and private organizations serving people with ophthalmological disorders.

Bibliographic Note

This volume contains documents and excerpts from publications issued by the following U.S. government agencies: Centers for Disease Control and Prevention (CDC); National Cancer Institute (NCI); National Eye Institute (NEI); National Human Genome Research Institute; National Institute of Diabetes, Digestive, and Kidney Diseases (NIDDK); National Institute of Neurological Disorders and Stroke (NINDS); National Institute on Aging (NIA); National Institutes of Health (NIH); Social Security Administration; U.S. Fire Administration; U.S. Food and Drug Administration (FDA); and the U.S. National Library of Medicine.

In addition, this volume contains copyrighted documents from the following organizations and individuals: Access Media Group, L.L.C.; A.D.A.M., Inc.; AMD Alliance International; American Academy of

Ophthalmology; American Foundation for the Blind; American Optometric Association; American Osteopathic Association; Association for Retinopathy of Prematurity and Related Diseases; Cleveland Clinic Cole Eye Institute; Denver Regional Council of Governments; Eye-Bank for Sight Restoration; Eye Surgery Education Council/American Society for Cataract and Refractive Surgery; Foundation Fighting Blindness; Glaucoma Research Foundation; Lighthouse International; Low Vision Centers of Indiana; The Macular Degeneration Partnership; National Federation of the Blind; National Keratoconus Foundation; National Rosacea Society; The Nemours Foundation; Prevent Blindness America; Sjögren's Syndrome Foundation; Trustees of the University of Pennsylvania; University of Connecticut Health Center; and the University of Illinois Eye Center.

Full citation information is provided on the first page of each chapter or section. Every effort has been made to secure all necessary rights to reprint the copyrighted material. If any omissions have been made, please contact Omnigraphics to make corrections for future editions.

Acknowledgements

Thanks go to the many organizations, agencies, and individuals who have contributed materials for this *Sourcebook* and to medical consultant Dr. David Cooke and document engineer Bruce Bellenir. Special thanks go to managing editor Karen Bellenir and research and permissions coordinator Liz Collins for their help and support.

About the Health Reference Series

The *Health Reference Series* is designed to provide basic medical information for patients, families, caregivers, and the general public. Each volume takes a particular topic and provides comprehensive coverage. This is especially important for people who may be dealing with a newly diagnosed disease or a chronic disorder in themselves or in a family member. People looking for preventive guidance, information about disease warning signs, medical statistics, and risk factors for health problems will also find answers to their questions in the *Health Reference Series*. The *Series*, however, is not intended to serve as a tool for diagnosing illness, in prescribing treatments, or as a substitute for the physician/patient relationship. All people concerned about medical symptoms or the possibility of disease are encouraged to seek professional care from an appropriate health care provider.

A Note about Spelling and Style

Health Reference Series editors use *Stedman's Medical Dictionary* as an authority for questions related to the spelling of medical terms and the *Chicago Manual of Style* for questions related to grammatical structures, punctuation, and other editorial concerns. Consistent adherence is not always possible, however, because the individual volumes within the *Series* include many documents from a wide variety of different producers and copyright holders, and the editor's primary goal is to present material from each source as accurately as is possible following the terms specified by each document's producer. This sometimes means that information in different chapters or sections may follow other guidelines and alternate spelling authorities. For example, occasionally a copyright holder may require that eponymous terms be shown in possessive forms (Crohn's disease *vs.* Crohn disease) or that British spelling norms be retained (leukaemia *vs.* leukemia).

Locating Information within the Health Reference Series

The *Health Reference Series* contains a wealth of information about a wide variety of medical topics. Ensuring easy access to all the fact sheets, research reports, in-depth discussions, and other material contained within the individual books of the *Series* remains one of our highest priorities. As the *Series* continues to grow in size and scope, however, locating the precise information needed by a reader may become more challenging.

A Contents Guide to the Health Reference Series was developed to direct readers to the specific volumes that address their concerns. It presents an extensive list of diseases, treatments, and other topics of general interest compiled from the Tables of Contents and major index headings. To access *A Contents Guide to the Health Reference Series*, visit www.healthreferenceseries.com.

Medical Consultant

Medical consultation services are provided to the *Health Reference Series* editors by David A. Cooke, M.D. Dr. Cooke is a graduate of Brandeis University, and he received his M.D. degree from the University of Michigan. He completed residency training at the University of Wisconsin Hospital and Clinics. He is board-certified in Internal Medicine. Dr. Cooke currently works as part of the University of Michigan Health System and practices in Ann Arbor, MI. In his free time, he enjoys writing, science fiction, and spending time with his family.

Our Advisory Board

We would like to thank the following board members for providing guidance to the development of this *Series*:

Health Reference Series *Update Policy*

The inaugural book in the *Health Reference Series* was the first edition of *Cancer Sourcebook* published in 1989. Since then, the *Series* has been enthusiastically received by librarians and in the medical community. In order to maintain the standard of providing high-quality health information for the layperson the editorial staff at Omnigraphics felt it was necessary to implement a policy of updating volumes when warranted.

Medical researchers have been making tremendous strides, and it is the purpose of the *Health Reference Series* to stay current with the most recent advances. Each decision to update a volume is made on an individual basis. Some of the considerations include how much new information is available and the feedback we receive from people who use the books. If there is a topic you would like to see added to the update list, or an area of medical concern you feel has not been adequately addressed, please write to:

Editor
Health Reference Series
Omnigraphics, Inc.
P.O. Box 31-1640
Detroit, MI 48231
E-mail: editorial@omnigraphics.com

Part One

Facts about the Eyes and Eye Diseases and Disorders

Chapter 1

How We See

Chapter Contents

Section 1.1

Eye Anatomy

"How We See," © 2004 University of Illinois Eye Center,
Department of Ophthalmology and Visual Sciences (www.uic.edu/com/eye).
Reprinted with permission.

We all know how important our eyes are, but we may not be familiar with the variety of eye diseases that exist or the terms used to describe them. The following text explains how the eye functions, the different eye diseases and their treatments, advances in ophthalmology, and the types of research being done in this field. This text discusses the basics of how we see.

The main function of the eye is to convert light from the outside world into electrical nerve impulses. These impulses then travel to the part of the brain responsible for vision, where they are interpreted as a visual scene. In the eye, light traverses through the tear film, cornea, anterior chamber, pupil, lens, and vitreous to the retina, which sends the nerve impulses through the optic nerve to the brain. Vision is decreased if any one of these structures is abnormal, is irregularly sized, is not functioning adequately, or is not properly positioned in relation to the others.

To see clearly, the outermost layer, the tear film, must be intact and adequately lubricate the cornea. If the amount of tears produced is less than normal (dry eyes), the eyes will be uncomfortable and vision will be affected. The inadequate production of tears is not uncommon; it may be caused by an isolated problem or by a disease process that affects the entire body.

Beneath the tear film is the cornea, which provides a clear stable structure for the passage of light. The rounded shape of the cornea causes the light rays to bend as they pass through to the anterior chamber. If the cornea is misshapen or becomes cloudy and cannot allow enough light to pass through, then vision is severely hampered.

The anterior chamber is a space between the cornea and the iris (colored part of the eye). It contains fluids that bathe the structures in the front (anterior) part of the eye. If the anterior chamber is too shallow, the iris can move forward and touch the back of the cornea.

4

This abnormal relationship changes the anterior chamber angle (where the cornea and iris meet) and impedes the flow of fluids between the anterior chamber (via the trabecular meshwork in the angle) and the anterior structures. If the fluid cannot enter and exit freely through the trabecular meshwork in the angle, pressure builds up in the eye and glaucoma develops.

In the center of the iris is the pupil, which is an opening that allows light through to the lens. The muscles of the iris regulate the size of the pupil. In bright light the muscles constrict and the pupil becomes smaller; in the dark, the muscles dilate and open the pupil larger to let more light come through. Certain drugs and diseases affect the ability of the pupil to open and close normally.

In back of the pupil is the lens, a clear, pliable structure that changes the angle of the light rays as they enter the eye to focus them on the retina. With aging, changes occur in the lens. It may lose its clarity, and a cataract develops. Commonly, the lens becomes less pliable in a person's early to mid-forties, affecting the ability of the lens

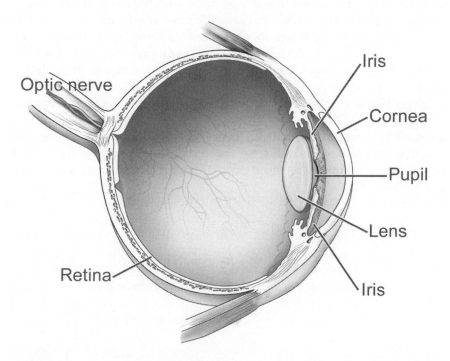

Figure 1.1. The parts and structures of the eye (Source: National Eye Institute, National Institutes of Health).

to focus the light rays, resulting in a need for reading glasses. It also has been shown that the lens helps to filter out ultraviolet light rays, which could damage the retina in the back of the eye.

Between the lens and the retina is another chamber, the vitreous cavity, which contains a clear jelly-like substance called the vitreous. Behind the vitreous is the retina, a paper-thin, delicate tissue that contains the photoreceptors that convert light into electrical signals, as well as other types of cells that process these electrical signals. The retina is often compared to the film in a camera: without it, the camera, or eye, is useless.

When light hits the retina, a photochemical reaction takes place. Electrical impulses develop in the light receptors (rods and cones), the impulses are processed by other cells within the eye, and then they are transmitted to the brain via the optic nerve, which is composed of a group of nerve fibers. When the impulses reach the brain, they are interpreted as a visual scene.

It is the ophthalmologist's job to assess the integrity of all these structures. If you have a specific eye problem, you will be asked to describe it. Many times important clues about your problem can be obtained as you report when the problem began and how it affects your vision. The ophthalmologist then will check your near and distant vision; look at all the structures of your eye to be sure that they are healthy; and check the pressure inside your eye to determine if glaucoma is present.

Even if you don't have a problem with your vision, regular checkups should be part of your normal health care. Examinations should be made by an ophthalmologist every two to three years to maintain healthy eyes. With the many research advances made in the past 20 years, more is able to be done now than in the past to preserve and maintain vision.

Section 1.2

Visual Acuity: What Is 20/20 Vision?

"Visual Acuity: What is 20/20 Vision?" © 2007 American Optometric Association (www.aoa.org). Reprinted with permission.

Visual acuity is only one in a series of factors that evaluate one's vision. 20/20 vision is a term used to express normal visual acuity (the clarity or sharpness of vision) measured at a distance of 20 feet. If you have 20/20 vision, you can see clearly at 20 feet what should normally be seen at that distance. If you have 20/100 vision, it means that you must be as close as 20 feet to see what a person with normal vision can see at 100 feet. 20/20 does not necessarily mean perfect vision. 20/20 vision only indicates the sharpness or clarity of vision at a distance. There are other important vision skills, including peripheral awareness or side vision, eye coordination, depth perception, focusing ability and color vision that contribute to your overall visual ability.

Some people can see well at a distance, but are unable to bring nearer objects into focus. This condition can be caused by hyperopia (farsightedness) or presbyopia (loss of focusing ability). Others can see items that are close, but cannot see those far away. This condition may be caused by myopia (nearsightedness).

A comprehensive eye examination by a doctor of optometry can diagnose those causes, if any, that are affecting your ability to see well. In most cases, your optometrist can prescribe glasses, contact lenses, or a vision therapy program that will help improve your vision. If the reduced vision is due to an eye disease, the use of ocular medication or other treatment may be used.

Chapter 2

Eye Care Facts and Myths

Chapter Contents

Section 2.1

Common Eye Care Myths

"Vision Facts and Myths" was provided by KidsHealth, one of the largest resources online for medically reviewed health information written for kids, teens, and parents. For more articles like this one, visit www.KidsHealth .org, or www.TeensHealth.org. © 2004 The Nemours Foundation. Reviewed by Sharon Lehman, M.D., May 2004.

Old wives' tales abound about the eyes. From watching TV to eating carrots, here's the lowdown on some vision facts and fiction.

MYTH: Sitting too close to the TV is bad for your child's eyes.

FACT: Although parents have been saying this ever since the television first found its way into our living rooms, there's no evidence that plunking down right in front of the television damages a child's eyes. The American Academy of Ophthalmology (AAO) says that kids can actually focus up close without eyestrain better than adults, so they often develop the habit of sitting right in front of the television or holding reading material close to their eyes. However, sitting too close to a TV may indicate that a child is nearsighted.

MYTH: If you cross your eyes, they'll stay that way.

FACT: No, contrary to the old saying, children's eyes will not stay that way if they cross them.

MYTH: If I have poor eyesight, my child will inherit that trait.

FACT: Unfortunately, this one is sometimes true. If you need glasses for good vision or have developed an eye condition (such as cataracts), your child may inherit that same trait. Discuss your family's visual history with your child's doctor.

MYTH: Children should eat carrots to improve their vision.

FACT: Although it's true that carrots are rich in vitamin A, which is essential for sight, many other foods (asparagus, apricots, nectarines, and milk, for example) also contain vitamin A. So, a well-balanced diet can provide the vitamin A needed for good vision, says the AAO.

MYTH: Using computers damages a child's eyes.

FACT: According to the AAO, working on computers won't harm your eyes. However, when using a computer for long periods of time, the eyes blink less than normal (like they do when reading or performing other close work). This makes the eyes dry, which may lead to a feeling of eyestrain or fatigue. So, it's a good idea to make sure your child takes frequent breaks from the computer or video games.

MYTH: Two blue-eyed parents can't produce a child with brown eyes.

FACT: Two blue-eyed parents can have a child with brown eyes, although it's very rare. Likewise, two brown-eyed parents can have a child with blue eyes, although this is also uncommon.

MYTH: Only boys can be color-blind.

FACT: It's estimated that up to 8% of boys have some degree of color blindness, whereas less than 1% of girls have the same condition.

Section 2.2

A Close Look at Eye Exercises

"The See Clearly Method: Do Eye Exercises Improve Vision?," by Rob Murphy, with updates by Marilyn Haddrill, is reprinted with permission from www.allaboutvision.com. © 2006 Access Media Group, LLC.

The first thing you want to know about a self-help program is whether it works. Before you spend time and money on a program of eye exercises such as the See Clearly Method, which once was widely advertised on radio stations and the Internet, you want to find out for yourself the likelihood that such methods might "eliminate or reduce your need for glasses and contacts."

In November 2006, an Iowa district court halted all sales of See Clearly Method kits that for several years were marketed as a way of using eye exercises to improve vision. The court ordered the Iowa company selling the kits to pay $200,000 into a restitution fund for consumers allegedly duped into buying the kits through misleading advertising. The Iowa Attorney General's office currently is developing a method of paying out restitution.

"We are confident this puts an end to this Iowa-based program of consumer fraud," Iowa Attorney General Tom Miller said in a press release. "It prevents there being any more victims, and it fences in the perpetrators so they cannot perpetrate similar consumer fraud in the future with respect to eye products or any other kind of products." (See more in the news update below)

On the See Clearly Method's website (seeclearlymethod.com), you searched in vain for any statement that the program actually worked. No word promoting the product—a regimen developed by four doctors from the American Vision Institute (AVI)—promised anything. (AVI licensed the See Clearly method to Vision Improvement Technologies, Inc., which in recent years marketed the program.)

Yet, the website also told you that the do-it-yourself vision-improvement plan was a "safe, healthy alternative to glasses, contacts, and even laser surgery." But then a disclaimer on the site noted, "The rate at which your eyesight improves as a result of the See Clearly Method and the extent of that improvement, if any, will vary among individuals." This was the most definite statement to be found on the site.

With no way of knowing whether it worked, purchasers bought the product on faith. The Iowa Attorney General's office said the company charged customers about $350 retail for each of the 5,000 to 10,000 kits sold monthly. People wanting to return the kits for a refund encountered difficulty getting through to a company representative. In the aftermath of the See Clearly Method investigation and details revealed about the company's business practices, even the most fervent of the faithful devoted to eye exercises would be well advised to learn all they can about any programs making similar claims without solid scientific basis.

News Alert: Iowa District Court Halts All Sales of See Clearly Method Kits

DES MOINES, Iowa, November 2006—An Iowa District Court has stopped all sales of See Clearly Method vision improvement kits, after hearing evidence in a consumer fraud lawsuit filed by Iowa Attorney General Tom Miller.

The court also ordered the company selling the See Clearly kits, Vision Improvement Technologies, Inc. in Fairfield, Iowa, to pay $200,000 into a restitution fund that will be used to repay customers who bought kits.

In the lawsuit, Miller accused the company marketing the See Clearly Method of making "dramatic claims for its product that could not be substantiated."

A Vision Improvements Technologies Inc. representative told AllAboutVision.com in early 2006 that the company was targeted after it became high profile, and that consumers have a right to know about natural alternatives for vision correction.

But Miller alleged in the lawsuit that the company "used a combination of misleading and unfair marketing tactics to sell their kits," including "exaggerated claims of effectiveness, false implications of scientific validity, and misleading consumer testimonials in advertising." People paid several hundred dollars each for the kits after, according to the lawsuit, "See Clearly telemarketers . . . made representations to prospective customers that grossly exaggerate the effectiveness of the method."

How Was the See Clearly Method Supposed to Work?

The basic version of the See Clearly Method included three videotapes, three audiotapes, an instruction manual, a daily progress chart, and other materials. The deluxe version included a CD-ROM.

You supposedly could get your money back within 30 days of your purchase if you were not satisfied. Presumably you were supposed to see some improvement by then.

A fundamental premise of vision therapy is that refractive disorders such as myopia (nearsightedness) and hyperopia (farsightedness) have both hereditary and environmental causes, such as nearpoint stress from reading. Certain eye exercises are designed to relieve so-called spasm of accommodation, believed to be an environmentally induced disruption of the eye's focusing capacity. Other exercises are said to improve the eyes' coordination or to straighten misaligned eyes. It's important to note that while many people think of such eye exercises as vision therapy, most vision therapists do not wish to be associated with self-directed programs.

The See Clearly Method had you do 30 minutes of exercises a day to strengthen and enhance the flexibility of the muscles that govern the eye's focusing power and control its movements. Six of the activities were described as "new visual habits." One, for example, had you hold a finger up as you varied your focus back and forth from the finger to a distant object.

Then there were 10 "booster techniques," designed to "address problems or encourage faster progress," according to the instruction manual. The "blur reading" technique, for example, had you turn a magazine upside-down at a distance from which the words were blurry. You were then supposed to select a word and run your gaze around it, and if you could pick out any letters, run your gaze around them. Each of the exercises might take two to four minutes. You recorded your progress in the journal that came with the kit.

The instruction manual recommended personal affirmations to help you along. You might remind yourself, for example, "I am seeing better each day." If you were having any doubts, you might declare, "I can see without my glasses." For a vaguer standard of success, you could simply say, "I feel positive changes in my vision taking place."

"Visualization" also came into play. Three of the booster techniques were holdovers from a vision-therapy regimen developed in the 1920s by maverick New York City ophthalmologist William Horatio Bates, M.D. Light therapy, a takeoff on Bates's technique of "sunning," has you sit with your eyes closed and your face six inches from an unshaded 150-watt bulb, just far enough to make your eyes "pleasantly warm but not too hot," according to the manual. Meanwhile, the manual suggested that you "repeat your affirmation and visualize your inner lens becoming more flexible and the ciliary muscle more powerful. Visualize the eyeball transforming into a better shape."

The "palming" technique had you close your eyes and rest them against your palms, while "hydrotherapy" had you alternately placing hot- and cold-water-soaked towels against your eyes. Affirmations and visualization were said to help with these techniques as well.

As (or if) your vision improved, you were encouraged to obtain progressively weaker corrective lenses until you no longer required correction or you enjoyed the maximum improvement. You were advised that patching one eye could be necessary if the fellow eye lagged in its expected improvement.

Does This Type of Eye Exercise Method Ever Work?

A long-standing criticism of eye exercises, coming from both mainstream optometrists as well as from eye surgeons, is the absence of reliable evidence that eye exercises can reduce your reliance on corrective lenses at all, let alone eliminate it. The medical literature lacks well-controlled clinical studies—with strict scientific criteria including carefully matched comparison populations—showing that they effectively treat myopia or hyperopia.

David W. Muris, O.D., one of the four doctors who developed the See Clearly Method, himself conducted what he called a "clinical evaluation" of the product in his Sacramento, California, practice during the fall of 1999. "The investors just wanted some due diligence and some people to actually go through this," Muris said in an interview. "They didn't want to require anything scientific."

According to Muris, the evaluation involved 21 people ages 14 to 80 with mild myopia (less than -3.00 diopters). After six weeks of therapy, nine of the 21 had "significant" improvement and 11 had "moderate" improvement in visual acuity. Seven eliminated their need for glasses or contacts, he said, while 11 had "reduced dependency," meaning they needed their corrective lenses for less time than before. AllAboutVision.com conducted its own decidedly unscientific evaluation of the See Clearly Method when a staffer gave it a try and experienced no vision improvement.

Defiantly Occupying the Fringe

Eye exercise programs occupy a nebulous space somewhere between medical science and folk remedy. Most optometrists and ophthalmologists are dismissive of them.

The See Clearly Method's advocates not only acknowledged the fringe status of the program, but they regarded that position as a virtue. From the instruction manual, we learned that, "In the history of medicine, new ideas have often been resisted by those schooled in traditional methods." We were told that the decision to wear glasses or contacts— for the present purposes defined as "crutches"—borders on the mentally unsound: "Certainly, except for diseases and injuries for which there is no cure, nobody in their right mind would willingly accept a condition that compromises the ability to function and enjoy life, or to be dependent on crutches forever."

The number of corrective-lens haters is open to debate, but Levi Meeske, a 25-year-old job-placement counselor in Atlanta, found his contact lenses sufficiently loathsome to give the See Clearly Method a try. Six weeks after starting the program, he was delighted, he said, with his visual improvement. The refractive error in his right eye had improved modestly from -3.25 to -3.00 diopters, while his left eye remained stable at -3.75 diopters.

Meeske still needed contacts lest his world appear blurry. "But when they are in, I can see farther—as I'm looking at buildings or at trees, the amount of detail that I'm able to pick up has greatly increased," he said. "Looking at grass, looking at flowers, the colors are much more vibrant."

Keep in mind, however, that the Iowa Attorney General's office found in company records that far more unhappy customers wrote in about their results, and that positive letters were "relatively scarce."

Learn to Temper Your Expectations about Eye Exercises

Anyone wishing to market a self-improvement program has to strike a delicate balance between attracting buyers and overselling the product's benefits. As a consumer, it pays to be careful. Do your homework by reading up on the program and others like it.

If you're interested in a home program like the See Clearly Method, it makes sense first to get an evaluation and professional opinion from an eye care practitioner to see if you might benefit from this approach.

The best advice with any self-directed eye exercise program may be to keep your expectations in check—and, as the court has directed in the case of See Clearly, your money in your wallet.

Chapter 3

Preparing for an Eye Exam: What You Need to Know

Eye care experts recommend that everyone have a complete eye exam every one to three years, depending on age, risk factors, and physical condition.

Children

Some experts estimate that approximately one in 20 preschool children and one in four school-aged children have an eye problem that could cause permanent vision loss if left untreated. Children without symptoms and who are at low risk for eye problems should have their eyes screened by six months of age, then examined at age three and again at the start of school. Risk-free children should then continue to have their eyes examined at least every two years throughout school.

Any child who does have risk factors for vision problems may need to have more frequent eye exams. Some examples of common risk factors include:

- prematurity;
- developmental delays;
- turned or crossed eyes;
- family history of eye disease;

"Preparing for an Eye Exam," by Dr. Jennifer Palombi, is reprinted with permission from www.allaboutvision.com. © 2007 Access Media Group, LLC.

- history of eye injury; or
- other physical illness or disease.

According to the American Optometric Association (AOA), children who wear eyeglasses or contact lenses need to be seen annually to keep their prescriptions current.

Adults

The AOA also recommends an annual eye exam for any adult who wears eyeglasses or contacts. If you don't normally need vision correction, you still need an eye exam every two to three years up to the age of 40, depending on your rate of visual change and overall health. Doctors often recommend more frequent examinations for adults with diabetes, high blood pressure, and other disorders, because many diseases can have an impact on the health of your eyes.

If you are over 40, it's a good idea to have your eyes examined every one to two years to check for common age-related eye problems such as presbyopia, cataracts, and macular degeneration.

Because the risk of eye disease continues to increase with advancing age, everyone over the age of 60 should be examined annually. The American Optometric Association provides general guidelines. Ask your eye care professional what interval is right for you.

Who Should I See for My Eye Exam?

There are three different kinds of eye care professionals: ophthalmologists, optometrists, and opticians. Who you should see depends on your needs.

Ophthalmologists are medical doctors (M.D.s or D.O.s) who specialize in eye care. Not only do they prescribe eyeglasses and contacts, but they also perform eye surgery and treat medical conditions of the eye. Ophthalmologists are doctors who have received 12 or more years of training.

Optometrists (O.D.s) are eye doctors who can prescribe glasses and contacts and treat medical conditions of the eye with eyedrops and other medicines. Optometrists generally receive eight or more years of training. Optometrists prescribe glasses, contacts, low-vision aids, vision therapy, and medication to treat eye diseases, as well as perform certain minor surgical procedures.

Opticians are not doctors, but eye care professionals who adjust and repair glasses, instruct patients in contact lens use, and grind and assemble spectacles. In some cases, specially trained opticians can determine your prescription and fit contact lenses. Opticians generally receive their training either "on the job" by apprenticeship or from technical schools.

Annual Exams: Here's Why

You may be surprised to know that there is no universal standard for the frequency of eye exams. Recommendations differ among individual eye doctors, as well as among the various professional associations (American Optometric Association, American Academy of Ophthalmology, etc.).

Those who advocate annual exams instead of less frequent ones do so because eyes can change very quickly, in ways that only an eye doctor may detect. And the earlier an eye condition is caught, the earlier treatment can begin.

All of these groups agree on this: everyone needs regular, comprehensive eye exams. Don't rely on vision screenings, because they are not complete. And don't let monetary considerations keep you from getting an exam. Programs are available to help pay for eye care.

How Much Does an Eye Exam Cost?

Eye exams are available everywhere, from discount outlets to surgical offices, so the fees can vary widely. Additionally, fees can vary depending upon the type of eye care professional that you are seeing and the type of services that you are requesting.

Generally speaking, contact lens exams cost more than eyeglass exams. Likewise, there is often an additional or higher fee for services such as laser surgery evaluations, specialty pediatric testing, and complex contact lens fits.

The best way to be an educated consumer is to ask your eye care professional what his or her fees are at the time you make your appointment. Be sure that you are getting a comprehensive eye exam for your money. A basic comprehensive eye examination should consist of the following:

- a review of personal and family health history;
- evaluation of your vision at distance and near (e.g., determining that you have 20/400 vision);
- evaluation for the presence of nearsightedness, farsightedness,

19

astigmatism, and presbyopia (e.g., determining the cause of your 20/400 vision and what prescription will correct it);

- evaluation of your eyes' ability to work together; and

- internal and external eye health examination.

Many insurance plans cover at least a portion of eye exam services. Check to see what your benefits are and what doctors participate in your plan before you make an appointment. Then be sure to let the doctor's office know that you'll be using insurance.

What Information Should I Take with Me to My Eye Exam?

It is important to have some basic information available at the time of your eye examination. First, be sure to have a copy of your vision insurance card if you will be using it for a portion of your fees. Additionally, the eye doctor will need some basic information in order to fully evaluate your eyes. Take your most recent prescription glasses and/or contact lenses with you.

The doctor will also need to know your complete health history as well as that of your family. Take a list of all prescription medications that you take, including dosages.

Finally, have a list of questions or concerns that you would like to discuss with the doctor and be sure to let him know at the start of the exam if you are interested in specialty services such as contact lens fitting or laser surgery evaluation.

Chapter 4

Financial Aid for Eye Care

Many state and national resources regularly provide aid to people with vision problems. The National Eye Institute, which supports eye research, does not help individuals pay for eye care. However, if you are in need of financial aid to assess or treat an eye problem, you might contact one or more of the following programs.

You may also contact a social worker at a local hospital or other community agency. Social workers often are knowledgeable about community resources that can help people facing financial and medical problems.

Eye Exams and Surgery

- **EyeCare America**, a public service foundation of the American Academy of Ophthalmology (AAO). Provides comprehensive eye exams and care for up to one year, often at no out-of-pocket expense to eligible callers through its seniors and Diabetes EyeCare Programs. Its Glaucoma EyeCare Program provides a glaucoma eye exam. The EyeCare America Children's EyeCare Program educates parents and primary care providers about the importance of early childhood (newborn through 36 months of age) eye care. Telephone: 800-222-EYES (3937). Website: www.eyecareamerica .org.

"Financial Aid for Eye Care," from the National Eye Institute (NEI, www.nei.nih.gov), part of the National Institutes of Health, February 2007.

- **VISION USA**, coordinated by the American Optometric Association (AOA), provides free eye care to uninsured, low-income workers and their families. Telephone: 800-766-4466. Website: www.aoa.org.

- **Lions Clubs International** provides financial assistance to individuals for eye care through local clubs. A local club can be found by using the "club locator" button found on their website at www.LionsClubs.org. If you are unable to find your local Lions club, contact the LCIF Grant Programs Department at (630) 571-5466 x393.

- **Mission Cataract USA**, coordinated by the Volunteer Eye Surgeons' Association, is a program providing free cataract surgery to people of all ages who have no other means to pay. Surgeries are scheduled annually on one day, usually in May. Telephone: 800-343-7265. Website: www.missioncataractUSA.org.

- **Knights Templar Eye Foundation** provides assistance for eye surgery for people who are unable to pay or receive adequate assistance from current government agencies or similar sources. Mailing address: 1000 East State Parkway, Suite I, Schaumburg, IL 60173. Telephone: (847) 490-3838. Website: www.knightstemplar.org/ktef.

- **National Keratoconus Assistance Foundation** provides financial support to patients who need surgical and optometric treatment for keratoconus and other corneal problems. This organization does not have a phone number available to the public. Website: www.nkcaf.org.

- **InfantSEE®** is a public health program designed to ensure early detection of eye conditions in babies. Member optometrists provide a free comprehensive infant eye assessment to children younger than one year. Telephone: 888-396-3937. Website: www.infantsee.org.

Eyeglasses

- **Sight for Students**, a Vision Service Plan (VSP) program, provides eye exams and glasses to children 18 years and younger whose families cannot afford vision care. Telephone: 888-290-4964. Website: www.sightforstudents.org.

- **New Eyes for the Needy** provides vouchers for the purchase of new prescription eyeglasses. Mailing address: 549 Millburn

Avenue, P.O. Box 332, Short Hills, NJ 07078-0332. Telephone: (973) 376-4903. E-mail: neweyesfortheneedy@verizon.net. Website: www.neweyesfortheneedy.org.

Prescription Drugs

- **The Medicine Program** assists people to enroll in one or more of the many patient assistance programs that provide prescription medicine free of charge to those in need. Patients must meet the sponsor's criteria. The program is conducted in cooperation with the patient's doctor. Mailing Address: P.O. Box 4182, Poplar Bluff, MO 63902-4182. Telephone: 866-694-3893. E-mail: help@themedicineprogram.com. Website: www .themedicineprogram.com.

- **Partnership for Prescription Assistance** offers a single point of access to more than 475 public and private patient assistance programs, including more than 150 programs offered by pharmaceutical companies. Telephone: 888-477-2669. Website: https://www.pparx.org.

Government Programs

Medicare Benefit for Eye Exams

- **For People with Diabetes:** People with Medicare who have diabetes can get a dilated eye exam to check for diabetic eye disease. Your doctor will decide how often you need this exam.

- **For People at Risk for Glaucoma:** Glaucoma is a leading cause of vision loss. People at high risk for glaucoma include those with diabetes or a family history of glaucoma, or African Americans age 50 or older. Medicare will pay for an eye exam to check for glaucoma once every 12 months. Patients must pay 20 percent of the Medicare-approved amount after the yearly Part B deductible. Telephone: 800-633-4227. Website: www.medicare.gov.

State Children's Health Insurance Program (SCHIP)

- For little or no cost, this insurance pays for doctor visits, prescription medicines, hospitalizations, and much more for children 18 years and younger. Most states also cover the cost of dental care, eye care, and medical equipment. Telephone: 877-

543-7669. Insure Kids Now! Website: www.insurekidsnow.gov/states.htm.

Chapter 5

All about Eye Care Professionals

Chapter Contents

Section 5.1

Eye Care Professionals:
Their Education, Training, and Practice

"Eye Care Professional: Their Education, Training, and Practice" is reprinted with permission from the Eye Surgery Education Council, an initiative of the American Society for Cataract and Refractive Surgery, © 2003.

Many patients and consumers are confused about the qualifications of the eye care professionals who serve them.

Perhaps the greatest area of confusion is the distinction between an optometrist and an ophthalmologist. In the simplest of terms, an ophthalmologist is a medical doctor who specializes in treating the eye. An optometrist is a non-medical practitioner who has completed a postgraduate study program to provide a variety of eye care services.

Differences in the education and training of health care professionals are important because they affect the quality and level of care patients receive. However, state-level lawmakers frequently determine the scope of practice—the variety of services a health care practitioner can provide, the range of drugs, therapies, and surgery, etc. Therefore, when considering their health care/eye care options, patients should be mindful of the provider's training and qualifications.

The following are more detailed descriptions drawn from the U.S. Department of Labor, Bureau of Labor Statistics (BLS), of the education, training and areas of practice of ophthalmologists, optometrists, and opticians.

Ophthalmologists

It takes many years of education and training to become a physician: 4 years of undergraduate school, 4 years of medical school, and 3 to 8 years of internship and residency, depending on the specialty selected.

Premedical students must complete undergraduate work in physics, biology, mathematics, English, and inorganic and organic chemistry.

Students also take courses in the humanities and the social sciences.

The minimum educational requirement for entry into a medical school is 3 years of college; most applicants, however, have at least a bachelor's degree. Acceptance to medical school is highly competitive.

Students spend most of the first 2 years of medical school in laboratories and classrooms, taking courses such as anatomy, biochemistry, physiology, pharmacology, psychology, microbiology, pathology, medical ethics, and laws governing medicine.

Ophthalmologists also learn to take medical histories, examine patients, and diagnose illnesses. During their last 2 years, students work with patients under the supervision of experienced physicians in hospitals and clinics, learning acute, chronic, preventive, and rehabilitative care. Through rotations in internal medicine, family practice, obstetrics and gynecology, pediatrics, psychiatry, and surgery, they gain experience in the diagnosis and treatment of illness.

Following medical school, almost all M.D.s enter a residency-graduate medical education in a specialty that takes the form of paid on-the-job training, usually in a hospital.

Physicians are licensed by the states. To be licensed, physicians must graduate from an accredited medical school, pass a licensing examination, and complete 1 to 7 years of graduate medical education. To maintain their license, they must fulfill continuing medical education requirements each year.

M.D.s seeking board certification in a specialty may spend up to 7 years in residency training, depending on the specialty. A final examination immediately after residency or after 1 or 2 years of practice also is necessary for certification by the American Board of Medical Specialists. There are 24 specialty boards, one of which is in ophthalmology. For certification in a subspecialty, physicians usually need another 1 to 2 years of residency.

Surgeons are physicians who specialize in the treatment of injury, disease, and deformity through operations. Using a variety of instruments, and with patients under general or local anesthesia, a surgeon corrects physical deformities, repairs tissue after injuries, or performs preventive surgeries on patients with debilitating diseases or disorders.

Although a large number perform general surgery, many surgeons choose to specialize in a specific area, one of which is ophthalmology. Like primary care and other specialist physicians, surgeons also examine patients, perform and interpret diagnostic tests, and counsel patients on preventive health care.

Optometrists

Optometrists, also known as doctors of optometry, or ODs, provide most primary vision care. Most optometrists complete a four-year bachelor's degree before beginning the four-year program at a college of optometry leading to the doctor of optometry (O.D.) degree. About 10 percent complete an additional resident or postgraduate program in a particular area of interest, according to the American Optometric Association (AOA). Optometrists do not attend a medical school, and they are not medical doctors.

Optometrists examine people's eyes to diagnose vision problems and eye diseases, and they test patients' visual acuity, depth and color perception, and ability to focus and coordinate their eyes. Optometrists prescribe eyeglasses and contact lenses and provide vision therapy and low-vision rehabilitation. Optometrists analyze test results and develop a treatment plan. Optometrists often provide preoperative and postoperative care to cataract patients, as well as patients who have had laser vision correction or other eye surgery. They also diagnose conditions due to systemic diseases such as diabetes and high blood pressure, referring patients to other health practitioners as needed. Most optometrists are in general practice, according to the BLS.

Optometrists administer drugs for diagnostic and therapeutic purposes, privileges they have obtained largely through legislative efforts over the past two decades. Some of their professional societies are seeking permission from state regulatory authorities to perform surgical therapies.

Opticians

Employers usually hire individuals with no eye care educational background as an optician or those who have worked as ophthalmic laboratory technicians. The employers then provide the required training.

Most dispensing opticians receive training on the job or through apprenticeships lasting 2 or more years. Some employers seek people with postsecondary (beyond high school) training in the field. In the 21 states that require dispensing opticians to be licensed, individuals without postsecondary training work from 2 to 4 years as apprentices. Apprenticeship or formal training is offered in most states as well. Formal training in the field is offered in community colleges and a few colleges and universities.

Dispensing opticians may apply to the American Board of Opticianry (ABO) and the National Contact Lens Examiners (NCLE) for certification, which must be renewed every 3 years through continuing education.

Training usually includes instruction in optical mathematics, optical physics, and the use of precision measuring instruments and other machinery and tools.

Under the supervision of an experienced optician, optometrist, or ophthalmologist, apprentices work directly with patients, fitting eyeglasses and contact lenses.

Section 5.2

Finding an Eye Care Professional

From the National Eye Institute (NEI, www.nei.nih.gov), part of the National Institutes of Health, December 2006.

The National Eye Institute does not provide referrals or recommend specific eye care professionals. However, you may wish to consider the following ways of finding a professional to provide your eye care. You can:

- Ask family members and friends about eye care professionals they use.

- Ask your family doctor for the name of a local eye care specialist.

- Call the department of ophthalmology or optometry at a nearby hospital or university medical center.

- Contact a state or county association of ophthalmologists or optometrists. These groups, usually called academies or societies, may have lists of eye care professionals with specific information on specialty and experience.

- Contact your insurance company or health plan to learn whether it has a list of eye care professionals that are covered under your plan.

At a bookstore or library, check on available journals and books about choosing a physician and medical treatment. A library reference specialist can help you identify books on finding health care professionals. Here are some examples:

- Most large libraries have the reference set *The ABMS Compendium of Certified Medical Professionals*, which lists board-certified ophthalmologists, each with a small amount of biographical information.

- Each year usually in August the magazine *U.S. News and World Report* features an article that rates hospitals in the United States.

- The *Consumer's Guide to Top Doctors* provides a state-by-state listing of medical specialists most frequently mentioned in a survey of doctors.

For More Information

- The American Academy of Ophthalmology coordinates Find an Eye MD, an online listing of member ophthalmologists practicing in the United States and abroad. This service is designed to help the general public locate ophthalmologists within a specific region. This service is available via the Internet at: http://www .aao.org/eyemd_disclaimer.cfm.

- The American Optometric Association offers Dr. Locator, an online listing of member optometrists. This service is designed to help the general public locate optometrists within a specific region. This service is available via the Internet at: http://www .aoa.org.

- The International Society of Refractive Surgery maintains comprehensive directory of surgeons around the world who are currently performing refractive surgery. Telephone: (415) 561-8581. Website: http://www.locateanisrsdoctor.com.

- Administrators in Medicine and the Association of State Medical Board Executive Directors have launched DocFinder, an online database that helps consumers learn whether any malpractice actions have been taken against a particular doctor. The site provides links to the licensing boards in the participating states. This service is available via the Internet: http://www.docboard.org.

- The American Association of Eye and Ear Hospitals (AAEEH) is comprised of the premier centers for specialized eye and ear procedures in the world. Association members are major referral centers that offer some of the most innovative teaching programs and routinely treat the most severely ill eye and ear patients. Telephone: 703-243-8848. A list of member facilities is available online at http://www.aaeeh.org/locations.html.

- The American Medical Association's Physician Select provides basic professional information on virtually every licensed physician in the United States and its territories. You can limit your search to include only ophthalmologists. This service is available via the Internet: http://www.ama-assn.org/aps/amahg.htm.

Section 5.3

Talking to Your Doctor

From the National Eye Institute (NEI, www.nei.nih.gov), part of the National Institutes of Health, August 2002. Reviewed by David A. Cooke, M.D., July 2007.

Today, patients take an active role in their health care. You and your doctor will work in partnership to achieve your best possible level of health. An important part of this relationship is good communication. Here are some questions you can ask your doctor to get your discussion started.

About My Disease or Disorder

- What is my diagnosis?
- What caused my condition?
- Can my condition be treated?
- How will this condition affect my vision now and in the future?
- Should I watch for any particular symptoms and notify you if they occur?
- Should I make any lifestyle changes?

About My Treatment

- What is the treatment for my condition?

- When will the treatment start, and how long will it last?

- What are the benefits of this treatment, and how successful is it?

- What are the risks and side effects associated with this treatment?

- Are there foods, drugs, or activities I should avoid while I'm on this treatment?

- If my treatment includes taking a medication, what should I do if I miss a dose?

- Are other treatments available?

About My Tests

- What kinds of tests will I have?

- What do you expect to find out from these tests?

- When will I know the results?

- Do I have to do anything special to prepare for any of the tests?

- Do these tests have any side effects or risks?

- Will I need more tests later?

Understanding your doctor's responses is essential to good communication. Here are a few more tips:

- If you don't understand your doctor's responses, ask questions until you do understand.

- Take notes, or get a friend or family member to take notes for you. Or, bring a recorder to assist in your recollection of the discussion.

- Ask your doctor to write down his or her instructions to you.

- Ask your doctor for printed material about your condition.

- If you still have trouble understanding your doctor's answers, ask where you can go for more information.

- Other members of your health care team, such as nurses and pharmacists, can be good sources of information. Talk to them, too.

Chapter 6

Eye Care and Vision Concerns in Children

Chapter Contents

Section 6.1

How Your Child's Vision Develops

The wonders of the world are often first encountered through the eyes of a child. Yet without good vision, a child's ability to learn about the world becomes more difficult. Vision problems affect one in 20 preschoolers and one in four school-age children. Since many vision problems begin at an early age, it is very important that children receive proper eye care. Untreated eye problems can worsen and lead to other serious problems as well as affect learning ability, personality, and adjustment in school.

Development of Vision

Newborns

The acuity (sharpness of vision) of newborns is less than fully developed. They usually prefer looking at close objects, and are especially attracted to faces and by objects that are brightly colored or of high contrast and moving.

Three Months

By this age, most babies can smoothly follow a moving object and can hold their eyes on it even when the object stops. The colors, details, and moving parts of mobiles in cribs fascinate infants and help stimulate their visual development.

Three to Six Months

By now, the retina of the eye is quite well developed, and the baby's visual acuity is good enough to permit small details to be seen. The infant is able to look from near to far and back to near again. Judgment of distances (depth perception) is also developing.

Six Months

At 6 months of age, the eye has reached about two thirds of its adult size. Usually by this stage, the two eyes are fully working together, resulting in good binocular vision. Distance vision and depth perception are still improving.

One Year Old

By the age of one, a child's vision is well on its way toward full development. Coordination of the eyes with the hands and body are naturally practiced by children and can be enhanced by games involving pointing, grasping, tossing, placing, and catching.

Two to Five Years Old

The preschooler is typically eager to draw and look at pictures. Stories connected to pictures, drawings, and symbols often captivate the child and help to coordinate hearing and vision.

Section 6.2

Overview of Children's Vision Concerns

"Your Child's Vision" was provided by KidsHealth, one of the largest resources online for medically reviewed health information written for kids, teens, and parents. For more articles like this one, visit www.KidsHealth.org, or www.TeensHealth.org © 2004 The Nemours Foundation. Reviewed by Sharon Lehman, M.D., May 2004.

There's nothing quite like looking into your child's eyes. But while you're busy gazing at your young one, be sure to pay attention to his or her eyesight. Early detection and treatment of eye problems are essential to a child's visual health.

Check It Out

Children don't have to be able to talk to have eye examinations. Most pediatric eye doctors (ophthalmologists and optometrists) use devices such as hand puppets to evaluate vision in young children. An ophthalmologist is a medical doctor who specializes in examining, diagnosing, and treating eyes and eye diseases, whereas an optometrist has been trained to diagnose and treat many of the same eye conditions as ophthalmologists, except for treatments involving surgery.

So when does your child need to have the first eye examination? The American Academy of Ophthalmology recommends the following:

- Newborns should be checked for general eye health by a pediatrician or family physician in the hospital nursery.

- High-risk newborns (including premature infants), those with a family history of eye problems, and those with obvious eye irregularities should be examined by an eye doctor.

- In the first year of life, all infants should be routinely screened for eye health during well-baby visits with their doctors.

- Around the age of 3½, children should undergo eye health screenings and visual acuity tests (or tests that measure sharpness of vision) with their doctors.

- Around the age of 5, children should have their vision and eye alignment evaluated by their doctors. Children who fail either test should be examined by an eye doctor.

- After age 5, further screening exams should be conducted at routine checks at school or at your child's doctor's office or after the appearance of symptoms such as squinting or frequent headaches. (Many times, a teacher will realize the child isn't seeing well in class.)

However, children who wear prescription glasses or contacts probably need annual checkups to screen for vision changes.

Signs that a young child may have vision problems include:

- constant eye rubbing;
- extreme light sensitivity;
- poor focusing;
- poor visual tracking (following an object);
- abnormal alignment or movement of the eyes (after 6 months of age);
- chronic redness of the eyes;

- chronic tearing of the eyes; or
- a white pupil instead of black.

In school-age children, watch for other signs such as:

- inability to see objects at a distance;
- inability to read the blackboard;
- squinting;
- difficulty reading; or
- sitting too close to the TV.

It's also a good idea to watch your child for evidence of poor vision or crossed eyes. If you detect any evidence of eye conditions, your child should be examined immediately so that the problem doesn't become permanent. If caught early, eye conditions can often be reversed.

Newborn Vision

It's difficult to measure how well a newborn can see, but it's esti-mated that a newborn's vision is quite blurry until about 6 months of age. After that, vision rapidly improves. Infants then develop what's called "stereo vision," that is, they combine the picture they see with one eye with the picture they see with their other eye. Babies will start developing depth perception by doing such things as looking directly at the faces of their parents.

Common Eye Problems

There are several eye conditions that may affect children. Most of them are detected by a vision screening using an acuity chart during the preschool years.

- **Amblyopia (lazy eye)** is poor vision in an eye that appears to be normal. Two common causes are crossed eyes and a difference in the refractive error between the two eyes. If untreated, amblyo-pia can cause irreversible visual loss in the affected eye. (By then, the brain's "programming" will ignore signals from that eye.) Am-blyopia is best treated during the preschool years.

- **Strabismus** is a misalignment of the eyes; they may turn in, out, up, or down. If the same eye is chronically misaligned, am-blyopia may develop in that eye. With early detection, vision can be restored by patching the properly aligned eye, which forces the misaligned one to work. Surgery or specially designed glasses may also help the eyes to align.

- **Refractive errors** mean that the shape of the eye doesn't refract, or bend, light properly, so images appear blurred. Refractive errors may also cause eyestrain and/or amblyopia. The most common form of refractive error is nearsightedness; others include farsightedness and astigmatism.

- **Nearsightedness** is poor distance vision (also called myopia), which is usually treated with glasses or contacts.

- **Farsightedness** is poor near vision (also called hyperopia), which is usually treated with glasses or contacts.

- **Astigmatism** is imperfect curvature of the front surface of the eye. It's usually treated with glasses if it causes blurred vision or discomfort.

Other eye conditions require immediate attention, such as **retinopathy of prematurity** (a disease that usually affects premature infants who were on a ventilator for a long period of time after birth) and those associated with a family history, including the following:

- **Retinoblastoma** is a malignant tumor that usually appears in the first 3 years of life. The affected eye may have visual loss and whiteness in the pupil.

- **Infantile cataracts** can occur in newborns. A cataract is a gradual clouding of the eye's lens.

- **Congenital glaucoma** in infants is a rare condition that may be inherited. It is the result of incorrect or incomplete development of the eye drainage canals during the prenatal period. Congenital glaucoma can be treated with medication and surgery.

- **Genetic or metabolic diseases of the eye**, such as inherited disorders that make a child more likely to develop retinoblastoma or cataracts, may make it necessary for a child to have an eye exam at an early age and regular screenings.

Be sure to talk to your child's doctor if your child is at risk for any of these conditions.

Glasses and Contacts

Children of all ages—even babies—can wear glasses and contacts. Keep these tips in mind for a child who wears glasses:

- Allow your child to pick his or her own frames.

- Plastic frames are best for kids younger than 2.

- If older children wear metal frames, make sure they have spring hinges, which are more durable.

- An elastic strap attached to the glasses will help keep them in place for active toddlers.

- Children with severe eye problems may need special lenses called high-index lenses that are thinner and lighter than plastic lenses.

- Polycarbonate lenses are recommended for children, especially those who play sports. Polycarbonate is a tough, transparent thermoplastic that's used to make thin, light lenses. However, although they're very impact-resistant, these lenses scratch more easily than plastic lenses.

Infants born with congenital cataracts may need to have their cataracts surgically removed during the first few weeks of life. Some children born with cataracts wear contact lenses at 6 months of age.

Around age 10, children may express a desire to get contact lenses for cosmetic purposes or convenience if they play sports. Allowing your child to wear contacts depends on his or her ability to insert and remove lenses properly, faithfully take them out as required, and clean them as recommended by the doctor. Soft lenses are easier to adapt to than hard lenses, but not all children are candidates for soft lenses. Talk to your child's eye doctor about what type of contact lens is best for your child.

Section 6.3

Vision, Learning, and Dyslexia

Excerpted from "Vision, Learning and Dyslexia: A Joint Policy Statement of the American Academy of Optometry and the American Optometric Association," © 1997 American Optometric Association (www.aoa.org). Reprinted with permission. Current as of August 2007.

Many children and adults continue to struggle with learning in the classroom and the workplace. Advances in information technology, its expanding necessity, and its accessibility are placing greater demands on people for efficient learning and information processing.

Learning is accomplished through complex and interrelated processes, one of which is vision. Determining the relationships between vision and learning involves more than evaluating eye health and visual acuity (clarity of sight). Problems in identifying and treating people with learning-related vision problems arise when such a limited definition of vision is employed.

This text addresses these issues, which are important to individuals who have learning-related vision problems, their families, their teachers, the educational system, and society.

Policy Statement

People at risk for learning-related vision problems should receive a comprehensive optometric evaluation. This evaluation should be conducted as part of a multidisciplinary approach in which all appropriate areas of function are evaluated and managed.

The role of the optometrist when evaluating people for learning-related vision problems is to conduct a thorough assessment of eye health and visual functions and communicate the results and recommendations. The management plan may include treatment, guidance, and appropriate referral.

The expected outcome of optometric intervention is an improvement in visual function with the alleviation of associated signs and symptoms. Optometric intervention for people with learning-related vision problems consists of lenses, prisms, and vision therapy. Vision therapy does not directly treat learning disabilities or dyslexia. Vision therapy is a treatment to improve visual efficiency and visual processing, thereby allowing the person to be more responsive to educational instruction. It does not preclude any other form of treatment and should be a part of a multidisciplinary approach to learning disabilities.

Pertinent Issues

Vision is a fundamental factor in the learning process. The three interrelated areas of visual function are:

1. Visual pathway integrity including eye health, visual acuity, and refractive status;

2. Visual efficiency including accommodation (focusing, binocular vision [eye teaming] and eye movements;

3. Visual information processing including identification and discrimination, spatial awareness, and integration with other senses.

To identify learning-related vision problems, each of these interrelated areas must be fully evaluated.

Educational, neuropsychological, and medical research has suggested distinct subtypes of learning difficulties. Current research indicates that some people with reading difficulties have co-existing visual and language processing deficits. For this reason, no single treatment, profession, or discipline can be expected to adequately address all of their needs.

Unresolved visual deficits can impair the ability to respond fully to educational instruction. Management may require optical correction, vision therapy, or a combination of both. Vision therapy, the art and science of developing and enhancing visual abilities and remediating vision dysfunctions, has a firm foundation in vision science, and both its application and efficacy have been established in the scientific literature. Some sources have erroneously associated optometric vision therapy with controversial and unfounded therapies, and equate eye defects with visual dysfunctions.

The eyes, visual pathways, and brain comprise the visual system. Therefore, to understand the complexities of visual function, one must look at the total visual system. Recent research has demonstrated that some people with reading disabilities have deficits in the transmission of information to the brain through a defective visual pathway. This creates confusion and disrupts the normal visual timing functions in reading.

Visual defects, such as a restriction in the visual field, can have a substantial impact on reading performance. Eye strain and double vision resulting from convergence insufficiency can be a significant handicap to learning. There are more subtle visual defects that influence learning affecting different people to different degrees. Vision is a multifaceted process and its relationships to reading and learning are complex. Each area of visual function must be considered in the evaluation of people who are experiencing reading or other learning problems. Likewise, treatment programs for learning-related vision problems must be designed individually to meet each person's unique needs.

Section 6.4

Signs of Eye Problems in Children

Below are general signs of eye problems in children. If you notice one or more of these signs, or if your child does or says any of the things listed here, take your child to an eye doctor right away.

How do your child's eyes look?

- Eyes don't line up; one eye appears crossed or looks out
- Eyelids are red-rimmed, crusted, or swollen
- Eyes are watery or red (inflamed)

How does your child act?

- Rubs eyes a lot

- Closes or covers one eye
- Tilts head or thrusts head forward
- Has trouble reading or doing other close-up work or holds objects close to eyes to see
- Blinks more than usual or seems cranky when doing close-up work
- Things are blurry or hard to see
- Squints eyes or frowns

What does your child say?

- "My eyes are itchy," "my eyes are burning," or "my eyes feel scratchy."
- "I can't see very well."
- After doing close-up work your child says, "I feel dizzy," "I have a headache," or "I feel sick/nauseous."
- "Everything looks blurry" or "I see double."

Remember, your child may still have an eye problem even if he or she does not complain or has not shown any unusual signs.

Section 6.5

Screening Young Children for Vision Disorders

"Trained Screeners Can Identify Preschoolers With Vision Disorders," by
the National Eye Institute (NEI, www.nei.nih.gov), part of the National
Institutes of Health, December 2006.

Specially trained nurses and lay people performed effectively when
using certain vision screening tests to identify preschoolers with vision disorders, according to a National Institutes of Health-funded
research study of more than 1,400 children.

In comparisons using selected vision screening tests, trained nurses
and lay people were able to correctly identify up to 68 percent of children with at least one of the most prevalent vision disorders of childhood: amblyopia (lazy eye), strabismus (eye misalignment), refractive
errors (poor vision that can be corrected with glasses or contact
lenses), or poor vision not associated with any obvious disorder. These
results demonstrate that trained lay people and nurses can achieve
similar results when using specific tests to screen preschool children
for vision disorders.

The purpose of the Vision In Preschoolers Study (VIP Study) is to
identify whether vision-screening tests can accurately identify preschool-aged children who would benefit from a comprehensive vision
examination. Study personnel evaluated selected children enrolled in
Head Start centers in Berkeley, CA; Boston, MA; Columbus, OH; Philadelphia, PA; and Tahlequah, OK. The VIP Study was funded by the
National Eye Institute (NEI), part of the National Institutes of Health.
Results from the second phase of this study are published in the August 2005 issue of the journal *Investigative Ophthalmology and Visual Science*. An earlier phase of the VIP Study found that four
commonly used vision screening tests were more effective than seven
other commercially available tests in recognizing vision problems in
preschool-aged children.

During the first phase of the study, published in the April 2004
issue of the journal *Ophthalmology*, licensed optometrists and ophthalmologists compared 11 commercially available screening tests for
diagnosing eye disorders in children. They tested 2,588 children in a

mobile van specially designed with four vision screening rooms. They also gave each child a full eye examination using established diagnostic examination procedures and tests.

The 11 tests varied widely in performance when they were administered by the eye care professionals. The best tests detected two thirds of children having at least one of the targeted vision disorders and nearly 90 percent of children with the most important conditions. Three tests that assessed refractive error (e.g., nearsightedness, farsightedness, or astigmatism) and one test that evaluated visual acuity were more accurate than others in detecting children with vision problems. These tests included two handheld autorefractors used to measure refractive error; retinoscopy, which uses light reflected off the back of the eye and handheld lenses to measure refractive error; and a visual acuity test in which children stand 10 feet away from a chart displaying symbols and name each symbol as the screener points to it.

"We are excited to have identified the best-performing tools for vision screening of preschool children, and to have found that trained lay screeners and nurses can use those tools effectively," said Paul A. Sieving, M.D., Ph.D., director of the NEI. "As early detection of childhood eye disease increases the likelihood of successful treatment, these results have important implications for the visual health of children."

For the second phase of the study, nurses and lay screeners administered four vision screening tests to 1,452 children at their Head Start centers. They screened all children who had failed a basic Head Start vision screening and a random sample of those children who passed the screening.

The screening tests included three of the tests that performed best in the first phase of the study: two handheld automated refractors to measure refractive error and a test of visual acuity in which children name or match symbols at a set distance. The screeners also administered a test for depth perception in which the children point to a three-dimensional image. All children screened also received a standardized, comprehensive eye examination by a licensed eye care professional in a specially equipped vision van at the child's Head Start Center.

The results demonstrated that trained nurses and lay screeners achieved similar accuracy rates administering the two automated refractors. Nurses correctly identified up to 68 percent of children with vision disorders while lay screeners correctly identified up to 62 percent of these children. Using these handheld instruments, nurses and lay screeners correctly identified more than 80 percent of children with conditions considered most severe.

Using charts displaying several symbols at one time at a distance of 10 feet, nurses and lay screeners were not able to correctly identify as many children with vision disorders. However, when lay screeners administered a simpler version of the symbols visual acuity test at a distance of five feet, they correctly identified 61 percent of children with vision problems. Nurses and lay screeners identified about the same percentage of children with vision problems (45 percent versus 40 percent) using the test of depth perception.

The researchers estimate that, nationwide, two to five percent of children ages three to five have amblyopia, three to four percent have strabismus, and 10 to 15 percent have significant refractive error.

"It is estimated that up to 15 percent of preschool children between the ages of three and five have an eye or vision condition that, if not corrected, can result in reduced vision," said Paulette P. Schmidt, O.D., M.S., chairperson of the VIP Study and a professor of optometry and vision science at the Ohio State University College of Optometry. "Unfortunately, many parents are unaware that their child has an eye problem because vision problems do not hurt and children do not know how well they should see."

"Accurate and efficient identification of preschool children with vision disorders has a significant impact on visual outcome," Schmidt said. "Parents should question which eye problems are being screened for, the accuracy of the tests, and how often serious eye conditions are missed by these tests," she said. "If results from a vision screening test indicate that a child should have a follow-up examination, parents should ask about next steps. Parents also should be aware that vision screening programs do not substitute for a comprehensive eye examination by a licensed eye care professional. However, vision screening may be a valuable way to detect children who would benefit most from an eye examination."

Planning is now underway for a third phase of the VIP Study.

Chapter 7

Eye Care and Vision Concerns in Adults

Chapter Contents

Section 7.1

Pregnancy and Your Vision

Pregnancy brings an increase in hormones that may cause changes in vision. In most cases, these are temporary eye conditions that will return to normal after delivery. It's important for expectant mothers to be aware of vision changes during pregnancy and know what symptoms indicate a serious problem.

Refractive Changes

During pregnancy, changes in hormone levels can alter the strength you need in your eyeglasses or contact lenses. Though this is usually nothing to worry about, it's a good idea to discuss any vision changes with an eye doctor who can help you decide whether or not to change your prescription. The doctor may simply tell you to wait a few weeks after delivery before making a change in your prescription.

Dry Eyes

Some women experience dry eyes during pregnancy. This is usually temporary and goes away after delivery. The good news is that lubricating or rewetting eye drops are perfectly safe to use while you are pregnant or nursing. They can lessen the discomfort of dry eyes. It's also good to know that contact lenses, contact lens solutions, and enzymatic cleaners are safe to use while you are pregnant. To reduce the irritation caused by a combination of dry eyes and contact lenses, try cleaning your contact lenses with an enzymatic cleaner more often. If dry, irritated eyes make wearing contacts too uncomfortable, don't worry. Your eyes will return to normal within a few weeks after delivery.

Puffy Eyelids

Puffiness around the eyes is another common side effect of certain hormonal changes women may have while pregnant. Puffy eyelids may interfere with side vision. As a rule of thumb, don't skimp on your water intake and stick to a moderate diet, low in sodium and caffeine. These healthy habits can help limit water retention and boost your overall comfort.

Migraine Headaches

Migraine headaches linked to hormonal changes are very common among pregnant women. In some cases, painful migraine headaches make eyes feel more sensitive to light. If you are pregnant and suffering from migraines, be sure to talk to your doctor before taking any prescription or non-prescription migraine headache medications.

Prenatal care helps keep both you and your unborn child healthy. Be sure to tell your doctor if you are having any problems. Keep your eye doctor up-to-date about your overall health. Tell him or her about any pre-existing conditions, and about any prescription and non-prescription medications you are taking.

Diabetes

Women who are diabetic before their pregnancy and those who develop gestational diabetes need to watch their vision closely. Blurred vision in such cases may indicate elevated blood sugar levels.

High Blood Pressure

In some cases, a woman may have blurry vision or spots in front of her eyes while pregnant. These symptoms can be caused by an increase in blood pressure during pregnancy. At excessive levels, high blood pressure can even cause retinal detachment.

Glaucoma

Women being treated for glaucoma should tell their eye doctor right away if they are pregnant or intend to become pregnant. While many glaucoma medications are safe to take during pregnancy, certain glaucoma medications such as carbonic anhydrase inhibitors can be harmful to the developing baby.

Just because you are expecting a baby doesn't mean you have to put off your regular eye exam! You can have your eyes safely dilated while you are pregnant. If you suffer from any pre-existing eye conditions, like glaucoma, high blood pressure, or diabetes, it's very important to tell your eye doctor that you are pregnant. Your eye doctor may watch closely for changes in your vision during this exciting time in your life.

Section 7.2

Aging and Your Eyes

From "Aging and Your Eyes," an *AgePages* publication by the National Institute on Aging (NIA, www.nia.nih.gov), part of the National Institutes of Health, October 2005.

Are you holding the newspaper farther away from your eyes than you used to? Join the crowd—age can bring changes that affect your eyesight. Some changes are more serious than others, but no matter what the problem, there are things you can do to protect your vision. The keys are regular eye exams and finding problems early.

Five Steps to Protect Your Eyesight

- Have your eyes checked every 1 or 2 years by an eye care professional. This can be an ophthalmologist or optometrist. He or she should put drops in your eyes to enlarge (dilate) your pupils. This is the only way to find some eye diseases, such as diabetic retinopathy, that have no early signs or symptoms. If you wear glasses, they should be checked, too.

- Find out if you are at high risk for eye disease. Are you over age 65? Are you African American and over age 40? Do you or people in your family have diabetes or eye disease? If so, you need to have a dilated eye exam.

- Have regular physical exams to check for diseases like diabetes and high blood pressure. These diseases can cause eye problems if not treated.

- See an eye care professional right away if you suddenly cannot see or everything looks dim or if you see flashes of light. Also see an eye care professional if you have eye pain, fluid coming from the eye, double vision, redness, or swelling of your eye or eyelid.

- Wear sunglasses that block ultraviolet (UV) radiation and a hat with a wide brim when outside. This will protect your eyes from too much sunlight, which can raise your risk of getting cataracts.

Eye Problems

Some eye problems do not threaten your eyesight. Others are more serious diseases and can lead to blindness.

Common Eye Problems

The following common eye complaints can be treated easily. Sometimes they can be signs of more serious problems.

- **Presbyopia** is a slow loss of ability to see close objects or small print. It is a normal process that happens as you get older. Holding the newspaper at arm's length is a sign of presbyopia. You might also get headaches or tired eyes when you read or do other close work. Reading glasses usually fix the problem.

- **Floaters** are tiny specks or "cobwebs" that seem to float across your eyes. You might notice them in well-lit rooms or outdoors on a bright day. Floaters can be a normal part of aging. Sometimes they are a sign of a more serious eye problem such as retinal detachment. If you see many new floaters and/or flashes of light, see your eye care professional right away. This is considered a medical emergency.

- **Tearing** (or having too many tears) can come from being sensitive to light, wind, or temperature changes. Protecting your eyes, by wearing sunglasses for example, may solve the problem. Sometimes, tearing may mean a more serious eye problem, such as an infection or a blocked tear duct. Your eye care professional can treat both of these conditions.

- **Eyelid problems** can come from different diseases or conditions. Common eyelid problems include red and swollen eyelids, itching, tearing, being sensitive to light, and crusting of eyelashes during sleep. This condition is called blepharitis and may be treated with warm compresses. Other less common eyelid problems, such as swelling or growths, can be treated with medicine or surgery.

Eye Diseases and Disorders

The following eye problems can lead to vision loss and blindness. Often they have few or no symptoms. Having regular eye exams is the best way to protect yourself. If your eye care professional finds a problem early there are things you can do to keep your eyesight.

- **Cataracts** are cloudy areas in the eye's lens causing loss of eyesight. Cataracts often form slowly without any symptoms. Some stay small and don't change eyesight very much. Others may become large or dense and harm vision. Cataract surgery can help. Your eye care professional can watch for changes in your cataract over time to see if you need surgery. Cataract surgery is very safe. It is one of the most common surgeries done in the United States.

- **Corneal diseases and conditions** can cause redness, watery eyes, pain, lower vision, or a halo effect. The cornea is the clear, dome-shaped "window" at the front of the eye. Disease, infection, injury, and other things can hurt the cornea. Some corneal conditions are more common in older people. Treatments for corneal problems can be simple. You may just need to change your eyeglass prescription and use eye drops. In severe cases, corneal transplantation is the treatment. It generally works well and is safe.

- **Dry eye** happens when tear glands don't work well. You may feel itching, burning, or have some vision loss. Dry eye is more common as people get older, especially among women. Your eye care professional may tell you to use a home humidifier, or special eyedrops (artificial tears) or ointments to treat dry eye. In serious cases special contact lenses or surgery may help.

- **Glaucoma** comes from too much fluid pressure inside the eye. Over time, the pressure can hurt the optic nerve. This leads to vision loss and blindness. Most people with glaucoma have no early symptoms or pain from the extra pressure. You can protect yourself by having regular eye exams through dilated pupils. Treatment may be prescription eyedrops, medicines that you take by mouth, laser treatment, or surgery.

- **Retinal disorders** are a leading cause of blindness in the United States. The retina is a thin tissue that lines the back of the eye and sends light signals to the brain. Retinal disorders that affect aging eyes include:

- **Age-related macular degeneration (AMD):** AMD affects the part of the retina (the macula) that gives you sharp central vision. Over time, AMD can ruin the sharp vision needed to see objects clearly and to do common tasks like driving and reading. In some cases, AMD can be treated with lasers. Photodynamic therapy uses a drug and strong light to slow the progress of AMD. Another treatment uses injections. Ask your eye care professional if you have signs of AMD. Also ask if you should be taking special dietary supplements that may lower your chances of its getting worse.

- **Diabetic retinopathy:** This is a problem that may appear if you have diabetes. It happens when small blood vessels stop feeding the retina as they should. It develops slowly and there are no early warning signs. Laser surgery and a treatment called vitrectomy can help. Studies show that keeping blood sugar under control can prevent diabetic retinopathy or slow its progress. If you have diabetes be sure to have an eye exam through dilated pupils at least once a year.

- **Retinal detachment:** This is when the retina separates from the back of the eye. When this happens, you may see more floaters or light flashes in your eye, either all at once or over time. Or it may seem as though there is a curtain in front of your eyes. If you have any of these symptoms, see your eye care professional at once. **This is a medical emergency.** With surgery or laser treatment, doctors often can bring back all or part of your eyesight.

Low Vision

Low vision affects some people as they age. Low vision means you cannot fix your eyesight with glasses, contact lenses, medicine, or surgery. It can get in the way of your normal daily routine. You may have low vision if you:

- have trouble seeing well enough to do everyday tasks like reading, cooking, or sewing;

- can't recognize the faces of friends or family;

- have trouble reading street signs; or

- find that lights don't seem as bright as usual.

If you have any of these problems, ask your eye care professional to test you for low vision. There are special tools and aids to help people with low vision read, write, and manage daily living tasks. Lighting can be changed to suit your needs. You also can try large-print reading materials, magnifying aids, closed-circuit televisions, audio tapes, electronic reading machines, and computers that use large print and speech.

Other simple changes also may help:

- Write with bold, black felt-tip markers.

- Use paper with bold lines to help you write in a straight line.

- Put colored tape on the edge of your steps to help you keep from falling.

- Install dark-colored light switches and electrical outlets that you can see easily against light-colored walls.

- Use motion lights that turn on by themselves when you enter a room. These may help you avoid accidents caused by poor lighting.

- Use telephones, clocks, and watches with large numbers; put large-print labels on the microwave and stove.

Chapter 8

Defining Vision Impairment and Low Vision

Chapter Contents

Section 8.1

What Is Vision Impairment?

Excerpted from "Vision Impairment," by the National Center on Birth
Defects and Developmental Disabilities, part of the Centers for Disease
Control and Prevention (CDC, www.cdc.gov), October 29, 2004.

Vision impairment means that a person's eyesight cannot be corrected to a "normal" level. Vision impairment may be caused by a loss of visual acuity, where the eye does not see objects as clearly as usual. It may also be caused by a loss of visual field, where the eye cannot see as wide an area as usual without moving the eyes or turning the head.

There are different ways of describing how severe a person's vision loss is. The World Health Organization defines "low vision" as visual acuity between 20/70 and 20/400, with the best possible correction, or a visual field of 20 degrees or less. "Blindness" is defined as a visual acuity worse than 20/400, with the best possible correction, or a visual field of 10 degrees or less. Someone with a visual acuity of 20/70 can see at 20 feet what someone with normal sight can see at 70 feet. Someone with a visual acuity of 20/400 can see at 20 feet what someone with normal sight can see at 400 feet. A normal visual field is about 160 to 170 degrees horizontally.

Vision impairment severity may be categorized differently for certain purposes. In the United States, for example, we use the term "legal blindness" to indicate that a person is eligible for certain education or federal programs. Legal blindness is defined as a visual acuity of 20/200 or worse, with the best possible correction, or a visual field of 20 degrees or less.

Visual acuity alone cannot tell you how much a person's life will be affected by their vision loss. It is important to also assess how well a person uses the vision they have. Two people may have the same visual acuity, but one may be able to use his or her vision better to do everyday tasks. Most people who are "blind" have at least some usable vision that can help them move around in their environment and do things in their daily lives. A person's functional vision can be evaluated by observing them in different settings to see how they use their vision. A functional vision evaluation can answer questions such as these:

• Can the person scan a room to find someone or something?

- What lighting is best for the person to do different tasks?
- How does the person use his or her vision to move around in a room or outside?

Vision impairment changes how a child understands and functions in the world. Impaired vision can affect a child's cognitive, emotional, neurological, and physical development by possibly limiting the range of experiences and the kinds of information a child is exposed to.

Nearly two thirds of children with vision impairment also have one or more other developmental disabilities, such as mental retardation, cerebral palsy, hearing loss, or epilepsy. Children with more severe vision impairment are more likely to have additional disabilities than are children with milder vision impairment.

Section 8.2

What You Should Know about Low Vision

The quiz "Do You Have Low Vision?" is from the National Eye Institute (NEI, www.nei.nih.gov), part of the National Institutes of Health, November 2006. The text following the heading "What You Should Know about Low Vision" is excerpted from a booklet by the same title, produced by NEI, January 2007.

Do You Have Low Vision?

Take this quiz and find out.

There are many signs that can signal vision loss. For example, even with your regular glasses, do you have difficulty:

Recognizing faces of friends and relatives?

- Yes　　- No

Doing things that require you to see well up close, like reading, cooking, sewing, or fixing things around the house?

- Yes　　- No

Picking out and matching the color of your clothes?

- Yes • No

Doing things at work or home because lights seem dimmer than they used to?

- Yes • No

Reading street and bus signs or the names of stores?

- Yes • No

If you answered "yes" to any of these questions, vision changes like these could be early warning signs of eye disease. Regular eye exams should be part of your routine health care. However, if you believe your vision has recently changed, you should see your eye care professional as soon as possible. Usually, the earlier your problem is diagnosed, the better the chance of keeping your remaining vision.

What You Should Know About Low Vision

This information will help people with vision loss and their families and friends better understand low vision. It describes how to get help and live more safely and independently.

What is low vision?

Low vision means that even with regular glasses, contact lenses, medicine, or surgery, people find everyday tasks difficult to do. Reading the mail, shopping, cooking, seeing the TV, and writing can seem challenging.

Millions of Americans lose some of their vision every year. Irreversible vision loss is most common among people over age 65.

Is losing vision just part of getting older?

No. Some normal changes in our eyes and vision occur as we get older. However, these changes usually don't lead to low vision.

Most people develop low vision because of eye diseases and health conditions like macular degeneration, cataract, glaucoma, and diabetes. A few people develop vision loss after eye injuries or from birth defects. While vision that's lost usually cannot be restored, many people can make the most of the vision they have.

Your eye care professional can tell the difference between normal changes in the aging eye and those caused by eye diseases.

How do I know when to get an eye exam?

Regular dilated eye exams should be part of your routine health care. However, if you believe your vision has recently changed, you should see your eye care professional as soon as possible.

A specialist in low vision is an optometrist or ophthalmologist who is trained to evaluate vision. This person can prescribe visual devices and teach people how to use them. There are a wide variety of devices that help people make the most of their remaining vision.

What can I do if I have low vision?

Many people with low vision are taking charge. They want more information about devices and services that can help them keep their independence.

It's important to talk with your eye care professional about your vision problems. Even though it may be difficult, ask for help. Find out where you can get more information about services and devices that can help you.

Many people require more than one visual device. They may need magnifying lenses for close-up viewing, and telescopic lenses for seeing in the distance. Some people may need to learn how to get around their neighborhoods.

If your eye care professional says, "Nothing more can be done for your vision," ask about vision rehabilitation.

These programs offer a wide range of services, such as low vision evaluations and special training to use visual and adaptive devices. They also offer guidance for modifying your home as well as group support from others with low vision.

Be persistent. Remember that you are your best health advocate. Investigate and learn as much as you can, especially if you have been told that you may lose more vision. It is important that you ask questions about vision rehabilitation and get answers. Many resources are available to help you.

Write down questions to ask your doctor, or take a tape recorder with you. Rehabilitation programs, devices, and technology can help you adapt to vision loss. They may help you keep doing many of the things you did before. Know that you can make the difference in living with low vision.

What can I do about my low vision?

Although many people maintain good vision throughout their lifetimes, people over age 65 are at increased risk of developing low vision. You and your eye care professional or specialist in low vision need to work in partnership to achieve what is best for you. An important part of this relationship is good communication.

Here are some questions to ask your eye care professional or specialist in low vision to get the discussion started. Questions to ask your eye care professional:

- What changes can I expect in my vision?

- Will my vision loss get worse? How much of my vision will I lose?

- Will regular eyeglasses improve my vision?

- What medical/surgical treatments are available for my condition?

- What can I do to protect or prolong my vision?

- Will diet, exercise, or other lifestyle changes help?

- If my vision can't be corrected, can you refer me to a specialist in low vision?

- Where can I get a low vision examination and evaluation? Where can I get vision rehabilitation?

Questions to ask your specialist in low vision:

- How can I continue my normal, routine activities?

- Are there resources to help me in my job?

- Will any special devices help me with daily activities like reading, sewing, cooking, or fixing things around the house?

- What training and services are available to help me live better and more safely with low vision?

- Where can I find individual or group support to cope with my vision loss?

Chapter 9

Vision Impairment and Blindness in the United States

Introduction

Vision impairment is one of the most feared disabilities. Although it is believed that half of all blindness can be prevented, the number of people in America who suffer vision loss continues to increase.

The leading causes of vision impairment and blindness in the United States are primarily age-related eye diseases. The number of Americans at risk for age-related eye diseases is increasing as the baby-boomer generation ages. These conditions, including age-related macular degeneration, cataract, diabetic retinopathy, and glaucoma, affect more Americans than ever before. Disturbingly, the number of Americans with age-related eye disease and the vision impairment that results is expected to double within the next three decades. As of the year 2000 census, there were more than 119 million people in the United States in this age group.

Awareness of vision impairment and its causes is important to all of us. We must be aware of our own personal risk of vision loss and take steps to preserve and protect our precious eyesight. Our communities must be informed so that they may prepare the treatment and rehabilitation services that will be needed. Most important, our nation's leaders must comprehend the scope of eye problems in our country so that adequate government resources can be devoted to research, treatment, and prevention.

Vision Problems in the U.S., now in its fourth edition, provides useful estimates of the prevalence of sight-threatening eye diseases in Americans age 40 and older. This text includes information on the prevalence of blindness and vision impairment, significant refractive error, and the four leading eye diseases affecting older Americans: age-related macular degeneration, cataract, diabetic retinopathy, and glaucoma.

Vision Impairment and Blindness

The term "blindness" can have many connotations and is difficult to define precisely. To many people, blindness refers to the complete loss of vision with no remaining perception of light. However, this ultimate form of complete blindness is rare. Far more people have a permanent loss of some, but not all, of their eyesight. The severity of vision loss can vary widely and may result in equally varying degrees of functional impairment.

"Legal blindness" represents an artificial distinction and has little value for rehabilitation, but it is significant in that it determines eligibility for certain disability benefits from the Federal Government. In the United States, it is typically defined as visual acuity with best correction in the better eye worse than or equal to 20/200 or a visual field extent of less than 20 degrees in diameter. These overly simple criteria for visual impairment are far from comprehensive in defining the visual function deficits that can cause difficulties for daily living tasks.

Vision impairment is defined as having 20/40 or worse vision in the better eye even with eyeglasses. People with the least degree of vision impairment may still face challenges in everyday life. For instance, people with vision worse than 20/40 cannot obtain an unrestricted driver's license in most states.

Almost everyone with blindness or vision impairment can benefit from vision rehabilitation that can help make the most of whatever vision remains.

Unfortunately, blindness and vision impairment represent a significant burden, not only to those affected by sight loss, but to our national economy as well. It is estimated that blindness and vision impairment cost the federal government more than $4 billion annually in benefits and lost taxable income.

Blindness, as defined above, affects more than one million Americans age 40 and older. The visually impaired, including those who are blind, total more than 3.4 million older Americans (see Tables 9.1 and 9.2). Blindness affects Blacks more frequently than Whites and Hispanics. Hispanics, however, have higher rates of visual impairment than other races. The prevalence of blindness and vision impairment increases rapidly in the later years, particularly after age 75.

Refractive Error

Refractive errors are the most frequent eye problems in the United States. They are optical defects that result in light not being properly focused on the eye's retina.

Nearsightedness (myopia) and farsightedness (hyperopia) are the most common refractive errors. People with myopia see near objects clearly, while distant ones are blurred. People with hyperopia experience just the opposite—distant objects are clear while near ones are blurred.

Why refractive errors develop is uncertain. Most infants have some degree of hyperopia, but vision becomes more normal with age, usually

Table 9.1. Estimated Number of Cases of Vision Impairment (Including Blindness) in the U.S. Population Age 40 and Older by State, Race, and Sex

Total	**3,406,280**
Female	2,253,866
Male	1,152,413
White	2,861,479
Black	265,277
Hispanic	170,462
Other	109,063
White Female	1,920,686
White Male	940,793
Black Female	169,088
Black Male	96,188
Hispanic Female	100,631
Hispanic Male	69,831
Other Female	63,461
Other Male	45,602

Table 9.2. Estimated Number of Cases of Blindness in the U.S. Population Age 40 and Older by State, Race, and Sex

Total	1,046,920
Female	712,171
Male	334,748
White	883,698
Black	111,877
Hispanic	23,170
Other	28,175
White Female	612,301
White Male	271,397
Black Female	70,335
Black Male	41,541
Hispanic Female	13,459
Hispanic Male	9,711
Other Female	16,076
Other Male	12,099

leveling off by age 6. However, some children remain farsighted or become so later in life. While some children may be nearsighted early in life, most myopia occurs later during adolescence. Refractive error can continue to change over our lifetime.

Other common refractive errors include astigmatism (uneven focus) and presbyopia (age-related problem with near focus). Fortunately, almost all refractive errors can be corrected by eyeglasses or contact lenses. It is estimated that more than 150 million Americans use corrective eyewear to compensate for their refractive error. Americans are estimated to spend over $15 billion each year on eyewear, supporting an optical industry in the United States worth more than $30 billion.

Refractive surgery is now another alternative for correcting problems such as myopia, hyperopia and astigmatism. The number of people seeking refractive surgery is increasing. However, the surgical procedures are not without some risk and the long-term effects of many of these procedures are still unknown.

Uncorrected or under-corrected refractive error can result in significant vision impairment. The magnitude of refractive error is measured in units called diopters. For each diopter of refractive error, a person may be unable to read the next smaller line of an eye chart. For instance, a person with more than two diopters of hyperopia might find it difficult to read this text.

Myopia is a very common disorder affecting more than 30.5 million Americans age 40 and older. Prevalence is greater in women through age 60 when rates become more comparable between genders. Myopia affects more Whites than other races, and is generally less frequent with age. Because of the higher threshold for significance, hyperopia is less common, affecting 12 million older Americans. Prevalence of hyperopia generally increases with age. It is most frequent in Whites, but also affects Hispanics more often than Blacks.

Age-Related Macular Degeneration

Age-related macular degeneration (AMD) is a condition that primarily affects the part of the retina responsible for sharp central vision. There are two forms:

1. **Dry AMD** (non-exudative) is the most common form of the disease. Early AMD involves the presence of drusen, fatty deposits under the light-sensing cells in the retina. Late cases of dry AMD may also involve atrophy of the supportive layer under the light-sensing cells in the retina that helps keep those cells healthy. Vision loss in early dry AMD is usually moderate and only slowly progressive. Atrophy in late cases of dry AMD can result in more significant vision loss.

2. **Wet AMD** (exudative) is less common, but is more threatening to vision. It's called wet AMD because of the growth of tiny new blood vessels (neovascularization) under the retina that leak fluid or break open. This distorts vision and causes scar tissue to form. All cases of the wet form are considered late AMD.

The exact cause of AMD is unknown, but risk factors for the disease include age (rarely affecting those under age 50), White race, and cigarette smoking. Research also suggests that long-term diets low in certain antioxidant nutrients may increase the risk of AMD. Because AMD often damages central vision, it is likely the most common cause of legal blindness and vision impairment in older Americans.

Unfortunately, there is no generally-accepted treatment for dry AMD. Laser therapies to destroy leaking blood vessels can help reduce the risk of advancing vision loss in many cases of wet AMD. Research has recently shown that certain doses of zinc, vitamins A and C, and beta-carotene can help control the advance of late AMD, but appear to have no effect in preventing the disease in otherwise healthy individuals.

Over 1.6 million Americans age 50 and older have late AMD. Age-specific prevalence rates are initially comparable between races, but advance more significantly for Whites after age 75. In Blacks, the disease is more prevalent in women until about age 75 as well.

Cataract

Cataract is a clouding of the eye's naturally clear lens. Most cataracts appear with advancing age. The exact cause of cataract is unclear, but it may be the result of a lifetime of exposure to ultraviolet radiation contained in sunlight, or may be related to other lifestyle factors such as cigarette smoking, diet, and alcohol consumption.

Cataract can also occur at any age as a result of other causes such as eye injury, exposure to toxic substances or radiation, or as a result of other diseases such as diabetes.

Congenital cataracts may even be present at birth due to genetic defects or developmental problems. Cataracts in infants may also result from exposure to diseases such as rubella during pregnancy.

According to the World Health Organization, cataract is the leading cause of blindness in the world. In the United States, cataract is sometimes considered a conquered disease because treatment is widely available that can eliminate vision loss due to the disease. However, cataract still accounts for a significant amount of vision impairment in the United States, particularly in older people who may have difficulty accessing appropriate eye care due to cost, availability, or other barriers.

Treatment of cataract involves removal of the clouded natural lens. The lens is usually replaced with an artificial intraocular lens (IOL) implant. Cataract removal is now one of the most commonly performed surgical procedures with more than a million such surgeries performed each year.

Surgery is not truly a cure for cataract, however, and its success in controlling vision loss comes with a price. It is estimated that the federal government spends more than $3.4 billion each year treating cataract through the Medicare program.

Ongoing research into the normal healthy functioning of the eye's lens may help us better understand the causes of cataract and how they might be prevented. Even partial achievement of this goal might save hundreds of millions of dollars in the annual costs of treating cataract.

Cataract affects nearly 20.5 million Americans age 40 and older, or about one in every six people in this age range. By age 80, more than half of all Americans have cataract.

Cataract is slightly more common in women than in men. It also affects Whites somewhat more frequently than other races, particularly with increasing age.

Diabetic Retinopathy

Diabetic retinopathy is a common complication of diabetes. It affects the tiny blood vessels of the retina. Retinal blood vessels can break down, leak, or become blocked—affecting and impairing vision over time. In some people with diabetic retinopathy, serious damage to the eye can occur when abnormal new blood vessels grow on the surface of the retina.

Diabetic retinopathy can affect almost anyone with diabetes. The U.S. Centers for Disease Control and Prevention (CDC) estimate that 10.3 million Americans have diagnosed diabetes, while an additional 5.4 million have diabetes that has not been diagnosed.

In general, the longer someone has diabetes, the greater the risk of developing diabetic retinopathy. Eventually, almost everyone with juvenile-onset diabetes will develop some signs of diabetic retinopathy. Those who acquire diabetes later in life are also at risk of diabetic retinopathy, although they are somewhat less likely to develop advanced diabetic retinopathy.

Diabetes also increases the risk of other eye diseases such as cataract and glaucoma. Because of its dangers to good vision, people with diabetes are urged to seek annual dilated eye exams.

Research suggests that the risk of diabetic retinopathy can be reduced through careful control of blood sugar. People with diabetes are also encouraged to control their blood pressure.

Laser treatment, called photocoagulation, has been shown to reduce the risk of sight loss in advanced cases of diabetic retinopathy. Focal photocoagulation can be used to destroy leaking blood vessels. Scatter photocoagulation, where a large number of spots are destroyed by the laser, is used to control the growth of abnormal blood vessels. In some cases vitrectomy, a surgical procedure to remove clouded fluid and gel from inside the eye, can help.

Because diabetes includes a form with juvenile onset, the information below reflects the prevalence of diabetic retinopathy in Americans age 18 and older. Approximately 209 million Americans are in this age group.

Diabetic retinopathy affects over 5.3 million Americans age 18 and older, or just over 2.5% of this population. Prior to age 40, diabetic retinopathy affects Whites more frequently than other races. In later decades, Hispanics are the most commonly affected by the disease.

Glaucoma

Glaucoma is a disease that causes a gradual degeneration of cells that make up the optic nerve which carries visual information from the eye to the brain. As the nerve cells die, vision is slowly lost, usually beginning in the periphery. Often, the loss of vision is unnoticeable until a significant amount of nerve damage has occurred. For this reason, as many as half of all people with glaucoma may be unaware of their disease.

The exact cause of primary open-angle glaucoma, the most common form of the disease, is uncertain. Other forms of glaucoma (such as angle-closure, secondary and congenital glaucoma) occur in relation to specific physical causes.

Elevated fluid pressure within the eye (intraocular pressure) seems related in some way to all cases of glaucoma. The majority of cases of glaucoma exhibit intraocular pressure outside normal limits at some time. However, even those cases with apparently normal pressure seem to benefit from treatment aimed at lowering pressure.

Most cases of glaucoma can be controlled and vision loss slowed or halted by treatment. Medications, laser treatments, and surgery can be used to lower intraocular pressure. However, any vision lost to glaucoma cannot be restored.

Unfortunately, glaucoma cannot be prevented. Factors that increase the risk of glaucoma include age, race, diabetes, eye trauma, and long-term use of steroid medications.

Glaucoma is traditionally defined by a triad of signs, including the presence of at least two of the following: elevated intraocular pressure, optic disc cupping, and visual field loss. However, case definitions used in the various epidemiologic studies of the disease have differed on specific criteria.

Glaucoma affects more than 2.2 million Americans age 40 and older, or about 1.9% of this population. Glaucoma prevalence is clearly related to age and race. In general, glaucoma is more common in Blacks, Hispanics and with increasing age.

In the 65–69 age group, the prevalence rate for White females is about 1.6%, while in Black females, the rate is three times higher at 4.8%. For those age 80 and older, glaucoma affects more than 10% of Black men and Hispanic women.

Glaucoma appears to be more common initially in women, but by age 65, prevalence becomes more comparable between the sexes.

Chapter 10

Vision Loss from Eye Diseases Will Increase as Americans Age

With the aging of the population, the number of Americans with major eye diseases is increasing, and vision loss is becoming a major public health problem. By the year 2020, the number of people who are blind or have low vision is projected to increase substantially. These findings appear in the April [2004] issue of *Archives of Ophthalmology*.

Blindness or low vision affects 3.3 million Americans age 40 and over, or one in 28, according to study authors. This figure is projected to reach 5.5 million by the year 2020. The study reports that low vision and blindness increase significantly with age, particularly in people over age 65. People 80 years of age and older currently make up eight percent of the population, but account for 69 percent of blindness. The study provides the most robust and up-to-date estimates available of the burden of visual impairment. It was sponsored by the National Eye Institute (NEI), part of the Federal government's National Institutes of Health (NIH).

"Blindness and low vision can lead to loss of independence and reduced quality of life," said Elias A. Zerhouni, M.D., Director of the NIH. "As our population lives longer, eye disease will be an ever greater concern. These data underscore NIH's commitment to the support of vision research that will prevent, delay, and possibly cure eye diseases."

From the National Eye Institute (NEI, www.nei.nih.gov), part of the National Institutes of Health, April 12, 2004.

The study identifies age-related macular degeneration (AMD), glaucoma, cataract, and diabetic retinopathy as the most common eye diseases in Americans age 40 and over. The leading cause of blindness among white Americans is AMD, accounting for 54 percent of all blindness. Among African Americans, the leading causes of blindness are cataract and glaucoma. Among Hispanics, glaucoma is the most common cause of blindness. The study authors emphasize the importance of annual comprehensive eye examinations in preventing and/ or delaying eye disease for those at higher risk for blindness, such as those over age 65, people with diabetes, or African Americans over age 40.

Study authors provide estimates of the number of Americans with each disease. The authors say that due largely to the aging of the population, the prevalence of low vision and blindness will increase markedly by 2020.

Table 10.1. Eye Disease Prevalence and Projections for Adults 40 Years and Older in the United States

	Current Estimates (in millions)	2020 Projections (in millions)
Advanced Age-Related Macular Degeneration (with associated vision loss)	1.8*	2.9
Glaucoma	2.2	3.3
Diabetic Retinopathy	4.1	7.2
Cataract	20.5	30.1

Note: Another 7.3 million people are at substantial risk for vision loss from AMD.

There were other significant findings from the study:

• AMD is strongly associated with increasing age, particularly after age 60. AMD rises dramatically in whites over age 80; more than one in 10 white Americans over age 80 has vision loss from AMD.

• Glaucoma is almost three times as common in African Americans as in whites.

• The prevalence of glaucoma rises rapidly in Hispanics over age 65.

- Cataract is the leading cause of low vision among all Americans, responsible for about 50 percent of all cases.

- One in every 12 people with diabetes age 40 and older has vision-threatening diabetic retinopathy.

"These data will help identify areas where we should direct our research efforts," said NEI Director Paul A. Sieving, M.D., Ph.D. "Also, health professionals and state and local agencies can use study data to prioritize public health programs emphasizing the importance of early detection and timely treatment. Developing blindness prevention strategies could help address the potentially devastating impact of the increased prevalence of eye diseases in the next few decades."

Frederick Ferris III, M.D., director of clinical research at the NEI, said that the estimates of low vision and blindness "are the first to take full advantage of information derived from several excellent eye disease studies reported since 1990. These data, collected from different populations, allow us to identify the most common eye diseases and give us good estimates of their relative magnitudes."

The study was conducted by the Eye Disease Prevalence Research Group, a consortium of principal investigators who have conducted population-based eye disease studies. The Eye Disease Prevalence Research Group produced prevalence estimates of blindness and low vision in people age 40 and over by analyzing standardized data from several high quality studies. The derived prevalence rates were then modeled to the U.S. population using 2000 census data, and projected to 2020 based on 2020 U.S. census estimates.

Chapter 11

Eye Care and Eye Diseases in Minority Populations

Chapter Contents

Section 11.1

Racial and Ethnic Factors That Affect the Receipt of Eye Care

Excerpted from "Identification of Variables That Influence the Receipt of Eye Care," a report of focus group findings by the National Eye Institute (NEI, www.nei.nih.gov), part of the National Institutes of Health, August 25, 2005.

What Are the Cultural Factors That Influence the Receipt of Eye Care?

The influence of culture on receiving eye care is noteworthy, although cultural factors are not reported by every racial and ethnic group. Nonetheless, several themes with cultural implications have been noted to directly influence the receipt of eye care. Cultural issues that influence the receipt of eye care are traditional, folk, and home remedy use, primarily by African Americans; an ideology to not use preventive medicine, embedded primarily within the Hispanic/ Latino culture; an ideology to "wait and see" among African Americans; and an ideology that African-American males are less likely to receive health care services. Also, undertones of perceived racial and ethnic discrimination and bias have been noted, particularly among the African American and Hispanic/Latino participants. These perceptions affect beliefs about the health care system, and in some instances, the receipt of care.

Traditional, folk, and home remedies were reportedly used to cure eye problems before going to see an eye care professional. In the majority of cases, these remedies were all the care received, as participants reported that these remedies cured any ailments they were experiencing with their eyes. Cultural factors, unlike factors such as communication and knowledge, appear to directly serve as barriers to the receipt of eye care.

Perhaps through better education, the influence of some of these cultural factors can be reduced. In many cases, "waiting it out" and not taking a preventive stance related to health care can have devastating consequences. Furthermore, gender issues in the receipt of care need to be addressed. What appears to be driving gender disparities in the receipt of care is that males do not want to seem dependent or weak. In some manner, this attitude must be confronted, such that if care is not received, they will indeed become dependent and weak. What will also pose a difficulty in increasing the receipt of eye care is that many of the traditional, folk, and home remedies were found to work. It is not the author's contention to downplay or dismiss the effectiveness of and trust certain cultures have in traditional therapies, however the consultation of an eye care professional should not be discounted if avenues in which to do so are available (i.e., insurance coverage).

Other Factors That Influence the Receipt of Eye Care

Outside of attitudes, knowledge, communication, and culture, a major factor reported to influence the receipt of eye care was cost. In every focus group, cost was reported as a barrier to receiving eye care services.

Cost was also mentioned as influencing whether followup and recommended services, such as prescriptions, were obtained. The cost of services is prohibitive, particularly when it comes to prescribing followup care. In many instances, followup care, even in the form of getting glasses, can be just as expensive, if not more, than the professional eye care services that were received. Eye drops, glasses, and lenses were reported to be very expensive. In many cases, eye care was just received from the local pharmacy or drug store, which meant that many participants were self-diagnosing their eye problems and identifying adequate prescription lenses on their own. This process completely circumvents the possibility of an eye care professional performing an eye exam and diagnosing other vision-related problems. The issue of cost also relates to the concerns of class and economic discrimination and bias that were raised by participants among each of the four racial/ethnic groups. Several participants were noted to perceive the health care system and doctors as being insensitive or discriminating, based on economic status and the ability to pay for health care services/type of insurance.

Lastly, the fact that many eye care services are not covered as a standard service in most general health plans was reported to be another factor that influences the receipt of eye care. Many participants discussed difficulty in receiving eye care services because of a lack of such services. Unfortunately, this lack of services also appeared to influence participants to think about eye care separately and not as a part of their general health. Also, many participants, particularly in Miami and San Francisco, stated that a referral was needed to seek eye care services. This referral process meant that additional time was required to make an appointment to see their primary care physician for a referral, and then to get an appointment to see an eye care professional. This process also contributes to additional cost outlays on behalf of the participants, as they have to pay two co-payments when their primary intention was to see just an eye care professional.

Factors That Influence the Receipt of Eye Care and Differ by Race/Ethnicity

The majority of the factors identified as influencing the receipt of eye care services for the 180 participants were reported to be factors affecting each of the four racial and ethnic groups studies. Each of the four racial and ethnic groups mentioned attitudes and knowledge as issues that influence the receipt of eye care. No significant differences in factors that influence the receipt of eye care were witnessed by the three focus group locations, with the exception of referrals, which were cited to influence the receipt of eye care slightly more in San Francisco and Miami than in Chicago.

The most differences were according to race and ethnicity when examining how culture and communication influence the receipt of eye care. Although the majority of participants felt good about the way their medical care provider explained health information to them, a few African-American and Hispanic/Latino participants reported that they have difficulty understanding medical terminology. Language, primarily among Hispanic/Latino and Asian participants, was also reported to impact communication and the level of understanding that patients and participants have about their health.

Cultural factors also influenced the receipt of eye care by race/ethnicity. African-American, Hispanic/Latino, and Asian participants used traditional, folk, or home remedies when they experience problems with their eyes before deciding to go to the doctor. Hispanic/Latino participants noted that within their community, preventive medicine is not practiced as it should be. Also, some of the Hispanic/Latino and African American participants mentioned that they are unlikely to go to the doctor unless their condition is really bad. Washing the eye out and taking a "wait and see" approach were reportedly done by African-American participants before contacting their primary care physician or eye doctor. African-American, Hispanic/Latino, and some Caucasian participants mentioned that males tend to not like going to the doctor. Lastly, undertones of perceived racial and ethnic discrimination and bias were present in several of the statements made by African-American and Hispanic/Latino participants, which may influence the receipt of eye care services.

Other factors that differed by race and ethnicity were fear and denial about receiving eye examinations and class discrimination and bias in the health care system. Fear and denial about receiving eye examinations were reported by all racial/ethnic groups with the exception of Asian participants. A number of participants, primarily those from racial and ethnic minority backgrounds, found doctors or the health care system to be insensitive and discriminating based on economic status and the ability to pay for health care services/type of insurance.

Section 11.2

U.S. Latinos Have High Rates of Eye Disease and Visual Impairment

From a press release by the National Eye Institute (NEI, www .nei.nih.gov), part of the National Institutes of Health, August 9, 2004.

Latinos living in the United States have high rates of eye disease and visual impairment, according to a research study, and a significant number may be unaware of their eye disease. This study, called the Los Angeles Latino Eye Study (LALES), is the largest, most comprehensive epidemiological analysis of visual impairment in Latinos conducted in the United States. It was funded by the National Eye Institute (NEI) and the National Center on Minority Health and Health Disparities (NCMHD), two components of the Federal government's National Institutes of Health (NIH). Study results were published in the June, July and August 2004 issues of the journal *Ophthalmology*.

Researchers found that Latinos had high rates of diabetic retinopathy, an eye complication of diabetes; and open-angle glaucoma, a disease that damages the optic nerve.

Study investigators gave a detailed health interview and clinical examination to more than 6,300 Latinos, primarily Mexican-Americans, aged 40 and older from the Los Angeles area, assessing their risk factors for eye disease and measuring health-related and vision-related quality of life. Each participant received a blood test for diabetes and a comprehensive eye exam that included photographs of the back of the eye.

"This research has provided much needed data on eye disease among the fastest growing minority group in the United States," said Elias A. Zerhouni, M.D., director of the NIH.

"Several epidemiological studies have been conducted on the prevalence and severity of major eye diseases in White and Black populations, however there have been relatively few such studies in Latino populations," said Paul A. Sieving, M.D., Ph.D., director of the NEI. "This study highlights the importance of providing health education and vision care to Latinos."

The researchers noted that many study participants did not know they had an eye disease. One in five individuals with diabetes was newly diagnosed during the LALES clinic exam, and 25 percent of these individuals were found to have diabetic retinopathy. Overall, almost half of all Latinos with diabetes had diabetic retinopathy. Among those with any signs of age-related macular degeneration (AMD), a condition that can lead to a loss of central vision, only 57 percent reported ever visiting an eye care practitioner, and only 21 percent did so annually. Seventy-five percent of Latinos with glaucoma and ocular hypertension (high pressure in the eye) were undiagnosed before participating in LALES.

"Because vision loss can often be reduced with regular comprehensive eye exams and timely treatment, there is an increasing need to implement culturally appropriate programs to detect and manage eye diseases in this population," said Rohit Varma, M.D., M.P.H., associate professor of ophthalmology and preventive medicine at the Keck School of Medicine's Doheny Eye Institute at the University of Southern California, and director of the study. "This is especially true when you consider that Latinos, compared with other ethnic groups in the United States, have a high prevalence of low vision, diabetic retinopathy, and glaucoma. Overall, Latinos were much more likely to have received general medical care than to have received eye care."

The study found that:

- Three percent of LALES participants were visually impaired, defined as best corrected visual acuity of 20/40 or worse in the better seeing eye, and 0.4 percent were blind, defined as best corrected visual acuity of 20/200 or worse in the better seeing eye. Prevalence rates of visual impairment in Latinos are higher than those reported in Whites and comparable to those reported in Blacks. Visual impairment increased with age. Those in their 70s and 80s were up to eight times more likely to have visual impairment than their younger counterparts. Other risk factors for visual impairment included female gender, low education, unemployment, a history of eye disease, and diabetes.

- Nearly half of all study participants with diabetes—almost a quarter of the LALES population—had some signs of diabetic retinopathy. Longer duration of diabetes was associated with a higher risk of retinopathy. In addition, more than 10 percent of participants with diabetes had macular edema (fluid buildup in the back of the eye), of whom 60 percent had cases severe enough to require laser treatment. Latinos had a higher rate of more severe vision-threatening diabetic retinopathy than Whites.

- The overall prevalence of open-angle glaucoma among Latinos in this study was nearly five percent. This rate increased with age from about eight percent for those in their 60s to 15 percent for those in their 70s. This is higher than the rate reported for Whites and similar to that for Blacks in this country. Nearly four percent of Latinos had ocular hypertension, a risk factor for glaucoma.

- About 10 percent of participants were considered to be at risk for progression to more advanced stages of AMD, and close to a quarter of these individuals had signs of AMD in both eyes. Only 25 individuals had advanced AMD, a prevalence rate of 0.5 percent. Age was a strong predictor for development of more advanced stages of AMD. While Latinos had the early signs of AMD at rates comparable to Whites, the rates of advanced AMD were lower than seen in Whites and comparable to Blacks.

- One in five adult Latinos had cataract. Half of Latinos with cataract or other clouding of the lens were visually impaired.

- Latinos with visual impairment based on the study eye examination reported lower visual function on a questionnaire. In particular, those whose vision had worsened by two lines or more on a standard eye chart were more likely to report a lower quality of life.

"Census 2000 data show that 12.5 percent of residents in this country, or 35 million people, are Latino," said John Ruffin, Ph.D., director of the NCMHD. "That number is projected to increase to 61.4 million by the year 2025. This study reaffirms the significance of eye disease and visual impairment among Latinos, and its importance to public health," Ruffin said.

Section 11.3

African Americans Experience Higher Rates of Blinding Eye Disease

"African-Americans and Glaucoma," © 1999 Glaucoma Research Foundation (www.glaucoma.org). Reprinted with permission. Reviewed by David A. Cooke, M.D., July 2007.

Primary open-angle glaucoma (referred to as glaucoma in the rest of this document) affects people of all ages and ethnicities. While glaucoma symptoms vary among black populations in different international regions, glaucoma clearly affects those of African heritage more.

Glaucoma occurs about five times more often in African Americans, and blindness from glaucoma is about six times more common. In addition to this higher frequency, glaucoma often occurs earlier in life in African Americans—on average, about 10 years earlier than in other ethnic populations.

Why is there a difference?

The reasons for the higher rate of glaucoma and subsequent blindness among African Americans are still unknown. However, researchers are becoming more and more certain that African Americans are genetically more likely to be susceptible to glaucoma, making early detection and treatment all the more important. For example, there may be a greater susceptibility to optic nerve damage, which causes vision loss, for blacks with glaucoma.

In studies such as the Baltimore Eye Survey and the Barbados Eye Study, researchers have been tracking how glaucoma affects different black populations. This information will be invaluable in better understanding the risk factors for blacks, and eventually, in developing more effective treatments and protocols.

Does glaucoma treatment differ?

Although treatment varies for all individuals, the overall goal is to prevent further damage and sight loss from glaucoma. One way that eye doctors seek to meet this goal is to aim for a target eye pressure. In African-Americans, glaucoma generally occurs earlier, often with a greater rate of vision loss. Because of this, an eye doctor may work with a patient to target an eye pressure that may be lower than for other glaucoma patients.

Initial results from the Advanced Glaucoma Intervention Study (AGIS) show that ethnicity may also be a factor in determining the better surgical treatment for glaucoma. Initially expecting both blacks and whites to have similar responses, researchers found that black patients with advanced glaucoma responded better to laser surgery than filtering (cutting) surgery. Now, an eye doctor's recommendation for surgery may consider the patient's race in addition to other important aspects of their individual health.

It is important to note, however, that treatments cannot be generalized. Each patient, regardless of race, should continue to be evaluated on the individual state of his or her disease, with a target pressure and treatment plan unique to each patient.

Although much still needs to be learned about why African Americans are more at risk for glaucoma, one thing is certain. Early diagnosis and treatment is key in preventing vision loss from glaucoma. The Glaucoma Research Foundation recommends that African Americans get a thorough check for glaucoma every one to two years after age 35. For more information on finding an eye doctor or getting an eye exam, please see the article at http://www.glaucoma.org/learn/diagnostic_test.html.

Thanks to Joanne Katz, ScD, Professor of International Health, Johns Hopkins School of Hygiene and Public Health, Baltimore, MD for contributing to this article. Dr. Katz was a co-investigator of the Baltimore Eye Survey.

This article appeared in the Winter 1999 issue of *Gleams*.

Chapter 12

Facts about Clinical Trials in Vision Research

The National Eye Institute (NEI) conducts or sponsors clinical trials to find new ways to treat or prevent eye disease and vision loss. Clinical trials in vision research have led to new medicines and surgeries that have saved or improved sight for thousands of people.

What is a clinical trial?

Clinical trials involve medical research with people. Most medical research begins with studies in test tubes and in animals. Treatments that show promise in these early studies may then be tried with people. The only sure way to find out whether a new treatment is safe, effective, and better than other treatments is to try it on patients in a clinical trial.

What kinds of clinical trials are there?

Clinical trials are carried out in three parts, or phases.

- **Phase I:** Researchers first conduct Phase I trials in small numbers of patients and healthy volunteers. If the new treatment is a medicine, researchers also want to find out how much of it can be given safely.

Excerpted from "Facts About Clinical Trials in Vision Research," by the National Eye Institute (NEI, www.nei.nih.gov), part of the National Institutes of Health, December 2006.

- **Phase II:** Researchers conduct Phase II trials in small numbers of patients to find out the effect of a new treatment on an eye disease or disorder.

- **Phase III:** Finally, researchers conduct Phase III trials to find out whether the new treatments work better, the same, or not as well as the standard treatments already being used. Phase III trials also help to determine if new treatments have any side effects. These trials—which may involve hundreds, perhaps thousands, of people around the country—can also compare new treatments with no treatment.

Where do clinical trials take place?

The NEI supports clinical trials at about 250 medical centers, hospitals, universities, and doctors' offices across the country. NEI researchers conduct other clinical trials at the National Institutes of Health in Bethesda, Maryland.

How is a clinical trial conducted?

At each facility taking part in the clinical trial, the principal investigator is the researcher in charge of the study. Most of the people who conduct clinical trials in eye disease are ophthalmologists or optometrists. The clinic coordinator knows all about how the study works and makes all the arrangements for your visits.

All doctors who take part in the study carefully follow a detailed treatment plan called a protocol. This plan fully explains how the doctors will treat you in the study. The protocol ensures that all patients are treated in the same way, no matter where they receive care.

- Clinical trials are controlled. This means that researchers compare the effects of the new treatment with those of the standard treatment. In some cases, when no standard treatment exists, the new treatment is compared with no treatment.

- Patients who get the new treatment are in the treatment group.

- Patients who get the standard treatment or no treatment are in the control group.

- In some clinical trials, patients in the treatment group get a new medicine and patients in the control group get a placebo. A placebo is a harmless substance—a "dummy" pill—that looks like the real treatment but has no effect on the eye disease or disorder. In other clinical trials, where a new surgery or device (not a medicine) is being tested, patients in the control group may receive a sham treatment. This treatment, like a placebo, has no effect on the eye disease or disorder and does not harm patients.

• Researchers assign patients randomly to the treatment or control group. This is like flipping a coin to decide which patients are in each group. Patients do not know ahead of time which group that is. The chance of any patient getting the new treatment is about 50 percent. Patients cannot request to receive the new treatment instead of the placebo or sham treatment. In some clinical trials, where the disease or disorder affects both eyes, one eye may be in the treatment group, and the other eye may be in the control group.

• Patients often do not know until the study is over whether they are in the treatment group or the control group. This is called a masked study. In some trials, neither doctors nor patients know who is getting what treatment. This is called a double masked study. These types of trials help to ensure that what patients or doctors might think about the treatment will not affect the study results.

What is expected of patients in a clinical trial?

Patients in a clinical trial are expected to have eye exams and other tests. You may also need to take medications and/or undergo surgery. Depending upon the treatment and the examination procedure, you may need a hospital stay.

You may have to go back to the medical facility later for followup examinations. These exams help find out how well the treatment is working. Followup studies can take months or years. However, the success of the clinical trial often depends on learning what happens to patients over a long period of time. Only patients who continue to return for followup examinations can provide this important long-term information.

What are the benefits of participating in a clinical trial?

Participating in a clinical trial can bring many benefits:

• There is the hope that a new treatment will be more effective than the current treatment for an eye disease or disorder. Only about half of the people in a clinical trial get the new treatment.

If the new treatment is effective and safer than the current treatment, those patients who do not receive the new treatment during the clinical trial may be among the first to benefit from the new treatment when the study is over.

- If the treatment is effective, it may help to improve vision and control or prevent eye disease or disorder.

- Clinical trial patients receive the highest quality medical care. Experts watch them closely during the study and may continue to follow them after the study is over.

- People who take part in these trials contribute to new knowledge that may help other people with the same eye problems. In cases where certain eye diseases or disorders run in families, your participation may lead to better care for family members.

What are the risks?

Clinical trials may involve risks as well as possible benefits.

- Whether or not a new treatment will work cannot be known ahead of time. There is always a chance that a new treatment may not work better than a standard treatment, may not work at all, or may be harmful.

- The treatment you receive may cause side effects that are serious enough to require medical attention.

How is patient safety protected?

Clinical trials can raise fears of the unknown. Understanding the safeguards that protect patients can ease some of these fears.

- Before a clinical trial begins, researchers must get approval from their hospital's Institutional Review Board (IRB), an advisory group that makes sure a clinical trial is designed to protect patient safety.

- During a clinical trial, doctors will closely watch you to see if the treatment is working and if you are having any side effects. All the results are carefully recorded and reviewed.

- A group of experts—the Data and Safety Monitoring Committee—carefully watches each clinical trial supported by the NEI. This group can recommend that a study be stopped at any time.

- Patients are asked to take part in a clinical trial only if they volunteer and understand the risks and benefits.

What are a patient's rights in a clinical trial?

Patients who are eligible for a clinical trial will be given information to help them decide whether to take part. As a patient, you have the right to:

- be told about all known risks and benefits of treatments involved in the study;
- know how the researchers plan to carry out the study, for how long, and where;
- know what is expected of you;
- know any costs involved for you or your insurers;
- be informed about any medical or personal information that may be shared with other researchers directly involved in the clinical trial; and
- talk openly with doctors and ask any questions.

After you join a clinical trial, you have the right to:

- leave the study at any time. Participation is strictly voluntary. However, you should not enroll if you do not plan to complete the study.
- receive any new information about the new treatment.
- continue to ask questions and get answers.
- maintain your privacy. Your name will not appear in any reports based on the study.
- be informed of your treatment assignment once the study is completed.

What about costs?

In some clinical trials, the medical facility conducting the research pays for treatment costs and some other expenses. You or your health insurance may have to pay for some things that are considered part of standard care. These things may include hospital stays, laboratory and other tests, and medical procedures. You also may need to pay for travel between your home and the clinic. For clinical trials conducted at the NEI's medical facility in Bethesda, Maryland, medical care is provided at no cost to patients. You should find out about costs ahead of time. If you have health insurance, find out exactly what it will cover. If you don't have health insurance, or if your insurance company will not cover your costs, talk to the clinic staff about other options for covering the cost of your care.

What questions should you ask before deciding to join a clinical trial?

Questions you should ask when thinking about joining a clinical trial include the following:

- What is the purpose of the clinical trial?

- What are the standard treatments for my disease or condition? Why do researchers think the new treatment may be better? What is likely to happen to me with or without the new treatment?

- What tests and treatments will I need? Will I need surgery? Medicines? Hospitalization?

- How long will the treatment last? How often will I have to come back for followup exams?

- What are the treatment's possible benefits to my condition? What are the short- and long-term risks? What are the possible side effects?

- Will the treatment be uncomfortable? Will it make me feel sick? If so, for how long?

- How will my health be monitored?

- Where will I need to go for the clinical trial? How will I get there?

- How much will it cost me to be in the study? What costs are covered by the study? How much will my health insurance cover?

- Will I be able to see my own doctor? Who will be in charge of my care?

- Will taking part in the study affect my daily life? Will I have the time to be in it?

- How do I feel about taking part in a clinical trial? Are there family members or friends who may benefit from my contributions to new medical knowledge?

What clinical trials are being held? Who can take part in them?

The NEI conducts or sponsors research on many eye diseases and disorders. Because funding for eye research goes to the medical areas that show promising research opportunities, it is not possible for the NEI to sponsor clinical trials in every eye disease and disorder at all times.

Not everyone can take part in a clinical trial for a specific eye disease or disorder. Each study enrolls patients with certain features, or eligibility criteria. These criteria may include the type and stage of disease or disorder, as well as the age and previous treatment history of the patient.

You or your doctor can contact the NEI to find out more about specific clinical trials and their eligibility criteria. If you are interested in joining a clinical trial, your doctor must contact one of the trial's investigators and provide details about your diagnosis and medical history.

The NEI's website (www.nei.nih.gov) lists the clinical trials the NEI is helping to support. Each trial description includes information on its background and purpose, as well as patient eligibility. There is information on how to participate in a trial and how to refer a patient to a trial.

Part Two

Refractive Problems and Procedures

Chapter 13

Understanding Refraction and Refractive Errors

Chapter Contents

Section 13.1

What Are Refractive Errors?

"Refraction and Refractive Errors: An Overview of How the Eye Sees," by Marilyn Haddrill, is reprinted with permission from www. allaboutvision.com. © 2006 Access Media Group, LLC.

When we have an eye examination, we may hear references to errors in the way our eye refracts light. This is because the eye's ability to refract or "bend" light is also its ability to focus light, which determines the sharpness of our vision.

The normal eye can refract or focus light without the help of any other lenses such as glasses or contacts. If the eye cannot focus an image sharply and requires another lens to assist it, then the eye is said to have a refractive error.

The procedure to determine a prescription for eyeglasses or contact lenses is called a refraction. Eye surgeons who use vision correction procedures are also referred to as refractive surgeons. But what does it really mean when we're told that our eye has a refractive error?

How Light Travels through the Eye

We all know that, in order to see, we must have light. While we don't fully understand all the different properties of light, we do have an idea of how light travels. A light ray can be deflected, reflected, bent, or absorbed, depending on the different substances it encounters.

When light travels through water or the curved glass of a lens, for example, its path is bent or refracted. Certain eye structures have refractive properties similar to water or lenses and can bend light rays into a precise point of focus essential for sharp vision. As the light rays are bent, so is the image from which they originate.

Most refraction in the eye occurs when light rays travel through the curved, clear front covering (cornea). The eye's natural (crystalline) lens also bends light rays. Even the eye's tear film and internal fluids (aqueous humor and vitreous) have certain refractive properties.

How the Eye Achieves Focus

Light rays from an image traveling through the eye's optical system are refracted and focused into a point of sharp focus that ideally should center on the retina. The retina is the tissue that lines the inside of the back of the eye, where light-sensitive cells (photoreceptors) capture images in much the same way that film in a camera does when exposed to light. These images then are transmitted through the eye's optic nerve to the brain for interpretation.

Just as a camera's aperture (called the diaphragm) is used to adjust the amount of light needed to expose film in just the right way, the eye's pupil widens or constricts to control the amount of light that reaches the retina. In dark conditions, the pupil widens. In bright conditions, the pupil constricts.

Refractive Errors in the Eye's Optical System

The eye's ability to refract or focus light sharply on the retina is based on two main anatomic features: the overall length of the eye and the curvature of the eye's surface or cornea.

- **Eye Length:** When the eye is too long, images mistakenly focused in front of the retina are out of focus by the time they actually hit the retina. Nearsightedness or myopia then results. When the eye is too short, images never have a chance to achieve focus by the time they hit the retina. This causes farsightedness or hyperopia.

- **Curvature of the Cornea:** If the cornea is not perfectly spherical, then the image is refracted or focused irregularly to create a condition called astigmatism. A person can be nearsighted or farsighted with or without an astigmatism.

As mentioned above, the tear film, crystalline lens, and internal fluids also play a role in focusing an image onto the retina. An irregularly shaped natural lens or defect in the way it functions also can cause focusing problems, leading to blurry or distorted vision.

These various defects in focusing can cause light rays to bend or refract at skewed angles, which means sharp focus cannot be achieved. When abnormalities of this type occur in the optical system, they are known as refractive errors.

More obscure vision errors, known as higher-order aberrations, also are related to flaws in the way light rays are refracted as they travel through our eye's optical system. These types of vision errors, which can create problems such as poor contrast sensitivity, are just now being detected through new technology known as wavefront analysis.

Vision Correction for Refractive Errors

A refraction from an eye care practitioner helps determine the type and degree of refractive error, which may be addressed with glasses, contacts, or refractive surgery.

Eyeglass lenses and contact lenses are fabricated with precise curvatures that help offset flaws in our eye's optical system. These lenses intercept and bend light rays, such that they achieve a more precise point of focus on our eye's retina.

Many vision correction surgeries such as LASIK also aim to correct refractive errors by changing the shape of our eye's front surface (cornea), so that light rays are bent into a more accurate point of focus.

Section 13.2

Questions and Answers about Refractive Errors

From the National Eye Institute (NEI, www.nei.nih.gov), part of the National Institutes of Health, December 2006.

Refractive errors include myopia, hyperopia, presbyopia, and astigmatism, eye conditions that are very common. Most people have one or more of them. Refractive errors can usually be corrected with eyeglasses or contact lenses.

What is myopia (nearsightedness)?

If you have myopia you can clearly see close objects, but distant objects are blurry. Myopia is caused by the eyeball being too long. Myopia occurs in different degrees from minimal to extreme. The more myopic you are the blurrier your vision is at a distance and objects will have to be closer to you so you can see them clearly.

What is hyperopia (farsightedness)?

If you have hyperopia, you can see distant objects clearly, but close ones are blurry. Hyperopia occurs when the eyeball is too short for the light rays to focus clearly on the retina.

What is astigmatism?

If you have an astigmatism, the surface of the eye (cornea) is not perfectly round, rather it is more oval and doesn't allow the eye to focus clearly. The cornea is very important in helping the eye focus light rays on the retina. Astigmatism rarely occurs alone. It is usually accompanies myopia or hyperopia.

What is presbyopia?

If you have presbyopia, you have the loss of the ability to focus up close that occurs as you age. Most people are between 40 and 50 years when they realize for the first time that they can't read objects close to them. The letters of the phonebook are "too small" or you have to hold the newspaper farther away from your eye to see it clearly. At the same time your ability to focus on objects that are far way remains normal.

Section 13.3

Eye Coordination Problems Often Improve When Refractive Errors Are Corrected

"Eye Coordination," © 2007 American Optometric Association (www.aoa.org). Reprinted with permission.

Eye coordination is a skill that must be developed. Eye coordination is the ability of both eyes to work together as a team. Each of your eyes sees a slightly different image and your brain, by a process called fusion, blends these two images into one three-dimensional picture. Good eye coordination keeps the eyes in proper alignment. Eye coordination is a skill that must be developed. Poor eye coordination results from a lack of adequate vision development or improperly developed eye muscle control. Although rare, an injury or disease can cause poor eye coordination.

Because the images seen by each eye must be virtually the same, a person usually compensates for poor eye muscle control by subconsciously exerting extra effort to maintain proper alignment of the eyes. In more severe cases, the muscles cannot adjust the eyes so that the same image is seen and double vision occurs. Because the brain will try to avoid seeing double, it eventually learns to ignore the image sent by one eye. This can result in amblyopia, a serious vision condition commonly known as lazy eye.

Some signs and symptoms that may indicate poor eye coordination include double vision, headaches, eye and body fatigue, irritability, dizziness and difficulty in reading and concentrating. Children may also display characteristics that may indicate poor eye coordination including covering one eye, skipping lines or losing their place while reading, poor sports performance, avoiding tasks that require close work and tiring easily.

Because poor eye coordination can be difficult to detect, periodic optometric examinations, beginning at age 6 months and again at age 3 years are recommended. A comprehensive examination by a doctor of optometry can determine the extent, if any, of poor eye coordination. Poor eye coordination is often successfully treated with eyeglasses and/or vision therapy. The success rate for achieving proper eye coordination is quite high. Sometimes, eye coordination will improve when other vision conditions like nearsightedness or farsightedness are corrected. In some cases, surgery may be necessary.

Chapter 14

All about Contact Lenses

Chapter Contents

Section 14.1

What Are the Different Types of Contact Lenses?

From "Contact Lenses," a publication of the Center for Devices and Radiological Health, a division of the U.S. Food and Drug Administration (FDA, www.fda.gov), February 2007.

Contact lenses are the number one choice for many people with vision correction needs. For many, contact lenses provide flexibility and convenience. There are many different lenses available for a variety of needs and preferences. Contact lenses can be used to correct a variety of vision disorders such as myopia (nearsightedness), hyperopia (farsightedness), astigmatism, and presbyopia (poor focusing with reading material and other near vision tasks).

You can buy contact lenses only if you have a current, valid prescription.

Types of Contact Lenses

There are two general categories of contact lenses—soft and rigid gas permeable (RGP). All contact lenses require a valid prescription.

Soft Contact Lenses

Soft contact lenses are made of soft, flexible plastics that allow oxygen to pass through to the cornea. Soft contact lenses may be easier to adjust to and are more comfortable than rigid gas permeable lenses. Newer soft lens materials include silicone-hydrogels to provide more oxygen to your eye while you wear your lenses.

Rigid Gas Permeable (RGP) Contact Lenses

Rigid gas permeable contact lenses (RGPs) are more durable and resistant to deposit buildup, and generally give a clearer, crisper vision. They tend to be less expensive over the life of the lens since they last longer than soft contact lenses. They are easier to handle and less likely to tear. However, they are not as comfortable initially as soft contacts and it may take a few weeks to get used to wearing RGPs, compared to several days for soft contacts.

Extended Wear Contact Lenses

Extended wear contact lenses are available for overnight or continuous wear ranging from one to six nights or up to 30 days. Extended wear contact lenses are usually soft contact lenses. They are made of flexible plastics that allow oxygen to pass through to the cornea. There are also a very few rigid gas permeable lenses that are designed and approved for overnight wear. Length of continuous wear depends on lens type and your eye care professional's evaluation of your tolerance for overnight wear. It's important for the eyes to have a rest without lenses for at least one night following each scheduled removal.

Disposable (Replacement Schedule) Contact Lenses

The majority of soft contact lens wearers are prescribed some type of frequent replacement schedule. "Disposable," as defined by the FDA, means used once and discarded. With a true daily wear disposable schedule, a brand new pair of lenses is used each day. Some soft contact lenses are referred to as "disposable" by contact lens sellers, but actually, they are for frequent/planned replacement. With extended wear lenses, the lenses may be worn continuously for the prescribed wearing period (for example, 7 days to 30 days) and then thrown away. When you remove your lenses, make sure to clean and disinfect them properly before reinserting.

Specialized Uses of Contact Lenses

Conventional contact lenses correct vision in the same way that glasses do, only they are in contact with the eye. Two types of lenses that serve a different purpose are orthokeratology lenses and decorative (plano) lenses.

Orthokeratology (Ortho-K): Orthokeratology, or Ortho-K, is a lens fitting procedure that uses specially designed rigid gas permeable (RGP) contact lenses to change the curvature of the cornea to temporarily improve the eye's ability to focus on objects. This procedure is primarily used for the correction of myopia (nearsightedness).

Overnight Ortho-K lenses are the most common type of Ortho-K. There are some Ortho-K lenses that are prescribed only for daytime wear. Overnight Ortho-K lenses are commonly prescribed to be worn while sleeping for at least eight hours each night. They are removed upon awakening and not worn during the day. Some people can go all day without their glasses or contact lenses. Others will find that their vision correction will wear off during the day.

The vision correction effect is temporary. If Ortho-K is discontinued, the corneas will return to their original curvature and the eye to its original amount of nearsightedness. Ortho-K lenses must continue to be worn every night or on some other prescribed maintenance schedule in order to maintain the treatment effect. Your eye care professional will determine the best maintenance schedule for you.

Currently, FDA requires that eye care professionals be trained and certified before using overnight Ortho-K lenses in their practice. You should ask your eye care professional about what lenses he or she is certified to fit if you are considering this procedure.

Decorative (Plano) Contact Lenses: Some contact lenses do not correct vision and are intended solely to change the appearance of the eye. These are sometimes called plano, zero-powered, or non-corrective lenses. For example, they can temporarily change a brown-eyed person's eye color to blue, or make a person's eyes look "weird" by portraying Halloween themes. Even though these decorative lenses don't correct vision, they're regulated by the FDA, just like corrective contact lenses. They also carry the same risks to the eye. These risks include:

- conjunctivitis (pink eye);

- corneal ulcers;

- corneal abrasion; or

- vision impairment or blindness.

FDA is aware that consumers without valid prescriptions have bought decorative contact lenses from beauty salons, record stores, video stores, flea markets, convenience stores, beach shops and the internet. Buying contact lenses without a prescription is dangerous.

If you're considering getting decorative contact lenses, you should:

- get an eye exam from a licensed eye care professional;

- get a valid prescription that includes the brand and lens dimensions;

- buy the lenses from an eye care professional or from a vendor who requires that you provide prescription information for the lenses; or

- follow directions for cleaning, disinfection, and wearing the lenses, and visit your eye care professional for follow-up eye exams.

Section 14.2

Understanding Your Contact Lens Prescription

From "Contact Lenses," a publication of the Center for Devices and Radiological Health, a division of the U.S. Food and Drug Administration (FDA, www.fda.gov), May 2006.

When you get an eye exam, you have the right to get a copy of your prescription. You can use this prescription at another vendor or to order contact lenses on the internet, over the phone, or by mail.

As defined by the Federal Trade Commission (FTC) regulations, a prescription should contain sufficient information for a seller to completely and accurately fill the prescription. This includes the following items:

- patient's name;

- examination date;

- date patient receives prescription after a contact lens fitting (issue date) and expiration date of prescription;

- name, address, phone number and fax number of prescriber;

- power;

- material and/or manufacturer of the prescribed contact lens;

- base curve or appropriate designation of the prescribed contact lens;

- diameter, when appropriate, of the prescribed contact lens; and

- for a private label contact lens, the name of the manufacturer, trade name of the private label brand, and if applicable, trade name of equivalent brand name.

Section 14.3

Buying Contact Lenses

From "Contact Lenses," a publication of the Center for Devices and Radiological Health, a division of the U.S. Food and Drug Administration (FDA, www.fda.gov), May 2006.

Contact lens sales are regulated by both the FDA and the Federal Trade Commission (FTC). Before you buy any contact lenses from someone other than your eye care professional, the FDA wants you to be a wise consumer. With a valid contact lens prescription, it is possible to purchase your contact lenses from stores, the internet, over the phone or by mail, The following questions and answers should help you take simple precautions to make your purchase safe and effective.

What do I need to consider when buying contact lenses?

- Is your contact lens prescription current? You should always have a current, valid prescription when you order contact lenses.

- If you have not had a checkup in the last one to two years, you may have problems with your eyes that you are not aware of, or your contact lenses may not correct your vision well.

- The expiration date for your prescription is currently set by your state. Some require a one-year renewal, some a two-year renewal. If your state has not set a minimum expiration date, federal regulation sets a one year date unless your eye care professional determines that there's a medical reason for less than one year.

- To be sure that your eyes remain healthy you should not order lenses with a prescription that has expired or stock up on lenses right before the prescription is about to expire. It's safer to be rechecked by your eye care professional.

Will I get in legal trouble if I buy contact lenses without a copy of my prescription?

You won't break any laws, but the company is selling you a pre-scription device as if it were an over-the-counter device. In legal terms, this misbrands the device. The company is also violating FTC regulations by selling you contact lenses without having your prescription. For more information, see the FTC website at www.ftc.gov.

What can I do to avoid serious problems when buying my contact lenses?

- Order your contact lenses from a supplier you are familiar with and know is reliable. Contact lenses are often more complex than they appear.

- Request the manufacturer's written patient information for your contact lenses. It will give you important risk/benefit information as well as instructions for use.

- Beware of attempts to substitute a different brand than you presently have. While this may be acceptable in some situations, there are differences in the water content and shape between different brands. The correct choice of which lens is right for you should be based only on an examination by your eye care professional, not over the phone.

- Carefully check to make sure the company gives you the
  - exact brand;
  - lens name;
  - power (sphere; cylinder, if any; axis, if any);
  - diameter;
  - base curve; and
  - peripheral curves, if any.

If you think you have received an incorrect lens, check with your eye care professional. Don't accept a substitution unless your eye care professional approves it.

Where can I report problems that I have when buying contact lenses?

- If you find a website you think is illegally selling contact lenses over the web, you should report it to FDA.

- If you do not get the exact lenses that you ordered, you should report the problem directly to the company that supplied them.

- To file a complaint about prescribing practices to FTC, use the FTC Consumer Complaint Form at www.ftc.gov.

Section 14.4

Risks of Contact Lenses

From "Contact Lenses," a publication of the Center for Devices and Radiological Health, a division of the U.S. Food and Drug Administration (FDA, www.fda.gov), May 2006.

Wearing contact lenses puts you at risk of several serious conditions including eye infections and corneal ulcers. These conditions can develop very quickly and can be very serious. In rare cases, these conditions can cause blindness.

You can not determine the seriousness of a problem that develops when you are wearing contact lenses. You have to get help from an eye care professional to determine your problem.

If you experience any symptoms of eye irritation or infection,

- remove your lenses immediately and do not put them back in your eyes.

- contact your eye care professional right way.

- don't throw away your lenses. Store them in your case and take them to your eye care professional.

He or she may want to use them to determine the cause of your symptoms. report serious eye problems associated with your lenses to the FDA's MedWatch reporting program at www.fda.gov/medwatch.

Symptoms of Eye Irritation or Infection

- discomfort
- excess tearing or other discharge
- unusual sensitivity to light
- itching, burning, or gritty feelings
- unusual redness
- blurred vision
- swelling
- pain

Serious Hazards of Contact Lenses

Symptoms of eye irritation can indicate a more serious condition. Some of the possible serious hazards of wearing contact lenses are corneal ulcers and eye infections.

Corneal ulcers are open sores in the outer layer of the cornea. They are usually caused by infections. You can reduce your chances of infection if:

- you replace your contact lens storage case every 3 to 6 months;
- you clean and disinfect your lenses properly;
- you always use fresh contact lens solution and avoid non-sterile water (distilled water and tap water are not sterile and should not be used);
- you never reuse contact lens solution; and
- you remove your contact lenses before swimming.

Any lenses worn overnight increase your risk of infection. Even lenses that are designed to be worn overnight (extended-wear contact lenses) increase your risk. When worn overnight, contact lenses reduce the amount of oxygen that gets to the cornea. This stresses and damages the surface of the cornea known as the epithelium. Germs can grow more rapidly in stressed corneas.

Other Risks of Contact Lenses

Other risks of contact lenses include:

- pink eye (conjunctivitis);

- corneal abrasions; and

- eye irritation.

Section 14.5

Everyday Eye Care

From "Contact Lenses," a publication of the Center for Devices and
Radiological Health, a division of the U.S. Food and Drug Administration
(FDA, www.fda.gov), March 2007.

Here are some safety tips you should follow if you wear contact
lenses. Make sure to:

- Get regular eye exams to assure the continued health of your
  eyes.

- Always have a back-up pair of glasses with a current prescription in the event that you have problems with your contact lenses.

- Always follow the directions of your eye care professional and
  all labeling instruction for proper use of contact lenses and lens
  care products.

- Always wash your hands before handling contact lenses to reduce the chance of getting an infection.

- Clean, rinse, and air-dry your lens case each time lenses are removed. Contact lens cases can be a source of bacterial growth.

- Remove the lenses immediately and consult your eye care professional if your eyes become red, irritated, or your vision changes.

- Ask your eye care professional about wearing glasses or contact
  lenses during sports activities to minimize your chance of injury.

- Always ask your eye care professional before using any medicine or using topical eye products, even those you buy without a
  prescription. Some medicines may affect your vision or irritate
  your eyes.

- Apply cosmetics after inserting lenses and remove your lenses before removing makeup.

- Apply any aerosol products (hairspray, cologne, and deodorant) before inserting lenses.

- Always inform your employer if you wear contact lenses. Some jobs may require the use of eye protection equipment or may require that you not wear lenses.

- Follow and save the directions that come with your lenses. If you didn't get a patient information booklet, request one from your eye care professional or look for one on the manufacturer's website.

- Replace contacts as recommended by your eye care professional. Throw away disposable lenses after recommended wearing period.

Do Not

- Sleep in daily wear lenses because it may increase your chance of infection or irritation.

- Purchase contact lenses from gas stations, video stores, record shops, or any other vendor not authorized by law to dispense contact lenses. Contact lenses are medical devices that require a prescription.

- Swap contact lens with another person. Swapping provides a way to transfer germs between people. Contact lenses are individually fitted. Incorrectly fitted lenses may cause permanent eye injury, infection, and may potentially lead to blindness.

- Smoke. Studies show that smokers who wear contact lenses have a higher rate of problems (adverse reactions) than non-smokers.

- Swim while wearing contact lenses. There is a risk of eye infection from bacteria in swimming pool water.

- Put your lenses in your mouth to wet them. Saliva is not a sterile solution.

- Use tap water, distilled water, or any homemade saline solution. Tap and distilled water have been associated with *Acanthamoeba* keratitis, a corneal infection that is resistant to treatment and cure.

- Transfer contact lens solutions into smaller travel size containers. This can affect the sterility of the solution which can lead to an eye infection. Transferring solutions into smaller size containers may also leave consumers open to accidentally using a solution not intended for the eyes.

- Rely on contact lenses to protect your eyes from the sun. Make sure to use sunglasses that block ultraviolet light.

Section 14.6

Tips for Keeping Your Eyes Healthy and Comfortable

From "Contact Lens Care," a fact sheet from the Office of Women's Health (www.fda.gov/womens), part of the U.S. Food and Drug Administration (FDA), August 2005.

Keep your eyes safe—take time to care for your contact lenses. Here are some tips for keeping your eyes healthy and comfortable while you wear contacts.

What to Do

- Wash and rinse your hands before touching your lenses.

- Use only the lens cleaners and eye drops that your eye doctor suggests.

- Follow the directions that came with your lenses, lens cleaner, and eye drops.

- Take care of your lens case. Clean, rinse, and dry it each time you take out the lenses. Get a new case every six months.

- Get your eye doctor's OK using any new or different medicines. Tell your doctor about things you can buy without a prescription, like eye drops or lens cleaners.

Table 14.1. Contact Lens Quick Guide

What kind of lens is it?	How long can I wear them?	When do I clean my lenses?
Disposable Lenses: Lenses that you throw away	You can wear the lenses for one day.	You don't need to clean them. You use new lenses each day.
Daily Wear Lenses: Lenses you use again and again	You can wear them for one day. Take them out when you go to bed or even take a nap.	Clean and rinse the lenses every time you take them out. Clean them if you have not worn the lenses in a long time.
Extended Wear Lenses: Lenses you can leave in for up to 30 days, even while you sleep	FDA has only approved these lenses to be worn all the time for up to 30 days.	After 30 days, you need to take the lenses out and clean them.
		They can increase your chances of getting small sores on the eyeballs.
		See your doctor right away if: your sight changes; your eyes get red; your eyes hurt or feel itchy; or you have a lot of tears.

113

- Use eye makeup that is safe for contact lens users.
- Take out your lenses and call your eye doctor right away if:
  - your vision changes.
  - your eyes are red.
  - your eyes hurt or feel itchy.
  - you have a lot of tears.

What Not to Do

- Never spit on your lenses to clean them.
- Never use tap water, bottled water, or salt water made at home to store or rinse your lenses. It can cause infections.
- Never mix different cleaners or drops.
- Never let lotions, creams, or sprays touch your lenses.
- Don't use eyeliner on the inside of your lower eyelid.
- Never wear lenses when you swim or go into a hot tub.
- Never wear your lenses when you are using cleaning products.
- Never wear daily-wear lenses when you sleep—not even during a nap.
- Never wear your lenses longer than your eye doctor tells you to.

If You Have a Problem

- Contact lenses may cause major eye problems.
- If you notice a problem, take out your lenses right away and see your doctor.
- Report the problems to FDA's MedWatch program. Call 800-FDA-1088.
- You can also fill out the form on the web. Go to www.fda.gov/medwatch. Always contact your doctor for medical advice. There are different kinds of lenses. Make sure you know which kind you have.

Section 14.7

Preventing Eye Infections Associated with Contact Lenses

Information under the heading "*Fusarium* Keratitis Infections Associated with Soft Contact Lens Use and Contact Lens Solution" is from "Investigation of Serious Eye Infections Associated With Soft Contact Lens Use and Contact Lens Solution," a press release from the U.S. Food and Drug Administration (FDA, www.fda.gov), April 10, 2006. Information under the heading "Contact Lens Solution and the Risk of *Acanthamoeba* Keratitis" is from "Recall: Complete MoisturePlus Contact Lens Solution," by the U.S. Food and Drug Administration (FDA, www.fda.gov), May 29, 2007.

Fusarium *Keratitis Infections Associated with Soft Contact Lens Use and Contact Lens Solution*

The U.S. Food and Drug Administration (FDA) and the Centers for Disease Control and Prevention (CDC) are alerting health care professionals and their patients who wear soft contact lenses to an increasing number of reports in the United States of rare but serious fungal infections in the eye that can cause permanent loss of sight. Some patients have reported a significant loss of vision, resulting in the need for a corneal transplant.

A fungus called *Fusarium* has been identified as the cause of the reported infections. As of April 9, 2006, 109 cases of suspected *Fusarium* keratitis are under investigation by CDC and public health authorities in 17 states of the United States.

"This is a serious infection and soft contact lens users should be mindful of the potential to develop this problem," said Dr. Daniel Schultz, director of the FDA's Center for Devices and Radiological Health. "We're advising consumers to practice good basic hygiene and follow manufacturers' instructions for proper use, cleaning and storage of their lenses, and report any signs of infection to their doctors."

Clinicians who evaluate patients with microbial keratitis should consider that a fungal infection may be involved and refer the patient to an ophthalmologist, if appropriate, to obtain a specimen for laboratory analysis. In addition, the FDA and CDC are urgently advising consumers to take precautions to prevent contamination of the soft lenses and the products used to maintain them. These preventive practices for contact lens wearers include the following:

- Wash hands with soap and water and dry (lint-free method) before handling lenses.

- Wear and replace lenses according to the schedule prescribed by the doctor.

- Follow the specific lens cleaning and storage guidelines from the doctor and the solution manufacturer.

- Keep the contact lens case clean and replace every 3 to 6 months.

- Remove the lenses and consult your doctor immediately if you experience symptoms such as redness, pain, tearing, increased light sensitivity, blurry vision, discharge, or swelling.

In addition, regardless of which cleaning/disinfecting solution used, wearers may want to consider performing a "rub and rinse" lens cleaning method, rather than a no-rub method, in order to minimize the number of germs and reduce the chances of infection.

Of the 30 patient cases fully investigated so far, 28 wore soft contact lenses and two reported no contact lens use. Twenty-six of the soft contact lens users who remembered which solution they used during the month prior to the infection onset reported using a Bausch & Lomb ReNu brand contact lens solution or a generic brand manufactured by the same company. Five case-patients reported using other solutions in addition to the ReNu brand, and 9 patients reported wearing contact lenses overnight, a known risk factor for microbial keratitis.

"It is important to note that some of the affected patients had used other solutions in addition to the ReNu brand, and that the source of this fungus has not yet been identified. But we're working with CDC and Bausch & Lomb—and we're investigating other possible causes—to prevent these infections," Dr. Schultz added.

Bausch and Lomb has informed FDA that they are voluntarily stopping shipment of the ReNu Moisture Loc product while they are continuing to investigate the cause of these infections. Soft contact lens users who have existing supplies of the ReNu Moisture Loc should use the product with caution and report any signs and symptoms of eye infection to their doctors.

Clusters of *Fusarium* keratitis were reported among contact lens users in Asia beginning in November 2005. In February 2006, Bausch & Lomb voluntarily suspended sales of its ReNu multipurpose solutions in Singapore and Hong Kong after multiple reports of the infection among contact lens users there. No other jurisdictions have taken similar action to date.

Fusarium species are normally found in many plants, soil, and tap water. The annual risk of contact lens-related microbial keratitis is estimated in most studies to be between four and 21 per 10,000 patients, depending on whether the lenses are worn only during the day or continuously overnight.

Fungal keratitis can be associated with trauma to the surface of the eye, immunodeficiencies, and contact lens use. Organisms associated with contact lens-related keratitis are usually bacteria rather than fungus, often arising from contamination of lens care products or from contact lens storage cases.

Contact Lens Solution and the Risk of Acanthamoeba Keratitis

FDA is alerting health care professionals and patients who wear soft contact lenses about a voluntary recall of Complete MoisturePlus Multi Purpose Solution. The company, Advanced Medical Optics of Santa Ana, California, is taking this action as a precaution because of reports of a rare but serious eye infection, *Acanthamoeba* keratitis, caused by a parasite.

"We believe the company acted responsibly in taking this voluntary action and support the decision to be proactive in the interest of public health," says Daniel Schultz, M.D., Director of FDA's Center for Devices and Radiological Health.

Steps for Consumers

If you wear soft contact lenses, you should:

- Stop using Complete MoisturePlus Contact Lens solution.

- Discard all partially used or unopened bottles.

- Replace your contact lenses and storage container.

- Ask your doctor about choosing an appropriate alternative cleaning/disinfecting product.

- Seek immediate treatment if you have symptoms of eye infection—eye pain or redness, blurred vision, light sensitivity, sensation of something in the eye, or excessive tearing. Early diagnosis is important for effective treatment.

If you believe that you have the recalled product, you may call the company at 888-899-9183.

About Acanthamoeba *Keratitis*

A serious eye infection: The symptoms of *Acanthamoeba* keratitis can be very similar to those of other more common eye infections and may include eye pain or redness, blurred vision, light sensitivity, sensation of something in the eye or excessive tearing but *Acanthamoeba* is more difficult to treat. *Acanthamoeba* keratitis may lead to vision loss with some patients requiring a corneal transplant. The infection primarily affects otherwise healthy people who wear contact lenses.

Recent increase in cases: The link between the solution and the infection was identified as a result of an investigation by the Centers for Disease Control and Prevention (CDC). It is estimated that *Acanthamoeba* keratitis infections occur in approximately 2 out of every 1 million contact lens users in the United States each year. But in a multi-state investigation to evaluate a recent increase in *Acanthamoeba* keratitis cases, CDC determined that the risk of developing *Acanthamoeba* keratitis was at least seven times greater for those consumers who used Complete MoisturePlus solution versus those who did not.

Ongoing investigation: FDA and CDC are working closely with the company to collect additional information and will continue to advise consumers as more information becomes available. Experts are collaborating to further understand whether usage or contamination of this solution led to these *Acanthamoeba* infections.

Measures to Help Prevent Eye Infections

All contact lens wearers should adhere to these measures to help prevent eye infections:

- Remove contact lenses before any activity involving contact with water, including showering, using a hot tub, or swimming.

- Wash hands with soap and water and dry them before handling contact lenses.

- Clean contact lenses according to manufacturer guidelines and instructions from an eye care professional.

- Use fresh cleaning or disinfecting solution each time lenses are cleaned and stored. Never reuse or top off old solution.

- Never use saline solution and rewetting drops to disinfect lenses. Neither solution is an effective or approved disinfectant.

- Schedule regular eye exams with your eye care professional.

- Wear and replace contact lenses according to the schedule prescribed by your eye care professional.

- Store lenses in a proper storage case. Storage cases should be irrigated with sterile contact lens solution (never use tap water) and left open to dry after each use.

- Replace storage cases at least once every three months.

Report Adverse Events

FDA and CDC want to gather information related to *Acanthamoeba* keratitis in contact lens users. Report adverse events related to these products to MedWatch, the FDA's voluntary reporting program: www.fda.gov/medwatch/report.htm; Phone: 800-332-1088; Fax: 800-332-0178; Mail: MedWatch, Food and Drug Administration, 5600 Fishers Lane, Rockville, MD, 20852-9787.

Chapter 15

All about Eyeglasses

Chapter Contents

Section 15.1

How to Read Your Eyeglasses Prescription

The numbers your Eye M.D. jots down during your eye exam describe what you're seeing, and what you're not seeing.

If you know how to read your prescription you can usually comparison shop for glasses over the phone, a good way to get a base price for the glasses of your choice. Don't forget that you will probably want lens enhancements, which will be an additional cost.

Whether your Eye M.D. writes your eye glass prescription on a preprinted form specifically for eyeglasses or on a blank sheet of paper, the numbers will read the same. O.D. (oculus dextrus) is your right eye and O.S. (oculus sinister) is your left. You might see the abbreviations RE and LE, or possibly no designation at all. If that is the case, you can safely assume that the first set of numbers is for your right eye.

The prescription in Table 15.1 reads, "Right eye, plus two point five zero, plus one point zero zero, axis 180. Left eye, plus one point seven five, plus one point five zero, axis one eighty. Plus two point zero zero add."

The "Sphere" column indicates how nearsighted or farsighted you are. "Cylinder" refers to the measurable degree of astigmatism of your central cornea. The cylindrical number describes the dioptric difference between your cornea's steepest and lowest curves.

If you have astigmatism, your cornea is shaped like the back of a spoon, curved more on one side than the other. The orientation of the

Table 15.1. What Your Prescription Means

	Sphere	Cylinder	Axis
O.D.	+2.50	+1.00	180
O.S.	+1.75	+1.50	180
	+2.00 add		

spoon shape can differ from person to person, for instance like a spoon standing on end or on it's side. The "Axis" column describes the orientation in degrees from horizontal. Most left and right eyes with astigmatism are symmetrical.

What Do the Numbers Mean?

Lens power is measured in units called diopters. Diopters are based on the extent light rays passing through the lens will be bent. As the power of the lens increases, so does the thickness of the lens. There are three different types of lenses:

- **Convex lenses** are thicker in the center than at the edges, like a magnifying glass. Light rays are gathered together towards a central point. Convex lenses are used in glasses for farsighted (hyperopic) eyes that can't bend light rays as much as they need to. Convex lenses are indicated with a plus (+) symbol on prescriptions.

- **Concave lenses** are thinner at the center than at the edges and spread light rays apart. These lenses are used for eyes that are nearsighted (myopic). Concave lenses are indicated with a minus (-) symbol.

- **Cylindrical lenses** are curved more in one direction than the other. To tell if your lenses are cylindrical, hold your glasses at arm's length and sight a straight line through the lens. Rotate the glasses clockwise and counterclockwise. If the line bends, it's a cylindrical lens. Cylindrical lenses, used for astigmatism, are usually part of a prescription for near- or farsightedness.

The prescription in Table 15.2 reads, "Right eye, minus one point two five, minus two point five zero, axis ninety. Left eye, minus zero point seven five, minus two point two five, axis ninety."

Table 15.2. How to Read a Prescription for Bifocals

	Sphere	Cylinder	Axis
O.D.	-1.25	-2.50	90
O.S.	-0.75	-2.25	90
	+1.50 add		

This means the patient's right eye has 1 1/4 diopters of nearsightedness with 2 1/2 diopters of astigmatism. The axis refers to the orientation of the cylindrical area of the lens. The axis can be anywhere from 1 to 180 degrees, with 90 being the vertical meridians. The left eye has 3/4 diopters of nearsightedness, 2 1/4 diopters of astigmatism, axis 90.

Bifocal prescriptions are indicated with numbers such as the "+1.50 add" above. This number indicates the strength of the lens. This patient will need 1 1/2 diopters of power for reading.

Section 15.2

Eyeglasses: Frequently Asked Questions

"Eyeglasses: Frequently Asked Questions," is reprinted with permission from www.allaboutvision.com. © 2006 Access Media Group, LLC.

Why should I bother to go to the eye doctor when I can simply pick up an inexpensive pair of eyeglasses at the store?

Some people do have good luck with drugstore reading glasses. However, you need to visit your eye care practitioner regularly for two reasons:

- Regular eye exams are the only way to catch "silent" diseases in their early stages, when they're more easily treated.

- One-size-fits-all reading glasses do not work well for people who have a different prescription in each eye, or whose eyes are not centered in the lens. Headaches are a common problem in those cases.

What's the secret to getting eyeglasses that look great on me?

First, decide which of the seven basic face shapes you have and read tips about frames that go well with your shape. Then, find out which colors suit your skin, eye, and hair colors.

How do I avoid annoying reflections on my eyeglasses?

Anti-reflective coating, also known as AR coating, helps you to see through your eyeglasses more easily, allows others to see your eyes better, and eliminates the annoying white glare spots in photos taken with a flash.

I'm interested in the glasses that change to sunglasses when you go outside. Can you tell me more about them?

These lenses are known as photochromic lenses. When they're exposed to ultraviolet light, they become darker or change to a different color. Most brands remain pretty light when you're driving, because windshields block UV light.

I find most eyeglasses to be too small for my head. Do you know of any brands that carry larger frames?

These days, most eyewear lines include at least one or two frames in larger-than-average sizes. But you might try styles from these collections, which have several larger styles for wider faces and/or people who need longer temple pieces:

- Cazal frames from Eastern States & Ultra Palm Eyewear
- Columbia Sportswear frames from L'Amy Group
- Prada frames from Luxottica Group
- Rodenstock frames
- Hart Schaffner Marx frames from Signature Eyewear
- Silhouette frames
- Harley-Davidson frames from Viva International Group
- Stetson, John Deere, Sophia Loren, and Gloria Vanderbilt frames from Zyloware

What are the warning signs that a child might need glasses?

- Consistently sitting too close to the TV or holding a book too close
- Losing her place while reading
- Using a finger to follow along while reading

- Squinting
- Tilting the head to see better
- Frequent eye rubbing
- Sensitivity to light
- Excessive tearing
- Closing one eye to read, watch TV, or see better
- Avoiding activities that require near vision, such as reading or homework, or distance vision, such as participating in sports or other recreational activities
- Complaining of headaches or tired eyes
- Receiving lower grades than usual

Schedule an appointment with your eye doctor if your child exhibits any of these signs.

How do I choose glasses that my child will actually wear without breaking the bank?

The most important factor in getting a child to wear glasses is to let him or her help pick them out.

I'm worried that my son's glasses could break while he's wearing them. What's the best way to protect his eyes?

Polycarbonate is usually recommended for children because it's very impact-resistant.

How can I prolong the life of my eyeglasses?

- If you're buying just one pair of glasses, avoid trendy frames that could go out of style quickly.
- If you're buying glasses for a child whose prescription changes often, ask to have new lenses put in the old frames, rather than buying new frames each time.
- Choose a style with spring hinges, which allow the temples to flex slightly outward without breaking the eyeglasses.
- Ask for scratch-resistant coating.
- Follow your eye care professional's instructions for the proper

care of your glasses. Improper care is a primary cause of damage to anti-reflective coating and can cause other problems as well.

How often should I get a new pair of glasses?

You should get a new pair if your prescription has changed; your doctor will let you know. Therefore, it's important to know how often to visit the eye doctor: it depends on many factors, but as a general rule, you should go once a year or once every two years. Your doctor can tell you what schedule is right for you.

If your prescription doesn't change very often, or at all, just get new glasses when you're tired of your old ones or they go out of style.

I can see fine to read or drive, but I'm having trouble with certain tasks, especially at work. What's wrong?

You should see your eye doctor if you're having any sort of problem with your vision. However, we can tell you some reasons this might be happening.

This is common problem for computer users who wear bifocals (which correct near and far vision) or reading glasses (which correct near vision), because computer monitors tend to be in your intermediate vision, neither near nor far. The solution is to ask your eye doctor about intermediate vision correction, either in the form of computer glasses, progressive lenses, or trifocals.

Sometimes, the problem is that the near-vision portion of your glasses is not compatible with what you're doing. Golfers, for example, benefit from having that portion placed very low and in the inside corner, so that it doesn't interfere with their game. Read more about these special types of multifocals, called occupational lenses.

I'm tired of my "Coke-bottle" lenses. Is there anything I can do?

You could ask your eye doctor about high-index lenses, which are compressed, or aspheric lenses, which have a flatter curve than regular lenses.

The anti-reflective coating on my glasses is smeary (or foggy). What causes that and what can I do about it?

Cleaning your eyeglasses improperly is a common cause of problems with anti-reflective coating. When you bought your eyeglasses, your eye doctor probably explained the best way to care for them; usually, you use lens spray and a certain type of cloth, like microfiber.

Sometimes, your eye doctor may be able to remove the damaged coating, but usually not. There's nothing you can do at home.

Do my glasses protect my eyes from the sun?

That depends. Many people have plastic lenses, which do not protect your eyes; you need to have UV coating for protection. Polycarbonate lenses have built-in UV protection. Glass lenses protect your eyes from harmful UVB rays, but not from UVA; some experts think UVA rays might have long-term, damaging effects on your eyes and skin.

What do all those numbers in my prescription mean?

An eyeglass prescription is written in a standardized format with standardized notation so it can be interpreted worldwide. Let's look at one and break it down:

$$-2.00 \ -1.00 \ \text{x} \ 180$$

The first number (-2.00) tells us the spherical refractive error (far-sightedness or nearsightedness). In this case, because there is a minus sign in front of the 2.00, this patient is nearsighted. A plus sign would indicate farsightedness.

The second number (-1.00) is the astigmatism. If there is no astigmatism, we generally write the letters DS or SPH after the first number to let the optician know that we didn't just forget to write in the astigmatism.

The final number (180) is the direction of the astigmatism. Astigmatism, a football-shaped eye, can be measured in any direction around the clock. We use the numbers from 90 to 180 to indicate the orientation of the football shape.

There may be additional numbers in a glasses prescription. For instance, if the basic prescription is followed by a small number with a superscript (1^) it indicates prism correction. There may be more than one set of prism numbers for each eye.

Lastly, there can also be numbers denoting the amount of near reading strength needed (bifocal or progressive). They usually go from +0.75 to +3.00, depending on age and visual need.

The letters OD and OS in front of a prescription let us know which eye each string of numbers is for. OD stands for right eye and OS for left eye, while OU means both eyes.

Section 15.3

Bifocals and Trifocals

"Bifocals & Trifocals: New Options for 'Short Arms,'"
by Liz DeFranco, A.B.O.C., N.C.L.C. is reprinted with permission from
www.allaboutvision.com. © 2007 Access Media Group, LLC.

Just as eyewear fashions have changed a lot recently, eyeglass lenses also have improved. As technology has advanced, more options have become available to multifocal wearers.

Not so long ago, anyone who needed a correction to see close-up had to wear the Franklin or Executive bifocal, with the line that goes all the way across the entire width of the lens. Then came the smaller, half-moon bifocal segment. And those who needed a correction in the intermediate zone (about arm's length away), had very few choices.

Nowadays, multifocal wearers have lots of options. They include special glasses for computers and other tasks that take place at the intermediate range, as well as lenses for reading distance and special combinations for unique work situations.

One Lens, Many Functions

Multifocals let you focus through different prescriptions at different distances through the same lens—hence the name. Bifocals (meaning a lens with two points of focus—usually one for distance and one for near) are the most commonly prescribed multifocal lenses.

Many people need some visual correction in order to read or see things close-up. Often, bifocals are necessary because people's arms "become shorter" (actually a condition called "presbyopia") as they enter middle age and things closer to them become more difficult to see. However, other conditions can cause people of any age to need more help seeing properly in the near range. Overconvergence, when the eyes work too hard to see close up, is one.

Regardless of the reason you need a prescription for near-vision correction, bifocals all work in the same way. A small portion of the eyeglass lens is reserved for the near-vision correction. The rest of the lens is usually a distance correction, but sometimes has no correction at all in it.

The segment that is devoted to near-vision correction can be in one of several shapes:

- A half-moon, also called a flat-top, straight-top, or D segment
- A round segment
- A narrow rectangular area, known as a ribbon segment
- A full bottom half of a lens, called the Franklin, Executive, or E style

Generally, you look up and through the distance portion of the lens when focusing on points farther away, and you look down and through the bifocal segment of the lens when focusing on reading material or detail work up to about 18 inches away.

Similar to bifocals are trifocals, or lenses with three points of focus—usually for distance, intermediate and near. Trifocals have an added segment above the bifocal for viewing things in the intermediate zone, which is farther than the near zone—about arm's length away. Computers are an excellent example of something that is in a person's intermediate zone. Motorists who need to see in the distance to drive, to see the gauges on the dashboard, and to read a map also would benefit from a trifocal. Flat-top and Executive lens styles are the most common trifocals.

How Multifocal Eyeglasses Are Fitted

Bifocals are typically placed so the line rests at the same height as the wearer's lower eyelid. As a bifocal wearer drops his eyes downward to read, the eyes naturally seek out the near-vision portion of the lens.

Trifocals are fitted a bit higher, with the top line of the intermediate area placed even with the pupil. A trifocal wearer focuses through the intermediate prescription area of the lens when looking at something between 18 and 24 inches away. The eyes gravitate straight ahead, or up and over the multifocal segments, when gazing at something in the distance.

Most bifocals and trifocals have lines, but there is a round bifocal segment called the E-Z-2-Vue, which is less obtrusive. It is blended into the distance portion of the lens so that it is not readily visible to the casual viewer.

A progressive lens is a special kind of no-line multifocal that incorporates all corrections, from distance to close-up, into one lens without any separation of the various visual zones by line.

Multifocal Occupational Lenses

Other multifocals are suited for performing a particular job or hobby and are not meant for everyday wear: Specialty multifocal lenses are designed to solve particular vision problems. If you have a special need because of your work, hobby, or favorite pastime, tell your eye care practitioner.

One occupational bifocal is a Double-D, which has a half-moon-shaped flat-top bifocal at the bottom of the lens and an upside-down flat-top at the top of the lens. The rest of the lens area is for distance correction. Car mechanics, who need to see well at the near point both looking down to read as well as looking up above their head to work on the undercarriage of a car on a lift, would benefit from a Double-D. Double-round segs are also occupational lenses that can be used for the same purposes as the Double-D.

An E-D trifocal has a distance correction along the top half of the lens, separated from the intermediate correction in the bottom half by a line that goes all the way across the width of the lens in the Executive bifocal style, and a D half-moon segment containing the near correction that resides within the lower half of the lens. The E-D trifocal is for someone who must see at the intermediate distance in a wide field of vision and who also must see clearly both close up and in the distance. A television production person, for example, who must keep an eye on several TV monitors spread out in front and to the sides while being able to read notes from a clipboard and recognize someone across the room, is a good candidate for this lens.

Sometimes a common multifocal can become an occupational lens by changing the way it is placed in the eyeglass frame. For example, instead of placing a long, narrow rectangular ribbon seg just at the bottom eyelid, where bifocals are normally situated, the ribbon seg can be moved to reside at your eye level. You would then look through the near vision correction rather than through the distance correction when standing or sitting in a normal position. While this wouldn't be ideal for everyday tasks such as driving, it would work for a pharmacist who must read the small print on labels right in front of her all day long.

For golf players, flat-top bifocals are often placed extremely low and in the inside corner of one lens of a pair of "golf glasses." Just enough

131

near vision correction is placed in the eyeglasses to allow the golfer to read and write on the scorecard without compromising the vision necessary to hit the sweet spot on the ball.

Chapter 16

Making a Decision about Laser Eye Surgery: Is It Right for You?

Introduction

Laser-assisted in situ keratomileusis, or LASIK, the most commonly performed type of laser surgery, is generally a safe and effective treatment for a wide range of common vision problems. Specifically, LASIK involves the use of a laser to permanently change the shape of the cornea, the clear covering of the front of the eye. LASIK is a quick and often painless procedure, and for the majority of patients, the surgery improves vision and reduces the need for corrective eyewear. However, as LASIK is a surgical procedure conducted on a delicate part of the eye, it is crucial that potential candidates are well educated on the benefits and risks of the procedure, understand the importance of a thorough screening by their physician, and maintain realistic expectations about the procedure's outcome.

Patient Profiles

Who is right for laser eye surgery? While many individuals are considered good candidates for LASIK, there are some who do not meet the generally accepted medical criteria to ensure a successful laser vision procedure. Individuals that are not deemed good candidates given today's technology may be able to have the surgery in the future, as technology advances and new techniques are refined. Anyone considering laser eye surgery must have a thorough examination by an ophthalmologist that will help determine, in consultation with the patient, whether or not the LASIK procedure is right for them. Based on various conditions and circumstances, all LASIK candidates will fall into one of the following three broad categories.

The Ideal LASIK Candidate

The ideal candidate includes those who:

- are over 18 years of age and have had a stable glasses or contact lens prescription for at least two years.

- have sufficient corneal thickness (the cornea is the transparent front part of the eye). A LASIK patient should have a cornea that is thick enough to allow the surgeon to safely create a clean corneal flap of appropriate depth.

- are affected by one of the common types of vision problems or refractive error—myopia (nearsightedness), astigmatism (blurred vision caused by an irregularly shaped cornea), hyperopia (farsightedness), or a combination thereof (e.g., myopia with astigmatism). Several lasers are now approved by the U.S. Food and Drug Administration (FDA) as safe and effective for use in LASIK, but the scope of each laser's approved indication and treatment range is limited to specified degrees of refractive error.

- do not suffer from any disease, vision-related or otherwise, that may reduce the effectiveness of the surgery or the patient's ability to heal properly and quickly.

- are adequately informed about the benefits and risks of the procedure. Candidates should thoroughly discuss the procedure with their physicians and understand that for most people, the goal of refractive surgery should be the reduction of dependency on glasses and contact lenses, not their complete elimination.

The 'Less Than Ideal' LASIK Candidate

Sometimes, factors exist that preclude a candidate from being ideal for LASIK surgery. In many cases, a surgeon may still be able to perform the procedure safely, given that the candidate and physician have adequately discussed the benefits and risks, and set realistic expectations for the results. Candidates in this category include those who:

- have a history of dry eyes, as they may find that the condition worsens following surgery.

- are being treated with medications such as steroids or immuno-suppressants, which can prevent healing, or are suffering from diseases that slow healing, such as autoimmune disorders.

- have scarring of the cornea.

More often, factors exist that may keep an individual from being a candidate immediately, but do not preclude the individual from being a candidate entirely. Candidates in this category include those who:

- are under age 18.

- have unstable vision, which usually occurs in young people. Doctors recommend that, prior to undergoing LASIK, candidates' vision has stabilized with a consistent glasses or contact lens prescription for at least two years.

- are pregnant or nursing.

- have a history of ocular herpes within one year prior to having the surgery. Once a year has passed from initial diagnosis of the disease, surgery can be considered.

- have refractive errors too severe for treatment with current technology. Although FDA-approved lasers are available to treat each of the three major types of refractive error—myopia, hyperopia, and astigmatism—current FDA-approved indications define appropriate candidates as those with myopia up to -12 D, astigmatism up to 6 D, and hyperopia up to +6 D. However, laser eye surgery technology is evolving rapidly, and doctors may be able to treat more severe errors in the future.

The Non-LASIK Candidate

Certain conditions and circumstances completely preclude individuals from being candidates for LASIK surgery. Non-candidates include individuals who:

- have diseases such as cataracts, advanced glaucoma, corneal diseases, corneal thinning disorders (keratoconus or pellucid marginal degeneration), or certain other pre-existing eye diseases that affect or threaten vision.

135

- do not give informed consent. It is absolutely necessary that candidates adequately discuss the procedure and its benefits and risks with their surgeon, and provide the appropriate consent prior to undergoing the surgery.

- have unrealistic expectations. It is critical for candidates to understand that laser eye surgery, as all surgical procedures, involves some risk. In addition, both the final outcome of surgery and the rate of healing vary from person to person and even from eye to eye in each individual.

Pre-LASIK Testing

What Types of Screening Exams Should Patients Expect?

Anyone considering LASIK should undergo a thorough examination by an eye care professional. The exam, and a follow-up consultation with the physician, can also identify ongoing health concerns that may affect the candidate's vision in the future, inform the candidate of potential outcomes of LASIK, frame expectations for what the procedure can do, and inform the candidate of his or her vision health status. A list of preliminary or screening tests that should be performed routinely appears below. Additional testing, depending on preliminary findings and the special needs of the candidate, may also be appropriate. If, after an evaluation, a patient has questions about why a test was included or omitted, he/she should discuss the matter with the eye care professional in question. Certainly a patient can and should question why a test was omitted. The patient should be satisfied with the explanation before proceeding.

Assessment of Eye Health History

- History of wearing glasses: It is important to determine if a candidate's vision has stabilized or is changing. If it is unstable, LASIK may not be appropriate at this time. The ideal candidate is at least 18 years of age with a stable glasses or contact lens prescription for at least 2 years.

- History of contact lens wear: Contact lenses may change the shape of the cornea (the clear front surface of the eye) or act in such a way as to prevent the ophthalmologist from determining a candidate's correct prescription. Most ophthalmologists require that soft contact lenses be discontinued at least 3 days and rigid contact lenses 2 to 3 weeks prior to the evaluation. If concern arises about contact lens-induced changes in the cornea, it may be necessary for a candidate to stop wearing contacts for as long as several months to allow the cornea to return to its natural contour, so that a surgical evaluation can be made.

- History of ocular or systemic diseases and medications: Some eye diseases and medications can affect the suitability of a candidate for LASIK.

- History of previous ocular problems such as lazy eyes, strabismus (eye misalignment caused by muscle imbalance), or the need for special glasses to prevent double vision.

- History of previous eye injury.

- Assessing vocational and lifestyle needs: The LASIK candidate's work or recreational activities and needs can influence vision correction strategies. For example, different strategies can affect depth perception and the ability to see near or far.

A Comprehensive Examination of the Eye

- Determination of uncorrected vision and vision as corrected by glasses or contacts.

- Determination of the magnitude of visual error in each eye to establish the amount of surgical correction that is needed and develop the appropriate surgical strategy.

- Assessment of the surface of the cornea by "mapping" its topography (corneal curvature or shape), to correlate its shape to errors in focusing (correlate corneal shape to refractive astigmatism), to find irregularities, if any, and to screen for disease states that may produce poor outcomes with LASIK.

- Measurement of pupil size in dim and room light. Pupil size is an important factor in counseling a candidate about night vision and planning the appropriate laser vision correction strategy.

- Assessment of motility to measure the ability of the muscles to align the eyes.

- Examination of the eyelids to see if they turn inward (possibly scratching the cornea) or outward and redirect tear flow away from the eye and other conditions.

- Examination of the conjunctiva, the transparent membrane that covers the outer surface of the eye and lines the inner surface of the eyelids, to see whether there are irritations, redness, irregular blood vessels, or other abnormalities.

- Examination of the cornea to determine if there are any abnormalities that could affect the outcome of surgery.

- Examination of the crystalline lens to determine if clouding of the lens (cataract) or other abnormalities are present.

- Measurement of corneal thickness (pachymetry). The amount of LASIK correction may be determined in part by corneal thickness.

- Measurement of intraocular pressure to detect glaucoma or preglaucomatous conditions. Glaucoma is a visual loss caused by damage to the optic nerve from excessively high pressures in the eye. It is a common cause of preventable vision loss.

- Assessment of the back (posterior segment) of the eye: The dilated fundus exam is used to assess the health of the inside back surface of the eye (retina), with the pupil fully open. Examination of the retina, optic nerve, and blood vessels screens for a number of eye and systemic disorders.

- Follow-up should include review of examination results by an ophthalmologist, discussion with the candidate, additional testing as necessary, and adoption of a plan for managing the candidate's eye-care needs.

Realistic Expectations: Why Are They Central to Patient Satisfaction?

The overwhelming majority of patients who have had LASIK surgery are fully satisfied with their results—having experienced the significant benefits of improved vision. However, as with any medical or surgical procedure, for certain patients the outcome of the procedure may not seem "ideal" or meet all of his/her expectations. A small minority of patients may also experience complications. Therefore, it is crucial that LASIK surgery candidates thoroughly discuss the procedure—its benefits, risks, and probable outcomes—with their physician prior to undergoing the surgery. Each patient should be fully informed and feel comfortable that they are making an educated decision based upon facts.

Candidates should be aware that:

- LASIK cannot provide perfect vision every time for every patient. However, for the majority of LASIK candidates, the surgery improves vision and reduces the need for corrective eyewear. In fact, the vast majority of patients with low to moderate nearsightedness achieve 20/40 vision or better, and many can expect to achieve 20/20 vision or better.

- Re-treatments (enhancements) may be required to achieve optimal outcomes. Fortunately, it is possible to repeat the laser treatment by lifting the flap, typically about three months after the original procedure. Even after enhancements, vision after LASIK may not be as good as it was with glasses or contact lenses before the procedure.

- There may be visual aberrations after LASIK—most commonly, glare and halos under dim lighting conditions. Usually, these are not significant, and resolve within several months of surgery. Occasionally, they are severe enough to interfere with normal activities.

- Monovision is a technique in which one eye is corrected for distance vision and the other is left nearsighted to focus on near objects without glasses. Today, it is the only way that LASIK candidates older than about 45 years can avoid reading glasses. LASIK will not cure presbyopia, the aging changes that prevent older people from seeing near objects through the same glasses that they use for viewing distant objects.

- LASIK surgery, as with all surgical procedures, has the risk of complications. Fortunately, the likelihood of visual loss with LASIK is very small. In the many millions of LASIK procedures done so far, less than one percent of patients have experienced serious, vision threatening problems. Most complications represent delays in full recovery and resolve within several months of surgery.

Initiating a Dialogue: What Should I Ask My Doctor?

The decision to have LASIK should be an informed one, made in close consultation with an eye care professional. In order to understand whether LASIK is right for them, patients considering the procedure should ask the following questions of their doctor:

- What type of testing will you do in order to determine whether I'm a candidate for LASIK?

- Has my glasses or contact lens prescription been consistent for at least two years?

- Does my nearsightedness, farsightedness, or astigmatism fall within the accepted levels established for surgery by the FDA?

- Are my corneas thick enough to perform LASIK surgery?

- Do I have cataracts, glaucoma, or other corneal diseases?

- Are my corneas scarred?

- Do I have any diseases that would affect the outcome of the surgery or my ability to heal properly?

- Are there any other reasons why I may not be a candidate for LASIK surgery?

- Am I at risk for complications?

- What can I expect during the procedure?

- What outcome can I expect from the surgery?

The Eye Surgery Education Council (ESEC) is an initiative established by the American Society of Cataract and Refractive Surgery (ASCRS), a professional society of ophthalmologists dedicated to raising the standards and skills of surgeons, who operate on the anterior (front) segment of the eye, through clinical education, and to work with patients, government, and the medical community to promote delivery of quality eye care. The ESEC, which is committed to helping patients make informed decisions about undergoing laser eye surgery, has two missions—to provide patients with accurate, accessible information, and to promote active physician/patient discussion about the benefits and risks of laser eye surgery procedures.

The information provided in these patient guidelines is intended to provide educational information to eye care professionals and is not intended to establish a particular standard of care, provide an exhaustive discussion of the subject of laser eye surgery, or serve as a substitute for the application of the individual physician's medical judgment in the particular circumstances presented by each patient care situation.

Candidates and prospective candidates for laser eye surgery should likewise understand that the information provided in these guidelines is educational in nature and is not intended to serve as a substitute for medical advice. The decision whether to undergo laser eye surgery must be made by each individual based on the relevant facts and circumstances acting in consultation with a qualified eye care professional.

Chapter 17

Laser-Assisted In Situ Keratomileusis (LASIK) Eye Surgery

Chapter Contents

Section 17.1

All about LASIK

Excerpted from "LASIK Eye Surgery," by the Centers for Devices
and Radiological Health (CDRH), part of the U.S. Food and Drug
Administration (FDA, www.fda.gov), July 12, 2006.

LASIK is a surgical procedure intended to reduce a person's dependency on glasses or contact lenses. LASIK stands for Laser-Assisted In Situ Keratomileusis and is a procedure that permanently changes the shape of the cornea, the clear covering of the front of the eye, using an excimer laser. A knife, called a microkeratome, is used to cut a flap in the cornea. A hinge is left at one end of this flap. The flap is folded back revealing the stroma, the middle section of the cornea. Pulses from a computer-controlled laser vaporize a portion of the stroma and the flap is replaced.

What Is LASIK?

The Eye and Vision Errors

The cornea is a part of the eye that helps focus light to create an image on the retina. It works in much the same way that the lens of a camera focuses light to create an image on film. The bending and focusing of light is also known as refraction. Usually the shape of the cornea and the eye are not perfect and the image on the retina is out of focus (blurred) or distorted. These imperfections in the focusing power of the eye are called refractive errors. There are three primary types of refractive errors: myopia, hyperopia, and astigmatism. Persons with myopia, or nearsightedness, have more difficulty seeing distant objects as clearly as near objects. Persons with hyperopia, or farsightedness, have more difficulty seeing near objects as clearly as distant objects. Astigmatism is a distortion of the image on the retina caused by irregularities in the cornea or lens of the eye. Combinations of myopia and astigmatism or hyperopia and astigmatism are common. Glasses or contact lenses are designed to compensate for the eye's imperfections. Surgical procedures aimed at improving the focusing power of the eye are called refractive surgery. In LASIK surgery, precise and controlled removal of corneal tissue by a special laser reshapes the cornea changing its focusing power.

Other Types of Refractive Surgery

Radial Keratotomy or RK and Photorefractive Keratectomy or PRK are other refractive surgeries used to reshape the cornea. In RK, a very sharp knife is used to cut slits in the cornea changing its shape. PRK was the first surgical procedure developed to reshape the cornea, by sculpting, using a laser. Later, LASIK was developed. The same type of laser is used for LASIK and PRK. Often the exact same laser is used for the two types of surgery. The major difference between the two surgeries is the way that the stroma, the middle layer of the cornea, is exposed before it is vaporized with the laser. In PRK, the top layer of the cornea, called the epithelium, is scraped away to expose the stromal layer underneath. In LASIK, a flap is cut in the stromal layer and the flap is folded back.

Another type of refractive surgery is thermokeratoplasty in which heat is used to reshape the cornea. The source of the heat can be a laser, but it is a different kind of laser than is used for LASIK and PRK. Other refractive devices include corneal ring segments that are inserted into the stroma and special contact lenses that temporarily reshape the cornea (orthokeratology).

What the FDA Regulates

In the United States, the Food and Drug Administration (FDA) regulates the sale of medical devices such as the lasers used for LASIK. Before a medical device can be legally sold in the United States, the person or company that wants to sell the device must seek approval from the FDA. To gain approval, they must present evidence that the device is reasonably safe and effective for a particular use, the "indication." Once the FDA has approved a medical device, a doctor may decide to use that device for other indications if the doctor feels it is in the best interest of a patient. The use of an approved device for other than its FDA-approved indication is called "off-label use." The FDA does not regulate off-label use or the practice of medicine.

The FDA does not have the authority to:

* regulate a doctor's practice. In other words, FDA does not tell doctors what to do when running their business or what they can or cannot tell their patients.

- set the amount a doctor can charge for LASIK eye surgery.

- insist the patient information booklet from the laser manufacturer be provided to the potential patient.

- make recommendations for individual doctors, clinics, or eye centers. FDA does not maintain nor have access to any such list of doctors performing LASIK eye surgery.

- conduct or provide a rating system on any medical device it regulates.

The first refractive laser systems approved by FDA were excimer lasers for use in PRK to treat myopia and later to treat astigmatism. However, doctors began using these lasers for LASIK (not just PRK), and to treat other refractive errors (not just myopia). Over the last several years, LASIK has become the main surgery doctors use to treat myopia in the United States. More recently, some laser manufacturers have gained FDA approval for laser systems for LASIK to treat myopia, hyperopia, and astigmatism and for PRK to treat hyperopia and astigmatism.

When Is LASIK Not for Me?

You are probably **not** a good candidate for refractive surgery if:

- **You are not a risk taker:** Certain complications are unavoidable in a percentage of patients, and there are no long-term data available for current procedures.

- **It will jeopardize your career:** Some jobs prohibit certain refractive procedures. Be sure to check with your employer/professional society/military service before undergoing any procedure.

- **Cost is an issue:** Most medical insurance will not pay for refractive surgery. Although the cost is coming down, it is still significant.

- **You required a change in your contact lens or glasses prescription in the past year:** This is called refractive instability. Patients who are in their early 20s or younger; whose hormones are fluctuating due to disease such as diabetes; who are pregnant or breastfeeding; or who are taking medications that may cause fluctuations in vision are more likely to have refractive instability and should discuss the possible additional risks with their doctor.

- **You have a disease or are on medications that may affect wound healing:** Certain conditions, such as autoimmune diseases (e.g., lupus, rheumatoid arthritis), immunodeficiency states (e.g., human immunodeficiency virus [HIV]) and diabetes, and some medications (e.g., retinoic acid and steroids) may prevent proper healing after a refractive procedure.

- **You actively participate in contact sports:** You participate in boxing, wrestling, martial arts, or other activities in which blows to the face and eyes are a normal occurrence.

- **You are not an adult:** Currently, no lasers are approved for LASIK on persons under the age of 18.

Precautions

The safety and effectiveness of refractive procedures has not been determined in patients with some diseases. Discuss with your doctor if you have a history of any of the following:

- herpes simplex or herpes zoster (shingles) involving the eye area

- glaucoma, glaucoma suspect, or ocular hypertension

- eye diseases, such as uveitis/iritis (inflammations of the eye)

- eye injuries or previous eye surgeries

- keratoconus

Other Risk Factors

Your doctor should screen you for the following conditions or indicators of risk:

- **Blepharitis:** Inflammation of the eyelids with crusting of the eyelashes, that may increase the risk of infection or inflammation of the cornea after LASIK.

- **Large pupils:** Make sure this evaluation is done in a dark room. Younger patients and patients on certain medications may be prone to having large pupils under dim lighting conditions. This can cause symptoms such as glare, halos, starbursts, and ghost images (double vision) after surgery. In some patients these symptoms may be debilitating. For example, a patient may no longer be able to drive a car at night or in certain weather conditions, such as fog.

- **Thin corneas:** The cornea is the thin clear covering of the eye that is over the iris, the colored part of the eye. Most refractive procedures change the eye's focusing power by reshaping the cornea (for example, by removing tissue). Performing a refractive procedure on a cornea that is too thin may result in blinding complications.

- **Previous refractive surgery (e.g., RK, PRK, LASIK):** Additional refractive surgery may not be recommended. The decision to have additional refractive surgery must be made in consultation with your doctor after careful consideration of your unique situation.

- **Dry eyes:** LASIK surgery tends to aggravate this condition.

What Are the Risks and How Can I Find the Right Doctor for Me?

Most patients are very pleased with the results of their refractive surgery. However, like any other medical procedure, there are risks involved. That's why it is important for you to understand the limitations and possible complications of refractive surgery.

Before undergoing a refractive procedure, you should carefully weigh the risks and benefits based on your own personal value system, and try to avoid being influenced by friends that have had the procedure or doctors encouraging you to do so.

- **Some patients lose vision:** Some patients lose lines of vision on the vision chart that cannot be corrected with glasses, contact lenses, or surgery as a result of treatment.

- **Some patients develop debilitating visual symptoms:** Some patients develop glare, halos, and/or double vision that can seriously affect nighttime vision. Even with good vision on the vision chart, some patients do not see as well in situations of low contrast, such as at night or in fog, after treatment as compared to before treatment.

- **You may be under treated or over treated:** Only a certain percent of patients achieve 20/20 vision without glasses or contacts. You may require additional treatment, but additional treatment may not be possible. You may still need glasses or contact lenses after surgery. This may be true even if you only required a very weak prescription before surgery. If you used reading glasses before surgery, you may still need reading glasses after surgery.

- **Some patients may develop severe dry eye syndrome:** As a result of surgery, your eye may not be able to produce enough tears to keep the eye moist and comfortable. Dry eye not only causes discomfort, but can reduce visual quality due to intermittent blurring and other visual symptoms. This condition may be permanent. Intensive drop therapy and use of plugs or other procedures may be required.

- **Results are generally not as good in patients with very large refractive errors of any type:** You should discuss your expectations with your doctor and realize that you may still require glasses or contacts after the surgery.

- **For some farsighted patients, results may diminish with age:** If you are farsighted, the level of improved vision you experience after surgery may decrease with age. This can occur if your manifest refraction (a vision exam with lenses before dilating drops) is very different from your cycloplegic refraction (a vision exam with lenses after dilating drops).

- **Long-term data are not available:** LASIK is a relatively new technology. The first laser was approved for LASIK eye surgery in 1998. Therefore, the long-term safety and effectiveness of LASIK surgery is not known.

Additional Risks of Other Techniques

Monovision: Monovision is one clinical technique used to deal with the correction of presbyopia, the gradual loss of the ability of the eye to change focus for close-up tasks that progresses with age. The intent of monovision is for the presbyopic patient to use one eye for distance viewing and one eye for near viewing. This practice was first applied to fit contact lens wearers and more recently to LASIK and other refractive surgeries. With contact lenses, a presbyopic patient has one eye fit with a contact lens to correct distance vision, and the other eye fit with a contact lens to correct near vision. In the same way, with LASIK, a presbyopic patient has one eye operated on to correct the distance vision, and the other operated on to correct the near vision. In other words, the goal of the surgery is for one eye to have vision worse than 20/20, the commonly referred to goal for LASIK surgical correction of distance vision. Since one eye is corrected for distance viewing and the other eye is corrected for near viewing, the two eyes no longer work together. This results in poorer quality vision and a decrease in depth perception. These effects of monovision are most noticeable in low lighting conditions and when performing tasks requiring very sharp vision. Therefore, you may need to wear glasses or contact lenses to fully correct both eyes for distance or near when performing visually demanding tasks, such as driving at night, operating dangerous equipment, or performing occupational tasks requiring very sharp close vision (e.g., reading small print for long periods of time).

Many patients cannot get used to having one eye blurred at all times. Therefore, if you are considering monovision with LASIK, make sure you go through a trial period with contact lenses to see if you can tolerate monovision, before having the surgery performed on your eyes. Find out if you pass your state's driver's license requirements with monovision.

In addition, you should consider how much your presbyopia is expected to increase in the future. Ask your doctor when you should expect the results of your monovision surgery to no longer be enough for you to see near-by objects clearly without the aid of glasses or contacts, or when a second surgery might be required to further correct your near vision.

Bilateral simultaneous treatment: You may choose to have LASIK surgery on both eyes at the same time or to have surgery on one eye at a time. Although the convenience of having surgery on both eyes on the same day is attractive, this practice is riskier than having two separate surgeries.

If you decide to have one eye done at a time, you and your doctor will decide how long to wait before having surgery on the other eye. If both eyes are treated at the same time or before one eye has a chance to fully heal, you and your doctor do not have the advantage of being able to see how the first eye responds to surgery before the second eye is treated.

Another disadvantage to having surgery on both eyes at the same time is that the vision in both eyes may be blurred after surgery until the initial healing process is over, rather than being able to rely on clear vision in at least one eye at all times.

Finding the Right Doctor

If you are considering refractive surgery, make sure you:

- Compare. The levels of risk and benefit vary slightly not only from procedure to procedure, but from device to device depending on the manufacturer, and from surgeon to surgeon depending on their level of experience with a particular procedure.

- Don't base your decision simply on cost and don't settle for the first eye center, doctor, or procedure you investigate. Remember that the decisions you make about your eyes and refractive surgery will affect you for the rest of your life.

- Be wary of eye centers that advertise "20/20 vision or your money back" or "package deals." There are never any guarantees in medicine.

- Read. It is important for you to read the patient handbook provided to your doctor by the manufacturer of the device used to perform the refractive procedure. Your doctor should provide you with this handbook and be willing to discuss his/her outcomes (successes as well as complications) compared to the results of studies outlined in the handbook.

Even the best screened patients under the care of most skilled surgeons can experience serious complications.

- **During surgery:** Malfunction of a device or other error, such as cutting a flap of cornea through and through instead of making a hinge during LASIK surgery, may lead to discontinuation of the procedure or irreversible damage to the eye.

- **After surgery:** Some complications, such as migration of the flap, inflammation or infection, may require another procedure and/or intensive treatment with drops. Even with aggressive therapy, such complications may lead to temporary loss of vision or even irreversible blindness. Under the care of an experienced doctor, carefully screened candidates with reasonable expectations and a clear understanding of the risks and alternatives are likely to be happy with the results of their refractive procedure.

Advertising

Be cautious about "slick" advertising and/or deals that sound "too good to be true." Remember, they usually are. There is a lot of competition resulting in a great deal of advertising and bidding for your business. Do your homework.

What Should I Expect before, during, and after Surgery?

What to expect before, during, and after surgery will vary from doctor to doctor and patient to patient. Discuss your expectations with your doctor.

Before Surgery

If you decide to go ahead with LASIK surgery, you will need an initial or baseline evaluation by your eye doctor to determine if you are a good candidate. This is what you need to know to prepare for the exam and what you should expect:

If you wear contact lenses, it is a good idea to stop wearing them before your baseline evaluation and switch to wearing your glasses full-time. Contact lenses change the shape of your cornea for up to several weeks after you have stopped using them depending on the type of contact lenses you wear. Not leaving your contact lenses out long enough for your cornea to assume its natural shape before surgery can have negative consequences. These consequences include inaccurate measurements and a poor surgical plan, resulting in poor vision after surgery. These measurements, which determine how much corneal tissue to remove, may need to be repeated at least a week after your initial evaluation and before surgery to make sure they have not changed, especially if you wear RGP (rigid gas permeable) or hard lenses. If you wear:

- soft contact lenses, you should stop wearing them for 2 weeks before your initial evaluation.

- toric soft lenses or RGP lenses, you should stop wearing them for at least 3 weeks before your initial evaluation.

- hard lenses, you should stop wearing them for at least 4 weeks before your initial evaluation.

You should tell your doctor:

- about your past and present medical and eye conditions; and

- about all the medications you are taking, including over-the-counter medications and any medications you may be allergic to.

Your doctor should perform a thorough eye exam and discuss:

- whether you are a good candidate;

- what the risks, benefits, and alternatives of the surgery are;
- what you should expect before, during, and after surgery; and
- what your responsibilities will be before, during, and after surgery.

You should have the opportunity to ask your doctor questions during this discussion. Give yourself plenty of time to think about the risk/benefit discussion, to review any informational literature provided by your doctor, and to have any additional questions answered by your doctor before deciding to go through with surgery and before signing the informed consent form.

You should not feel pressured by your doctor, family, friends, or anyone else to make a decision about having surgery. Carefully consider the pros and cons.

The day before surgery, you should stop using:

- creams;
- lotions;
- makeup; and
- perfumes.

These products as well as debris along the eyelashes may increase the risk of infection during and after surgery. Your doctor may ask you to scrub your eyelashes for a period of time before surgery to get rid of residues and debris along the lashes.

Also before surgery, arrange for transportation to and from your surgery and your first follow-up visit. On the day of surgery, your doctor may give you some medicine to make you relax. Because this medicine impairs your ability to drive and because your vision may be blurry, even if you don't drive make sure someone can bring you home after surgery.

During Surgery

The surgery should take less than 30 minutes. You will lie on your back in a reclining chair in an exam room containing the laser system. The laser system includes a large machine with a microscope attached to it and a computer screen.

A numbing drop will be placed in your eye, the area around your eye will be cleaned, and an instrument called a lid speculum will be used to hold your eyelids open. A ring will be placed on your eye and very high pressures will be applied to create suction to the cornea. Your vision will dim while the suction ring is on and you may feel the pressure and experience some discomfort during this part of the procedure. The microkeratome, a cutting instrument, is attached to the suction ring. Your doctor will use the blade of the microkeratome to cut a flap in your cornea. Microkeratome blades are meant to be used only once and then thrown out.

The microkeratome and the suction ring are then removed. You will be able to see, but you will experience fluctuating degrees of blurred vision during the rest of the procedure. The doctor will then lift the flap and fold it back on its hinge, and dry the exposed tissue.

The laser will be positioned over your eye and you will be asked to stare at a light. This is not the laser used to remove tissue from the cornea. This light is to help you keep your eye fixed on one spot once the laser comes on. **Note:** If you cannot stare at a fixed object for at least 60 seconds, you may not be a good candidate for this surgery.

When your eye is in the correct position, your doctor will start the laser. At this point in the surgery, you may become aware of new sounds and smells. The pulse of the laser makes a ticking sound. As the laser removes corneal tissue, some people have reported a smell similar to burning hair. A computer controls the amount of laser energy delivered to your eye. Before the start of surgery, your doctor will have programmed the computer to vaporize a particular amount of tissue based on the measurements taken at your initial evaluation. After the pulses of laser energy vaporize the corneal tissue, the flap is put back into position.

A shield should be placed over your eye at the end of the procedure as protection, since no stitches are used to hold the flap in place. It is important for you to wear this shield to prevent you from rubbing your eye and putting pressure on your eye while you sleep, and to protect your eye from accidentally being hit or poked until the flap has healed.

After Surgery

Immediately after the procedure, your eye may burn, itch, or feel like there is something in it. You may experience some discomfort, or in some cases, mild pain and your doctor may suggest you take a mild pain reliever. Both your eyes may tear or water. Your vision will probably be hazy or blurry. You will instinctively want to rub your eye, but don't! Rubbing your eye could dislodge the flap, requiring further treatment. In addition, you may experience sensitivity to light, glare, starbursts or haloes around lights, or the whites of your eye may look red or bloodshot. These symptoms should improve considerably within the first few days after surgery. You should plan on taking a few days off from work until these symptoms subside. You should contact your doctor immediately and not wait for your scheduled visit, if you experience severe pain, or if your vision or other symptoms get worse instead of better.

You should see your doctor within the first 24 to 48 hours after surgery and at regular intervals after that for at least the first six months. At the first postoperative visit, your doctor will remove the eye shield, test your vision, and examine your eye. Your doctor may give you one or more types of eyedrops to take at home to help prevent infection and/or inflammation. You may also be advised to use artificial tears to help lubricate the eye. Do not resume wearing a contact lens in the operated eye, even if your vision is blurry.

You should wait one to three days following surgery before beginning any non-contact sports, depending on the amount of activity required, how you feel, and your doctor's instructions.

To help prevent infection, you may need to wait for up to two weeks after surgery or until your doctor advises you otherwise before using lotions, creams, or makeup around the eye. Your doctor may advise you to continue scrubbing your eyelashes for a period of time after surgery. You should also avoid swimming and using hot tubs or whirlpools for 1 to 2 months.

Strenuous contact sports such as boxing, football, karate, etc. should not be attempted for at least four weeks after surgery. It is important to protect your eyes from anything that might get in them and from being hit or bumped.

During the first few months after surgery, your vision may fluctuate.

- It may take up to three to six months for your vision to stabilize after surgery.

- Glare, haloes, difficulty driving at night, and other visual symptoms may also persist during this stabilization period. If further correction or enhancement is necessary, you should wait until your eye measurements are consistent for two consecutive visits at least 3 months apart before re-operation.

- It is important to realize that although distance vision may improve after re-operation, it is unlikely that other visual symptoms such as glare or haloes will improve.

- It is also important to note that no laser company has presented enough evidence for the FDA to make conclusions about the safety or effectiveness of enhancement surgery.

Contact your eye doctor immediately, if you develop any new, unusual, or worsening symptoms at any point after surgery. Such symptoms could signal a problem that, if not treated early enough, may lead to a loss of vision.

Section 17.2

LASIK for Monovision Aids Nearsighted Adults

"First LASIK Device for Monovision," is from the U.S.
Food and Drug Administration (FDA, www.fda.gov), July 2007.

FDA has approved for marketing the first LASIK device designed for treating one eye to see faraway objects and the other eye for close-up vision. The device is called CustomVue Monovision LASIK.

LASIK, or Laser-Assisted In Situ Keratomileusis, is a procedure in which the surgeon cuts a flap in the outer layers of the clear covering of the front of the eye (cornea), removes a small amount of the tissue beneath it with the laser, and then replaces the flap.

Monovision is a corrective technique used to treat people with presbyopia, which is normal age-related loss of the ability to focus on near objects. The intent is for the person to use one eye for distance viewing and one eye for near viewing.

"Unlike traditional LASIK, Monovision LASIK may reduce the need for reading glasses in some people over 40," says Daniel Schultz, M.D., Director of FDA's Center for Devices and Radiological Health.

Who It's for

CustomVue Monovision LASIK produces monovision correction in nearsighted (myopic) adults, with or without an abnormal curve of the cornea (astigmatism), ages 40 years or older with presbyopia.

154

How It Works

The CustomVue device is designed to correct all nearsightedness in a person's dominant eye and only part of the nearsightedness in the non-dominant eye. This allows the person to use the fully corrected eye for distance vision and the under-corrected eye for seeing close up. After a period of time, the brain adjusts to the difference in perception between the two eyes.

Factors to Consider

People considering CustomVue Monovision LASIK should first wear monovision contact lenses for at least a week to determine if they can tolerate having one eye under-corrected. Following monovision surgery, both eyes may not work together as well as they did before in some people, especially in dim light or when performing tasks requiring very sharp vision or fine depth perception. Patients may need to wear glasses or contact lenses for some activities such as night driving or reading small type.

Side Effects

CustomVue Monovision LASIK is a permanent operation to the cornea. Side effects may include:

- glare from bright lights;
- rings around lights (halos);
- light sensitivity;
- night driving glare;
- ghost images;
- double vision; or
- visual fluctuation.

Follow-up Study

FDA based its approval on the review of a clinical study of safety and effectiveness outcomes submitted by the manufacturer, AMO/VISX Inc., Santa Clara, California.

At FDA's request, AMO/VISX will conduct a post-approval study. The study will follow 500 people for six months after surgery to estimate the proportion of monovision LASIK patients who experience visual disturbances that are severe enough to limit activities or adversely affect their quality of life.

Chapter 18

Wavefront-Guided LASIK: A Promising New Technology

Wavefront-guided LASIK [laser-assisted in situ keratomileusis] is a promising new technology that provides an advanced method for measuring optical distortions in the eye. Measuring and treating these distortions goes beyond nearsighted, farsighted, and astigmatism determinations that have been used for centuries. As a result, physicians can now customize the LASIK procedure according to each individual patient's unique vision correction needs. The treatment is unique to each eye, just as a fingerprint is unique. Wavefront systems work by measuring how light is distorted as it passes into the eye and then is reflected back. This creates an optical map of the eye, highlighting individual imperfections.

Wavefront technology functions as a roadmap for LASIK surgery, providing benefits to the patient during both the evaluation and treatment process.

- During the patient evaluation process, wavefront provides the physician comprehensive individual diagnostic information, not available using earlier technologies. Thus, before surgery even begins, the surgeon is better able to determine the appropriate course of treatment.

"Wavefront Diagnostics & Custom Treatment," is reprinted with permission from the Eye Surgery Education Council, an initiative of the American Society for Cataract and Refractive Surgery, © 2003.

- During treatment, wavefront allows the surgeon to tailor the laser beam settings, making the surgical procedure itself more precise. In this way, wavefront technology offers the patients sharper, crisper, better quality vision, as well as a reduction in nighttime vision difficulties, such as halos and glare.

Wavefront technology is an adjunct tool used to enhance an already safe and effective procedure. As the most common form of vision correction surgery, LASIK has already benefited millions of patients. The increased safety and the improved quality of vision benefits of customized procedures are an important technological advancement for patients and physicians alike.

Visual Errors

For purposes of this discussion, there are two categories of visual errors or "aberrations:" second-order and higher-order.

Conventional forms of optical correction have been limited to measuring the best spherical and cylindrical visual errors (second-order aberrations), which result in myopia (shortsightedness) or hyperopia (farsightedness) and regular astigmatism (blurriness), and prescribing spherocylindrical lenses in the form of spectacles, contact lenses, and conventional refractive (LASIK) surgery to correct them. Correcting second-order aberrations has the highest impact on acuity, which is the eye's ability to distinguish object details and shape. At the same time that conventional refractive surgery corrects major, second-order spherical errors, in many cases, it also induces some degree of minor spherical aberrations.

However, about 17 percent of optical errors are higher-order aberrations. If these are minimized, image contrast and special detail are increased. Minimizing higher-order aberrations with wavefront technology by reducing the naturally occurring ones is achievable and may be particularly beneficial to individuals with unusually large amounts of higher-order aberrations.

How Wavefront Works: The Wavefront Aberrometer

Light can be thought of as traveling in a series of flat sheets, known as wavefronts. To clarify the confusion about light traveling as waves instead of rays, waves are just perpendicular to light rays. These light waves are wrinkled or distorted as they pass through imperfections in the eye. These errors can be displayed on a color map of the wavefront image, which is the tool that is used to diagnose, and then determine corrections, for aberrations in the eye.

There are several ways of analyzing the optical system of the eye using wavefront technology. The most common, the Hartmann-Shack wavefront sensing method, deals with light waves as they exit the eye. In this system, the surgeon or other professional shines a small, low-intensity laser into the eye, and the patient focuses on the light. As that light scatters off of the retina (the rear-most portion of the eye) it passes through the lens, the rear surface of the cornea (the clear, crystalline front part of the eye) and the front surface of the cornea. Thus, the emerging waves of light are distorted by the imperfections in the total visual system of the eye. After leaving the eye, the light passes through an array of many small lenses in the sensing device (called an aberrometer), and is focused into spots, which are recorded by a special camera. The deviation of the spots from their ideal location provides information about focusing imperfections in the visual system.

Wavefront-Guided Treatment

The goal of wavefront-guided laser treatment is to make corrections in the surface of the cornea that compensate for errors in the total visual system. Thus, the amount of wrinkle or error in the wavefront reflected from the back of the eye, as compared to the reference wavefront that was projected into it, defines the compensating optical correction. If the wavefront is retarded in relation to the reference wavefront, the laser must remove more tissue from the part of cornea related to that pattern. If the wavefront is advanced (in front of the referenced wavefront), the laser must remove less tissue. It should be noted that wavefront treatment does induce some minor second-order spherical errors, but to a significantly lesser extent than conventional refractive surgery.

In this way, a wavefront-guided treatment is customized to the characteristics of each eye and intended to minimize higher-order aberrations so that the greatest quality of vision can be achieved.

Wavefront technology is relatively new to the United States. The U.S. Food and Drug Administration (FDA) issued its first approval of a wavefront system in August 2002, and other major U.S. laser manufacturers are expected to receive their approvals. As the FDA approves systems and they become widely available, patients will have greater access to wavefront technology and treatment.

Chapter 19

Phakic Intraocular Lenses

What are phakic lenses?

Phakic intraocular lenses, or phakic lenses, are lenses made of plastic or silicone that are implanted into the eye permanently to reduce a person's need for glasses or contact lenses. Phakic refers to the fact that the lens is implanted into the eye without removing the eye's natural lens. During phakic lens implantation surgery, a small incision is made in the front of the eye. The phakic lens is inserted through the incision and placed just in front of or just behind the iris.

What do they treat?

Phakic lenses are used to correct refractive errors, errors in the eye's focusing power. Currently all phakic lenses approved by the FDA are for the correction of nearsightedness (myopia).

The cornea and natural lens of the eye focus light to create an image on the retina, much like the way the lens of a camera focuses light to create an image on film. The bending and focusing of light is also known as refraction. Imperfections in the focusing power of the eye, called refractive errors, cause images on the retina to be out of focus or blurred.

Excerpted from "Learning about Phakic Intraocular Lenses," by the Center for Devices and Radiological Health, U.S. Food and Drug Administration (FDA, www.fda.gov), April 22, 2005.

People that are nearsighted have more difficulty seeing distant objects than near objects. For these people, the images of distant objects come to focus in front of the retina instead of on the retina.

Ideally, phakic lenses cause light entering the eye to be focused on the retina providing clear distance vision without the aid of glasses or contact lenses.

Surgery is not required to correct nearsightedness. You can wear glasses or contact lenses instead to correct your vision. Depending on how nearsighted you are, and other conditions of your eye, other refractive surgery (surgery to correct refractive errors) options may be available to you, including PRK (photorefractive keratectomy) and LASIK (laser assisted in-situ keratomileusis).

Can they be removed?

Phakic lenses are intended to be permanent. While the lenses can be surgically removed, return to your previous level of vision or condition of your eye cannot be guaranteed.

What is the difference between phakic intraocular lenses and intraocular lenses following cataract surgery?

Phakic intraocular lenses are implanted in the eye without removing the natural lens. This is in contrast to intraocular lenses that are implanted into eyes after the eye's cloudy natural lens (cataract) has been removed during cataract surgery.

Are phakic lenses for you?

You are probably **not** a good candidate for phakic lenses if:

- You are not an adult. There are no phakic lenses approved by the FDA for persons under the age of 21.

- You are not a risk taker. Certain complications are unavoidable in a percentage of patients, and there are no long-term data available for phakic lenses.

- You required a change in your contact lens or glasses prescription in the last 6 to 12 months in order to obtain the best possible vision for you. This is called refractive instability. Patients who are:

  - in their early 20s or younger;

- whose hormones are fluctuating due to disease such as diabetes;

- who are pregnant or breastfeeding; or

- who are taking medications that may cause fluctuations in vision

are more likely to have refractive instability and should discuss the possible additional risks with their doctor.

- You may jeopardize your career. Some jobs prohibit certain refractive procedures. Be sure to check with your employer/professional society/military service before undergoing any procedure.

- Cost is an issue. Most medical insurance will not pay for refractive surgery.

- You have a disease or are on medications that may affect wound healing. Certain conditions, such as autoimmune diseases (e.g., lupus, rheumatoid arthritis), immunodeficiency states (e.g., HIV) and diabetes, and some medications (e.g., retinoic acid and steroids) may prevent proper healing after intraocular surgery.

- You have a low endothelial cell count or abnormal endothelial cells. If the cells that pump the fluid out of your cornea, the endothelial cells, are low in number relative to your age, or if your endothelial cells are abnormal, you have a higher risk of developing a cloudy cornea and requiring a corneal transplant.

- You actively participate in sports with a high risk of eye trauma. Your eye may be more susceptible to damage should you receive a blow to the face or eye, such as a blow to the head during boxing or hit in the eye by a ball during baseball. Your eye may be more susceptible to rupture or retinal detachment, and the phakic lens may dislocate.

- You only have one eye with potentially good vision. If you only have one eye with good vision with glasses or contact lenses, due to disease, irreparable damage, or amblyopia (eye with poor vision since childhood that cannot be corrected with glasses or contact lenses), you and your doctor should consider the risk of possible damage and/or loss of vision to your better eye as a result phakic lens implantation.

- You have large pupils. If your pupil dilates in low lighting conditions to a size that is larger than the size of the lens, you have a higher risk of experiencing visual disturbances after surgery that may affect your ability to function comfortably or normally under such conditions (e.g., while driving at night).

- You have a shallow anterior chamber. If the space between the cornea and the iris, the anterior chamber, is narrow, you have a higher risk of developing complications, such as greater endothelial cell loss, due to implantation of the phakic lens.

- You have an abnormal iris. If your pupil is irregularly shaped you have a higher risk of developing visual disturbances.

- You have had uveitis. If you have had inflammation in your eye, you may have a recurrence or worsening of your disease and/or may develop additional complications, such as glaucoma, as a result of surgery.

- You have had problems with the posterior part of your eye. If you have had any problems in the back part of your eye or are at risk for such problems, for example, proliferative diabetic retinopathy (growth of abnormal vessels in the back of the eye due to diabetes) or retinal detachment, you may not be a good candidate for phakic lens implantation. The phakic lens may not allow your eye doctor to get a clear view of the back part of your eye, preventing or delaying detection of a new or worsening problem, and/or the phakic lens may prevent or make treatment of a problem in the back of your eye more difficult.

The safety and effectiveness of phakic lenses have NOT been studied in patients with certain conditions. If any of the following apply to you, make sure you discuss them with your doctor:

- You have glaucoma (damage to the nerve of the eye resulting in loss of peripheral and then central vision due to too high pressure inside the eye), ocular hypertension (high eye pressure), or glaucoma suspect (some indications, but not clear, that patient has glaucoma). You may have a higher risk of developing or worsening of glaucoma as a result of phakic lens implantation.

- You have pseudoexfoliation syndrome (abnormal deposits of material in the eye visible on the structures in the front part of the eye, such as on the front of the natural lens and the back of the cornea). This syndrome is associated with glaucoma and weakness of the structures holding the natural lens in place (the zonules). You may have a higher risk of surgical complications and/or complications after surgery if you have this syndrome.

- You have had an eye injury or previous eye surgery.

- Your need for visual correction is outside the range for which the phakic lens has been approved. Ask your eye doctor if the phakic lens that he or she recommends for you has been approved to treat your refractive error and/or check FDA-Approved Phakic Lenses for the approved refractive range.

- You are over the age of 45 years old. Some phakic lenses have not been studied in patients over the age of 45.

What are the risks?

Implanting a phakic lens involves a surgical procedure. As in any other medical procedure, there are risks involved. That's why it is important for you to understand the limitations and potential risks of phakic intraocular lens implant surgery.

Before undergoing surgery for implantation of a phakic intraocular lens, you should carefully weigh the risks and benefits and try to avoid being influenced by other people encouraging you to do it.

- You may lose vision. Some patients lose vision as a result of phakic lens implant surgery that cannot be corrected with glasses, contact lenses, or another surgery. The amount of vision loss may be severe.

- You may develop debilitating visual symptoms. Some patients develop glare, halos, double vision, and/or decreased vision in situations of low level lighting that can cause difficulty with performing tasks, such as driving, particularly at night or under foggy conditions.

- You may need additional eye surgery to reposition, replace, or remove the phakic lens implant. These surgeries may be necessary for your safety or to improve your visual function. If the lens power is not right, then a phakic lens exchange may be needed. You may also have to have the lens repositioned, removed, or replaced, if the lens does not stay in the right place, is not the right size, and/or causes debilitating visual symptoms. Every additional surgical procedure has its own risks.

- You may be under treated or over treated. A significant proportion of treated patients do not achieve 20/20 vision after surgery. The power of the implanted phakic lens may be too strong or too weak. This is because of the difficulties with determining exactly what power lens you need. This means that you will probably still need glasses or contact lenses to perform at least some tasks. For example, you may need glasses for reading, even if you did not need them before surgery. This also means that you may need a second surgery to replace the lens with another, if the power of the originally implanted lens was too far from what you needed.

- You may develop increased intraocular pressure. You may experience increased pressure inside the eye after surgery, which may require surgery or medication to control. You may need long-term treatment with glaucoma medications. If the pressure is too high for too long, you may lose vision.

- Your cornea may become cloudy. The endothelial cells of your cornea are a thin layer of cells responsible for pumping fluid out of the cornea to keep it clear. If the endothelial cells become too few in number, the endothelial cell pump will fail and the cornea will become cloudy, resulting in loss of vision. You start with a certain number of cells at birth, and this number continuously decreases as you age, since these cells are not replenished. Normally, you die from old age before the number of endothelial cells becomes so low that your cornea becomes cloudy. Some lens designs have shown that their implantation causes endothelial cells to be lost at a faster rate than normal. If the number of endothelial cells drops too low and your cornea becomes cloudy, you will lose vision and you may require a corneal transplant in order to see more clearly.

- You may develop a cataract. You may get a cataract, clouding of the natural lens. The amount of time for a cataract to develop can vary greatly. If the cataract develops and progresses enough to significantly decrease your vision, you may require cataract surgery during which both the natural and the phakic lenses will have to be removed.

- You may develop a retinal detachment. The retina is the tissue that lines the inside of the back of your eyeball. It contains the light-sensing cells that collect and send images to your brain, much like the film in a camera. The risk of the retina becoming detached from the back of the eye increases after intraocular surgery. It is not known at this time by how much your risk of retinal detachment will increase as a result of phakic intraocular lens implantation surgery.

- You may experience infection, bleeding, or severe inflammation (pain, redness, and decreased vision). These are rare complications that can sometimes lead to permanent loss of vision or loss of the eye.

- Long-term data is not available. Phakic lenses are a new technology and have only recently been approved by the FDA. Therefore, there may be other risks to having phakic lenses implanted that we don't yet know about.

Is surgery right for me?

To help you decide whether phakic lenses are right for you, talk to your doctor about your expectations and whether there are elements of your medical history, eye history, or eye examination that might increase your risk or prevent you from having the outcome you expect.

Before you sign an informed consent document (a form giving permission to your doctor to operate on your eye), you should discuss with your doctor:

- whether you are a good candidate;
- what are the risks, benefits and alternatives of the surgery;
- what you should expect before, during and after surgery; and
- what your responsibilities will be before, during, and after surgery.

You should have the opportunity to ask your doctor questions during this discussion. Ask your doctor for the Patient Labeling of the lens that he or she recommends for you. Give yourself plenty of time to think about the risk/benefit discussion, to review any informational literature provided by your doctor, and to have any additional questions answered by your doctor before deciding to go through with surgery and before signing the informed consent document. You should not feel pressured by anyone to make a decision about having surgery. Carefully consider the pros and cons.

Part Three

Cataracts

Chapter 20

Facts about Cataracts

Cataract Defined

What is a cataract?

A cataract is a clouding of the lens in the eye that affects vision. Most cataracts are related to aging. Cataracts are very common in older people. By age 80, more than half of all Americans either have a cataract or have had cataract surgery.

A cataract can occur in either or both eyes. It cannot spread from one eye to the other.

What is the lens?

The lens is a clear part of the eye that helps to focus light, or an image, on the retina. The retina is the light-sensitive tissue at the back of the eye.

In a normal eye, light passes through the transparent lens to the retina. Once it reaches the retina, light is changed into nerve signals that are sent to the brain.

The lens must be clear for the retina to receive a sharp image. If the lens is cloudy from a cataract, the image you see will be blurred.

From "Cataract," a resource guide by the National Eye Institute (www.nei.nih.gov), part of the National Institutes of Health, December 2006.

Are there other types of cataract?

Yes. Although most cataracts are related to aging, there are other types of cataract:

- **Secondary cataract:** Cataracts can form after surgery for other eye problems, such as glaucoma. Cataracts also can develop in people who have other health problems, such as diabetes. Cataracts are sometimes linked to steroid use.

- **Traumatic cataract:** Cataracts can develop after an eye injury, sometimes years later.

- **Congenital cataract:** Some babies are born with cataracts or develop them in childhood, often in both eyes. These cataracts may be so small that they do not affect vision. If they do, the lenses may need to be removed.

- **Radiation cataract:** Cataracts can develop after exposure to some types of radiation.

Causes and Risk Factors

What causes cataracts?

The lens lies behind the iris and the pupil. It works much like a camera lens. It focuses light onto the retina at the back of the eye, where an image is recorded. The lens also adjusts the eye's focus, letting us see things clearly both up close and far away. The lens is made of mostly water and protein. The protein is arranged in a precise way that keeps the lens clear and lets light pass through it.

But as we age, some of the protein may clump together and start to cloud a small area of the lens. This is a cataract. Over time, the cataract may grow larger and cloud more of the lens, making it harder to see.

Researchers suspect that there are several causes of cataract, such as smoking and diabetes. Or, it may be that the protein in the lens just changes from the wear and tear it takes over the years.

How can cataracts affect my vision?

Age-related cataracts can affect your vision in two ways.

Clumps of protein reduce the sharpness of the image reaching the retina: The lens consists mostly of water and protein. When the protein clumps up, it clouds the lens and reduces the light that reaches the retina. The clouding may become severe enough to cause blurred vision. Most age-related cataracts develop from protein clumpings.

When a cataract is small, the cloudiness affects only a small part of the lens. You may not notice any changes in your vision. Cataracts tend to "grow" slowly, so vision gets worse gradually. Over time, the cloudy area in the lens may get larger, and the cataract may increase in size. Seeing may become more difficult. Your vision may get duller or blurrier.

The clear lens slowly changes to a yellowish/brownish color, adding a brownish tint to vision: As the clear lens slowly colors with age, your vision gradually may acquire a brownish shade. At first, the amount of tinting may be small and may not cause a vision problem. Over time, increased tinting may make it more difficult to read and perform other routine activities. This gradual change in the amount of tinting does not affect the sharpness of the image transmitted to the retina.

If you have advanced lens discoloration, you may not be able to identify blues and purples. You may be wearing what you believe to be a pair of black socks, only to find out from friends that you are wearing purple socks.

When are you most likely to have a cataract?

The term "age-related" is a little misleading. You don't have to be a senior citizen to get this type of cataract. In fact, people can have an age-related cataract in their 40s and 50s. But during middle age, most cataracts are small and do not affect vision. It is after age 60 that most cataracts steal vision.

Who is at risk for cataract?

The risk of cataract increases as you get older. Other risk factors for cataract include:

- certain diseases such as diabetes;
- personal behavior such as smoking and alcohol use; and
- the environment such as prolonged exposure to sunlight.

What can I do to protect my vision?

Wearing sunglasses and a hat with a brim to block ultraviolet sunlight may help to delay cataract. If you smoke, stop. Researchers also believe good nutrition can help reduce the risk of age-related cataract.

They recommend eating green leafy vegetables, fruit, and other foods with antioxidants.

If you are age 60 or older, you should have a comprehensive dilated eye exam at least once every two years. In addition to cataract, your eye care professional can check for signs of age-related macular degeneration, glaucoma, and other vision disorders. Early treatment for many eye diseases may save your sight.

Symptoms and Detection

What are the symptoms of a cataract?

The most common symptoms of a cataract are:

- cloudy or blurry vision;

- colors seem faded;

- glare (Headlights, lamps, or sunlight may appear too bright. A halo may appear around lights.);

- poor night vision;

- double vision or multiple images in one eye (This symptom may clear as the cataract gets larger.);

- frequent prescription changes in your eyeglasses or contact lenses;

These symptoms also can be a sign of other eye problems. If you have any of these symptoms, check with your eye care professional.

How is a cataract detected?

Cataract is detected through a comprehensive eye exam that includes:

- **Visual acuity test:** This eye chart test measures how well you see at various distances.

- **Dilated eye exam:** Drops are placed in your eyes to widen, or dilate, the pupils. Your eye care professional uses a special magnifying lens to examine your retina and optic nerve for signs of damage and other eye problems. After the exam, your close-up vision may remain blurred for several hours.

- **Tonometry:** An instrument measures the pressure inside the eye. Numbing drops may be applied to your eye for this test.

Your eye care professional also may do other tests to learn more about the structure and health of your eye.

Treatment

How is a cataract treated?

The symptoms of early cataract may be improved with new eyeglasses, brighter lighting, anti-glare sunglasses, or magnifying lenses. If these measures do not help, surgery is the only effective treatment. Surgery involves removing the cloudy lens and replacing it with an artificial lens.

A cataract needs to be removed only when vision loss interferes with your everyday activities, such as driving, reading, or watching TV. You and your eye care professional can make this decision together. Once you understand the benefits and risks of surgery, you can make an informed decision about whether cataract surgery is right for you. In most cases, delaying cataract surgery will not cause long-term damage to your eye or make the surgery more difficult. You do not have to rush into surgery.

Sometimes a cataract should be removed even if it does not cause problems with your vision. For example, a cataract should be removed if it prevents examination or treatment of another eye problem, such as age-related macular degeneration or diabetic retinopathy. If your eye care professional finds a cataract, you may not need cataract surgery for several years. In fact, you might never need cataract surgery. By having your vision tested regularly, you and your eye care professional can discuss if and when you might need treatment.

If you choose surgery, your eye care professional may refer you to a specialist to remove the cataract.

If you have cataracts in both eyes that require surgery, the surgery will be performed on each eye at separate times, usually four to eight weeks apart.

Many people who need cataract surgery also have other eye conditions, such as age-related macular degeneration or glaucoma. If you have other eye conditions in addition to cataract, talk with your doctor. Learn about the risks, benefits, alternatives, and expected results of cataract surgery.

What are the different types of cataract surgery?

There are two types of cataract surgery. Your doctor can explain the differences and help determine which is better for you.

Phacoemulsification, or phaco: A small incision is made on the side of the cornea, the clear, dome-shaped surface that covers the front of the eye. Your doctor inserts a tiny probe into the eye. This device emits ultrasound waves that soften and break up the lens so that it can be removed by suction. Most cataract surgery today is done by phacoemulsification, also called "small incision cataract surgery."

Extracapsular surgery: Your doctor makes a longer incision on the side of the cornea and removes the cloudy core of the lens in one piece. The rest of the lens is removed by suction.

After the natural lens has been removed, it often is replaced by an artificial lens, called an intraocular lens (IOL). An IOL is a clear, plastic lens that requires no care and becomes a permanent part of your eye. Light is focused clearly by the IOL onto the retina, improving your vision. You will not feel or see the new lens.

Some people cannot have an IOL. They may have another eye disease or have problems during surgery. For these patients, a soft contact lens, or glasses that provide high magnification, may be suggested.

What are the risks of cataract surgery?

As with any surgery, cataract surgery poses risks, such as infection and bleeding. Before cataract surgery, your doctor may ask you to temporarily stop taking certain medications that increase the risk of bleeding during surgery. After surgery, you must keep your eye clean, wash your hands before touching your eye, and use the prescribed medications to help minimize the risk of infection. Serious infection can result in loss of vision.

Cataract surgery slightly increases your risk of retinal detachment. Other eye disorders, such as high myopia (nearsightedness), can further increase your risk of retinal detachment after cataract surgery. One sign of a retinal detachment is a sudden increase in flashes or floaters. Floaters are little "cobwebs" or specks that seem to float about in your field of vision. If you notice a sudden increase in floaters or flashes, see an eye care professional immediately. A retinal detachment is a medical emergency. If necessary, go to an emergency service or hospital. Your eye must be examined by an eye surgeon as soon as possible. A retinal detachment causes no pain. Early treatment for retinal detachment often can prevent permanent loss of vision. The sooner you get treatment, the more likely you will regain good vision. Even if you are treated promptly, some vision may be lost.

Talk to your eye care professional about these risks. Make sure cataract surgery is right for you.

Is cataract surgery effective?

Cataract removal is one of the most common operations performed in the United States. It also is one of the safest and most effective types of surgery. In about 90 percent of cases, people who have cataract surgery have better vision afterward.

What happens before surgery?

A week or two before surgery, your doctor will do some tests. These tests may include measuring the curve of the cornea and the size and shape of your eye. This information helps your doctor choose the right type of IOL.

You may be asked not to eat or drink anything 12 hours before your surgery.

What happens during surgery?

At the hospital or eye clinic, drops will be put into your eye to dilate the pupil. The area around your eye will be washed and cleansed.

The operation usually lasts less than one hour and is almost painless. Many people choose to stay awake during surgery. Others may need to be put to sleep for a short time.

If you are awake, you will have an anesthetic to numb the nerves in and around your eye.

After the operation, a patch may be placed over your eye. You will rest for a while. Your medical team will watch for any problems, such as bleeding. Most people who have cataract surgery can go home the same day. You will need someone to drive you home.

What happens after surgery?

Itching and mild discomfort are normal after cataract surgery. Some fluid discharge is also common. Your eye may be sensitive to light and touch. If you have discomfort, your doctor can suggest treatment. After one or two days, moderate discomfort should disappear.

For a few days after surgery, your doctor may ask you to use eyedrops to help healing and decrease the risk of infection. Ask your doctor about how to use your eyedrops, how often to use them, and what effects they can have. You will need to wear an eye shield or eyeglasses to help protect your eye. Avoid rubbing or pressing on your eye.

When you are home, try not to bend from the waist to pick up objects on the floor. Do not lift any heavy objects. You can walk, climb stairs, and do light household chores.

In most cases, healing will be complete within eight weeks. Your doctor will schedule exams to check on your progress.

Can problems develop after surgery?

Problems after surgery are rare, but they can occur. These problems can include infection, bleeding, inflammation (pain, redness, swelling), loss of vision, double vision, and high or low eye pressure. With prompt medical attention, these problems can usually be treated successfully.

Sometimes the eye tissue that encloses the IOL becomes cloudy and may blur your vision. This condition is called an after-cataract. An after-cataract can develop months or years after cataract surgery.

An after-cataract is treated with a laser. Your doctor uses a laser to make a tiny hole in the eye tissue behind the lens to let light pass through. This outpatient procedure is called a YAG laser capsulotomy. It is painless and rarely results in increased eye pressure or other eye problems. As a precaution, your doctor may give you eyedrops to lower your eye pressure before or after the procedure.

When will my vision be normal again?

You can return quickly to many everyday activities, but your vision may be blurry. The healing eye needs time to adjust so that it can focus properly with the other eye, especially if the other eye has a cataract. Ask your doctor when you can resume driving.

If you received an IOL, you may notice that colors are very bright. The IOL is clear, unlike your natural lens that may have had a yellowish/brownish tint. Within a few months after receiving an IOL, you will become used to improved color vision. Also, when your eye heals, you may need new glasses or contact lenses.

What can I do if I already have lost some vision from cataract?

If you have lost some sight from cataract or cataract surgery, ask your eye care professional about low vision services and devices that may help you make the most of your remaining vision. Ask for a referral to a specialist in low vision. Many community organizations and agencies offer information about low vision counseling, training, and other special services for people with visual impairments. A nearby school of medicine or optometry may provide low vision services.

Current Research

What research is being done?

The National Eye Institute is conducting and supporting a number of studies focusing on factors associated with the development of age-related cataract.
These studies include:

- The effect of sunlight exposure, which may be associated with an increased risk of cataract.

- Vitamin supplements, which have shown varying results in delaying the progression of cataract.

- Genetic studies, which show promise for better understanding cataract development.

Chapter 21

Frequently Asked Questions about Cataracts

What are cataracts?

A cataract is an opacification (clouding) of the natural lens inside of the eye. The lens helps us focus on objects at different distances. As a part of the normal aging process, changes in the lens can cause it to become cloudy. Left untreated, a cataract can become so dense that it causes blindness. In fact, cataracts are the leading cause of blindness in the world. The original meaning of "cataract" is "waterfall," and the name was chosen because distorted vision caused by a cataract reminded people of the distorted view that is obtained when looking through a waterfall.

Who gets cataracts?

Most people who develop cataracts are older than 60 years. Cataracts in older people are so common they can be regarded as normal part of the aging process. Among the major conditions related to cataracts are diabetes or injury to the eye. Medications such as steroids can also cause cataract formation.

In rare cases, congenital cataracts are present at birth. These cataracts are usually related to the mother having German measles,

"Cataract FAQ" is reprinted with permission from the Eye Surgery Education Council, an initiative of the American Society for Cataract and Refractive Surgery, © 2003.

chickenpox, or other infectious diseases during pregnancy or to the child having certain syndromes (e.g., Marfan's). Some cataracts are inherited.

What are the symptoms of a cataract?

Typical symptoms include:

- cloudy, fuzzy, foggy, or filmy vision;
- changes in the perception of colors;
- problems driving at night because headlights seem too bright;
- problems with glare from lamps or the sun;
- frequent changes in your eyeglass prescription; and
- double vision.

These symptoms can also be signs of other eye problems. If you have any of them, consult an ophthalmologist for an eye examination.

How do I decide to have surgery?

Most people have plenty of time to decide about cataract surgery. Your doctor cannot make the decision for you, but talking with your doctor can help you decide.

Tell your doctor how your cataract affects your vision and your life. Read the statements below, see which ones apply to you, and tell your doctor if:

- I need to drive, but there is too much glare from the sun or headlights.
- I do not see well enough to do my best at work.
- I do not see well enough to do the things I need to do at home.
- I do not see well enough to do things I like to do (for example, read, watch TV, sew, hike, play cards, and go out with friends).
- I am afraid I will bump into something or fall.
- Because of my cataract, I am not as independent as I would like to be.
- I cannot see well enough with my glasses.
- My eyesight bothers me a lot.

You may also have other specific problems you want to discuss with your eye doctor.

How can cataracts be treated?

The natural lens of the eye that has been damaged by a cataract is surgically removed and then replaced with a clear artificial lens. During the surgery, usually done on an outpatient basis, a tiny incision is made in the eye and the cataract-damaged natural lens is removed through the incision. An artificial lens is then inserted through the same incision. Most patients have significantly improved vision after the procedure.

Can a cataract return?

A cataract cannot return because the entire lens has been removed. However, in as many as half of all people who have extracapsular surgery or phacoemulsification, the lens capsule (the tissue bag that supports the replacement lens) becomes cloudy. This cloudiness can develop months or years after surgery. It can cause the same vision problems as the original cataract.

The treatment for this condition is a procedure called a YAG laser capsulotomy, which is named for the material used to generate the laser energy (yttrium-aluminum-garnet). The doctor uses a laser (light) beam to make a small opening in the capsule through which light can pass unimpeded. This surgery is painless and does not require a hospital stay. Most people see well after a YAG capsulotomy. Your doctor will discuss the risks with you.

What are the benefits of cataract surgery?

Cataract surgery restores quality vision for millions of patients each year. Good vision is vital to an enjoyable lifestyle. Numerous research studies show that cataract surgery restores quality-of-life functions including reading, working, moving around, hobbies, safety, self-confidence, independence, daytime and nighttime driving, community and social activities, mental health, and overall life satisfaction.

What are the risks of cataract surgery?

Cataract surgery is performed millions of times every year in the United States. In fact, it is the most commonly performed surgery in the United States. About 98 percent of patients have a complication-free experience that results in improved vision. Nevertheless, cataract surgery has risks and complications. Most complications resolve in a matter of days to months. In rare cases, patients lose some degree of vision permanently as a result of the surgery.

Is it still necessary to wear thick glasses after cataract surgery?

No. Today, cataract patients who have artificial or intraocular lenses (IOLs) implanted during surgery may only need reading glasses for close vision. Patients who do not receive IOLs wear contact lenses for distance vision and reading glasses for close vision. Some patients choose to wear multifocal contact lenses for all distances.

How successful is cataract surgery?

Cataract surgery has an overall success rate of 98 percent. Continuous innovations in techniques and instruments allow cataract surgeons to treat more patients while keeping costs down and improving quality of patient care.

Are lasers used to treat cataracts?

In general, no. In some cases, the bag-like capsule membrane that supports the artificial lens that replaces the damaged cataractous natural lens may become clouded several months after cataract surgery. In that case, a YAG laser may be used to make a clear opening in the lens-containing membrane.

What kind of doctor performs cataract surgery?

Medical doctors, M.D.s, who, after completing medical school and an internship, have had 3 or more years of special training in eye diseases and surgery, are called ophthalmologists. Only ophthalmologists who have had special training in eye surgery are allowed to perform cataract surgery.

Chapter 22

All about Cataract Surgery

Chapter Contents

Section 22.1

What Happens during Cataract Surgery?

"All about Cataract Surgery" was provided courtesy of, and is copyrighted, by Lighthouse International, www.Lighthouse.org, a leading non-profit organization that helps people of all ages overcome the challenge of vision loss. © 2007.

When Should a Cataract Be Surgically Removed?

Although cataract removal may be recommended because of the appearance of the lens or specific eye problems, it is important that you understand the options in treating cataracts.

Occasionally, your ophthalmologist may say "your cataract is not ripe enough" or it "is too ripe." These expressions refer to chemical changes the cataract undergoes as it ages. As the condition progresses, the protein of the lens slowly changes, frequently becoming very hard (nuclear) or very soft (cortical). Your ophthalmologist will suggest surgery before the cataract is allowed to age too long (get too ripe), in order to allow greater safety in the surgical procedure.

When a cataract has been diagnosed, consider how your vision affects your quality of life and ability to do the things you ordinarily do. Unless a cataract interferes with work, driving, reading or leisure activities, there is usually no urgent need to remove it, particularly if the condition affects only one eye. There's no harm in waiting if you keep regular appointments with your eye doctor to evaluate how the cataract is progressing and whether or not surgery can be safely postponed. When glasses or magnifiers no longer help, or both eyes develop a cataract, surgery in the eye with the worst acuity is the only option. There is no medicine or other treatment that can dissolve or remove the cataract.

Once the decision to have surgery is made, your ophthalmologist will discuss your chances of achieving a good visual result based on the results of preoperative tests.

The benefits of surgery depend on the health of your retina and optic nerve at the time the procedure is performed. For the majority of people having cataract surgery, vision is restored, perhaps requiring only glasses for distance or reading and sunglasses. If you have other eye conditions, you may still need special optical devices, like magnifiers, after the surgery. However, you may be able to use optical devices with less magnification and find it easier to see without the haze and blur caused by the cataract.

Routine Preoperative Procedures

A-Scan

The A-scan is an ultrasonic probe that measures the length of the eyeball and provides the data to calculate the power of optical correction of the lens implant. Although the use of a multifocal or bifocal type of plastic lens implant is slowly becoming the preferred choice as lenses are developed that are technically superior, most doctors still use a plastic or silicone implant set for distance vision. Within certain limits, it's possible to choose the type of sight you prefer. For example, a very nearsighted person may choose to be less nearsighted (to see at a distance without glasses) as long as the vision in the operated eye still closely matches the nonoperated eye. Otherwise, the inequality of vision will result in visual confusion. This consideration is particularly important if the cataract is only in one eye. Similarly, people who wear glasses to correct farsightedness (hyperopia) may elect to see at a distance without glasses. In this instance, reading glasses will be needed for close work.

Medical Evaluation

It is customary to have a medical checkup within the two-week period prior to surgery. If you have high blood pressure, a heart condition, or diabetes, it's important to consult your internist before surgery in case your medication schedule needs to be modified before and/or on the day of surgery. This is particularly true with diabetic medication or with heart conditions requiring blood thinners.

Informed Consent

Your ophthalmologist is required to review possible complications with you regardless of their low incidence. Complications often sound frightening but their probability is rare in these days of modern technology and skill.

Optional Preoperative Tests

Some preoperative tests are recommended only in special situations (see Table 22.1).

187

Table 22.1. Optional Preoperative Tests before Cataract Surgery

Condition: Glaucoma
Test: Visual field
Purpose: To determine the presence of visual field defects

Condition: Macular degeneration, diabetic retinopathy
Test: Fluorescein angiography
Purpose: To determine if the macula or any area of the retina is leaking fluid

Condition: Corneal dystrophy or for those with previous intracapsular cataract surgery who are being evaluated for a secondary lens implant
Test: Corneal cell count
Purpose: To determine if there are enough corneal cells to withstand a surgical procedure

Condition: High myopia or previous retinal detachment/injury
Test: B-scan ultrasonography
Purpose: To rule out ocular pathology that can't be seen through a dense cataract

What Surgical Procedures Are Used to Remove the Cataract?

Performed by an ophthalmologist in a hospital or surgical center, cataract surgery is an elective outpatient procedure. During surgery, the lens is removed and replaced with an artificial one (implant) that performs the same function.

Two types of surgical procedures are commonly performed: extracapsular extraction and phacoemulsification. The extracapsular method has been the standard for over a decade, but with advancing technology in surgical equipment and intraocular lens implants for both methods, phacoemulsification has gradually become the procedure of choice in the majority of cases. The ophthalmologist usually makes the decision at the time of the diagnostic evaluation based on the dilation of the pupil, the state of the lens, the effect of other eye problems such as glaucoma on the mechanics of the eye, and the history of previous eye surgery.

Not all cataracts can be removed by phacoemulsification. If a pupil is too small and doesn't dilate, the lens is too hard, the cataract is too advanced, the eyeball is too deep set or the brow too prominent, then the extracapsular method, which requires stitches, is preferred.

Eventually, after about six weeks and once stitches are removed, post-operative vision is comparable with either method.

What Does Cataract Surgery Entail?

Extracapsular Extraction

1. Incision at the border of the cornea and sclera of about 1/2 inch

2. Opening of the lens capsule to expose nucleus

3. Lens nucleus removed from capsular bag in one piece

4. Cortical material removed by aspiration (suction)

5. Plastic lens implant placed in the capsular bag

6. Eye sutured with seven to nine nylon stitches (Postoperative astigmatism will result from stitches)

7. Removal of some of the stitches after six or more weeks to reduce astigmatism

8. Corrective glasses after stitches are removed, or when astigmatism subsides (usually six to seven weeks after surgery)

Pros

- Very few complications
- Complete control of nucleus removal

Cons

- Larger incision/more stitches
- Temporary postoperative astigmatism usually exists until stitches are removed
- Longer recovery time of vision (weeks)

Phacoemulsification

1. Small corneal incision of 3/16 inch or rarely a small tunnel incision of 3/16 inch under a conjunctival flap in the sclera or directly in the cornea into the anterior chamber

2. Opening of the lens capsule to expose nucleus

3. Lens nucleus fragmented and removed from capsular bag by ultrasonic emulsification and suction

4. Cortical material removed by aspiration (suction)

5. Plastic lens implant placed in the capsular bag

6. No stitch or, in some cases, one stitch to close the small incision

7. Little or no astigmatism

8. No stitches to remove. If there's one stitch, it remains there without any ill effect

9. Corrective glasses if needed after the eye stabilizes, usually a few weeks after surgery

Pros

- One or no stitch
- Less postoperative astigmatism
- Rapid recovery of vision (days)

Cons

- Difficult when the eye is deep set, nucleus is hard, or pupil is small (does not dilate)

What Kind of Anesthesia Can I Expect?

In the majority of cases, the doctor performs cataract surgery under local anesthesia instilled directly into the eye and light sedation. However, general anesthesia is appropriate in special situations: a very tense or apprehensive person, a person who cannot cooperate.

Local anesthesia and preparation of the eye is the same regardless of which surgical procedure is used. Your pupil is dilated an hour before surgery with several types of dilating drops applied to the eye at approximately 10- to 15- minute intervals. Dilation allows a wider exposure to the front surface of the lens. If your pupil does not dilate well, the iris opening may be enlarged at the time of surgery or your ophthalmologist may elect to do extracapsular surgery, which does not require maximum dilation.

An intravenous needle is inserted into an arm vein to infuse saline or sugar solution. This allows the anesthesiologist to give you additional sedation or medication if needed. Since you are not asleep, you will be able to tell the ophthalmologist if you experience any discomfort. The anesthesiologist monitors your breathing rate and blood pressure throughout the surgery.

Most people can go home after a few hours, although it is required that they be accompanied by a family member or friend. In special circumstances, a person may be admitted to the hospital overnight. However, the latter is more the exception than the rule.

What Is Stitchless Surgery?

Stitchless surgery is a relatively recent development. The wide incision of the extracapsular method, which requires seven to nine stitches, causes postoperative astigmatism for several weeks. To reduce this recovery period and to attain an almost instant visual recovery, a different technique was developed.

By entering the eye either in the sclera or at the border of the cornea, a narrow opening is made through the sclera or cornea into the eye. This allows a small ultrasonic probe to be easily inserted into the eye to emulsify the cataract. The folded lens implant is then inserted through the tunnel into the capsular bag behind the iris where it unfolds and locks itself into place behind the iris. Saline is injected to raise the eye pressure until the eye seals itself shut. Although the slanted incision is watertight and does not require a stitch, some ophthalmologists place one stitch at the opening of the incision as a precaution.

What about Stitches and Astigmatism?

Astigmatism is a normal optical variation (an unequal curvature) in the shape of the cornea, which is correctable with special astigmatic or cylindrical lenses. After phacoemulsification, there is little or no change in astigmatism. However, with extracapsular surgery, there is a temporary increase in astigmatism due to the stitches. Ordinarily, six to eight weeks after surgery, stitches are removed if it's necessary to reduce the astigmatism. Usually, one to three stitches are released under local anesthetic drops. There is no pain associated with this office procedure.

Only enough stitches are removed to reduce astigmatism to the lowest possible level. Any remaining nonreactive nylon stitches may be left in the eye without ill effect. Occasionally, a stitch left in place will come to the surface causing irritation. At this point, make an appointment with your ophthalmologist. Removing the stitch is a minor procedure that can be done during a brief office visit.

What Is a Surgical Microscope?

One of the significant advances in instrument development is the surgical microscope that provides a uniform light level and magnifies the details of the eye. Modern surgery could not be done without it. The ophthalmologist looks through a binocular eyepiece with an internal light source. The surgeon controls the suction or phacoemulsification machine with a foot pedal leaving both hands free to hold the surgical instruments. The surgical assistant has a separate eye piece to observe the procedure and assist the surgeon as directed.

Are Lens Implants Safe?

The plastic lens implant (intraocular lens) that replaces the cloudy lens is the most important part of cataract surgery. The plastic is nonreactive and cannot cause an allergic reaction. Rejection of an implant is rare and caused only by some extraneous factor unrelated to the lens material itself. Lens implants are permanent and safe unless there is a complication that prevents the safe introduction of a lens at the time of surgery. In those situations, an implant can be introduced as a secondary procedure at a later date.

What Is a Secondary Lens Implant?

Over two decades ago, when the entire lens, including the capsule, was removed (intracapsular extraction), one had to wear corrective contact lenses or thick "cataract" glasses. Now, many of these people can be evaluated for a special lens implant (secondary lens implant) by their ophthalmologist. Not everyone is a good candidate and only your ophthalmologist can tell you if a secondary implant is right for you. This outpatient surgical procedure is simple, done under minimal local anesthesia, and usually takes about 10 minutes.

Will I Still Need to Wear Eyeglasses after Surgery?

During the immediate postoperative period, it is customary for most people to continue using their current eyeglass prescription.

A recent development in intraocular lenses is a lens that can focus for distance, intermediate and near range using special optical designs. As the lens is perfected, this "focusing" implant will probably be the lens of choice in most cases. At present, at the end of the healing period, new corrective glasses are generally prescribed. A person who chose to have distance vision without glasses would require only reading glasses. A nearsighted (myopic) person who preferred to remain moderately nearsighted may now read without glasses and continue to wear corrective glasses for distance. Some people choose to wear a bifocal, trifocal or progressive lens as they always did.

Generally, the choice is a matter of personal preference but it may also depend on the optical situation. For example, a myopic or hyperopic (farsighted) person with a cataract in only one eye must continue to be myopic or hyperopic in the operated eye to maintain the balance between the eyes. The power of the intraocular lens is determined by the results of the A-scan test performed on both eyes prior to surgery.

What Can I Expect after Cataract Surgery?

Although surgical instruments and procedures have become increasingly sophisticated, resulting in little or no discomfort after the surgery, you must remember that you have had an operation. Depending on the type of surgical procedure performed, recovery takes time, usually a few days to a few weeks. In addition, your ophthalmologist may need to remove stitches.

Your eyes will be examined the day after surgery. A glaucoma test will be done and you receive a prescription for antibiotic drops or a combination of antibiotic and steroid drops to be taken several times a day to prevent infection and an anti-inflammatory drop to reduce inflammation. You may need to wear an eye shield at night to protect your eye and your doctor may suggest that you wear sunglasses out of doors. You will be warned not to take aspirin or products containing aspirin for a short time. If you have high blood pressure, diabetes or glaucoma, your doctor will also tell you when to resume taking your medication for these conditions. In some situations, your doctor may also recommend that you avoid bending (e.g., changing linens on your bed) or lifting (e.g., groceries, vacuum cleaner, laundry basket) for a specified period of time, depending on your condition.

If you are active, tell the doctor before resuming your regular routine:

- Alert your doctor to activities, such as swimming, jogging, yoga, tennis or lifting weights.

- Ask your doctor about restrictions on sexual activity.

- In the days following surgery, taking a shower is fine but shampoo and soap may irritate the operated eye.

- Likewise, in the early stages of wound healing, swimming in chlorinated water—with goggles—can be risky. Once wound healing is complete, wearing goggles in a chlorinated pool provides some protection and can also prevent accidental injury to the eye.

- You can resume driving if your postoperative visual acuity is within the legal limit. Your vision is tested after surgery, so ask your doctor if you may drive. With phacoemulsification, the visual acuity in the operated eye is often excellent within a few days. With extracapsular surgery, the nonoperated eye must have sufficient vision to operate a vehicle.

- If you must take a plane shortly after surgery, discuss it with your doctor. You may be advised to plan your surgery after a vacation or business trip.

- Don't be surprised if you feel tired, have low energy or even feel mildly depressed or let down. Some people may feel hyper. Either reaction can be related to the anesthesia or can be your way of dealing with the anticipation and stress of the surgery. It is normal to experience mild to moderate apprehension with any type of surgical procedure.

Depending on the visual results, some people may be disappointed or even angry that their vision is not what they thought it would be. This is particularly true when cataract surgery is performed on people with other eye conditions such as glaucoma, diabetic retinopathy, macular degeneration or retinitis pigmentosa, where the visual outcome depends on the severity of the underlying condition.

That's why it is extremely important to discuss visual outcomes with your ophthalmologist prior to the surgery. If you're not happy with the results, discuss your disappointment, anger or frustration with your ophthalmologist during one of your post-surgery follow-up visits. Your ophthalmologist may recommend that you be evaluated for additional optical devices and may suggest the benefits of joining a support group in your locale.

Since each situation is different, it is essential to follow your ophthalmologist's advice and not rely solely on information from other sources.

Can a Cataract Come Back?

A cataract can't come back, but a "secondary membrane" or thickening of the elastic lens capsule can form within weeks or months or years after surgery. This causes your vision to become slightly cloudy. It occurs in about 20% of cases and is easily and permanently removed through a procedure called a YAG capsulotomy, which uses a special cutting laser. The procedure takes approximately five minutes and is done with anesthetic drops on an outpatient basis by an ophthalmologist. In this procedure, a small opening is made in the capsule behind the lens implant so that light can again reach the retina. The procedure is painless but you need to have your eye pressure checked the next day. In addition, you must use eyedrops for a few days. Your eyeglass prescription will not change.

What Can Go Wrong?

Although cataract surgery is technically successful in over 98% of those treated, visual outcome will vary from person to person, particularly for those with multiple eye conditions. As with any surgery, there are risks. That's why doctors do surgery only on one eye at a time.

The Agency for Healthcare Research and Quality (AHRQ; formerly, Agency for Health Care Policy and Research [AHCPR]) lists the following potential complications to be discussed with your ophthalmologist as part of informed consent:

- drooping eyelid;
- infection inside the eye;
- swelling or clouding of the cornea;
- bleeding;
- high eye pressure (postoperative glaucoma);
- nucleus of the lens falling into the vitreous;
- retinal detachment;
- artificial lens dislocation;
- loss of the eye; and
- blindness.

Keep in mind that the precautions observed both prior to and during surgery, as well as postoperative treatments, are all designed to minimize infection, bleeding, glaucoma, malfunction of equipment, or any of the other complications listed.

However, if you experience itching, redness, pain, swelling, or any change in your vision after the surgery, call your ophthalmologist right away. Prompt treatment is important and may prevent additional problems.

—by Eleanor E. Faye, M.D., FACS;
Bruce P. Rosenthal, O.D., FAAO; and
Carol J. Sussman-Skalka, CSW, MBA

Section 22.2

Questions to Ask before Cataract Surgery

"Questions to Ask About Cataract Surgery" was provided courtesy of, and is copyrighted, by Lighthouse International, www.Lighthouse.org, a leading non-profit organization that helps people of all ages overcome the challenge of vision loss. © 2007.

Although your doctor will usually tell you what to expect, think about your specific concerns and your situation. You may wish to write down your questions to take with you to your visit. Consider bringing a family member or friend with you to help you understand all your options. We've all had the experience of not being able to absorb everything we hear in a doctor's office. Your concerns are important, so be sure your ophthalmologist has addressed them. Some doctors provide informational videos to assist in preparing you for the surgery. Among the questions you should ask:

Preparing for Surgery

- Is it safe for me to postpone cataract surgery? If so, for how long?

- What are the risks of cataract surgery with my present medical condition? Will you consult with my internist, cardiologist, or other specialist?

- Will cataract surgery affect my other medical problems?

- What improvements in my vision can I realistically expect?

- Will surgery be done on an outpatient basis or require an overnight stay?

- Will I receive local or general anesthesia?

- What surgical procedure will be used, extracapsular extraction or phacoemulsification? Will an intraocular lens be used?

- How long will the procedure take?

- Will the incision require stitches? Will they need to be removed?

- When is the last time I should eat or drink prior to surgery?

- May I take my regular medications on the day of surgery?

- Will I have any discomfort or pain during or after the surgery?

After Surgery

- How long will I have to use eyedrops after surgery? Will I need to take any other medications?

- Will I have to wear a shield over my eye and, if so, for how long?

- What eyeglasses can I wear during the healing period? Will I eventually need a new prescription?

- Is it advisable to wear sunglasses indoors as well as outdoors?

- What activity restrictions will there be and for how long?

- When may I return to work?

- When will I be able to read, drive, take a shower, swim, fly on a plane, or take a vacation?

- When will my vision return to normal?

- Should I anticipate any emotional or psychological reactions?

- How can I best prepare myself and my family for whatever assistance I may need in the days following surgery?

—by Eleanor E. Faye, M.D., FACS;
Bruce P. Rosenthal, O.D., FAAO; and
Carol J. Sussman-Skalka, CSW, MBA

Section 22.3

Protecting Your Eyes from Sunlight after Cataract Surgery

"Protecting Your Eyes From Sunlight After Cataract Surgery" was provided courtesy of, and is copyrighted, by Lighthouse International, www .Lighthouse.org, a leading non-profit organization that helps people of all ages overcome the challenge of vision loss. © 2007.

Excessive light may be harmful to the retina after cataract surgery. This is because the natural lens has been removed and ultraviolet (UV) light is now focused on the macula through the plastic implant. The lens of the eye protects the retina by absorbing specific wavelengths of ultraviolet light and by focusing visible wavelengths onto the retina. Although the implant lens contains ultraviolet blocking agents, it doesn't provide the same degree of protection to the macula as the natural lens.

During surgery, your cornea is covered with a special translucent disk to protect the retina from operating room lights.

Following surgery, your ophthalmologist may give you a tinted wrap-around ultraviolet protective shield or advise you to wear your sunglasses outside in bright light. After the postoperative healing period, if your eyes still feel uncomfortable on a sunny day, be sure to tell your doctor. A variety of ultraviolet protective lenses are available, including glasses that automatically darken when exposed to light, plastic tinted lenses, and wrap-around sunglasses that can be worn over your own glasses.

The National Weather Service publishes the Ultraviolet Potential Index (UPI) to alert the public to the dangers of ultraviolet rays. In fact, exposure to ultraviolet B light rays (UVB) has been associated with cataract formation. These studies and the UPI underscore the importance of wearing ultraviolet protective lenses.

In addition to the ultraviolet protection, many absorptive lenses eliminate the blue light that is associated with glare. Individuals with cataracts should, therefore, discuss glare and ultraviolet protection with their optometrist or ophthalmologist.

In fact, it is recommended that people of all ages, including infants, protect their eyes with sunglasses, hats or visors. It's important to be informed about sunwear protection and the quality and nature of the lenses you purchase. Just because a lens is dark does not mean it filters out ultraviolet rays. You need to read the labels on sunwear, and it is recommended that you wear sunglasses that filter 99 to 100 percent of ultraviolet (UV) light. Some labels say, "UV absorption up to 400 nm," which is equivalent to 100% UV protection. The label "Meets ANSI UV requirements" means the sunwear blocks at least 99% of UV light.

—by Eleanor E. Faye, M.D., FACS;
Bruce P. Rosenthal, O.D., FAAO; and
Carol J. Sussman-Skalka, CSW, MBA

Chapter 23

Intraocular Lens Implantation

Chapter Contents

Section 23.1

What Is Intraocular Lens Implantation?

"Intraocular Lens Implantation," © 2006 The Cleveland Clinic Cole Eye Institute, 9500 Euclid Avenue Mail Stop W14, Cleveland, OH 44195, www.clevelandclinic.org/eye. Additional information is available from the Cleveland Clinic Health Information Center, 216-444-3771, toll-free 800-223-2273 extension 43771, or at http://www.clevelandclinic.org/health.

What is an intraocular lens?

The eye contains a lens that focuses light so we can see. Sometimes the natural lens of the eye turns cloudy (which is called a cataract), and the only way to let light into the eye is to remove the whole lens. The natural lens is almost always replaced with an implantable medical device called an intraocular lens.

Why do people need intraocular lenses?

When natural lenses are removed from the eyes in cataract surgery, the eyes are left like cameras with no lenses. Even though light can get through, it will not make a clear image—just a fuzzy blur. The eyes need some kind of replacement lenses to be able to focus again.

Are there any alternatives to intraocular lenses?

Before intraocular lenses were invented, doctors could only prescribe eyeglasses or contact lenses after cataract surgery. Usually, the eyeglasses had to be very thick ("Coke-bottle" glasses) in order to match the strength of the eye's natural lens. But vision is not very good when eyeglass lenses are so thick, and thick contact lenses are not a much better option. Intraocular lenses were invented to solve these problems.

About 2 million people per year in the United States have cataract surgery, and almost all of them receive an intraocular lens. There are many different kinds of intraocular lenses. Your doctor can decide which lens is right for you only after a careful examination of your eye.

Intraocular lenses can be divided into two main groups: non-foldable and foldable. Intraocular lenses were originally made from a hard plastic material, but materials were later invented to make soft lenses that could be folded in half. This type of intraocular lens can be inserted through a smaller opening in the eye, which can be better for the patient because smaller incisions usually heal faster than larger ones.

What happens in the operation to implant intraocular lenses?

Intraocular lenses are usually implanted during cataract surgery, which is usually performed with local anesthesia. That is, the patient is awake but does not feel the procedure. In a few cases, the surgeon will use general anesthesia (the patient is "asleep").

The surgeon will make a very small opening in the front of the eye so the cloudy lens can be removed. There are two ways to remove the lens. One way is to remove it whole and the other is to use a special instrument to break the lens into pieces, then remove those pieces through a small incision.

Most cataract surgery is done with an instrument that breaks up lenses with ultrasound: sound waves that are too high in frequency for humans to hear. The energy from these ultrasound waves breaks up the lens in a process called phacoemulsification.

After the natural lenses have been removed, the intraocular lenses are placed into the eye. Usually, the intraocular lens goes where the natural lens had been. This area of the eye is called the posterior chamber. Sometimes, however, that might not be the best place for the intraocular lens so some lenses are designed to be placed in the anterior chamber, the area in front of the colored iris of the eye. Both types of lenses work well at putting the eye back into focus. Depending on which method of lens removal is used, the opening in the eye might not even need stitches. The patient is usually ready to go home about an hour after surgery.

Cataract surgery is sometimes performed without implanting intraocular lenses. It is usually possible to implant an intraocular lens at a later time. Surgeons often recommend the anterior chamber type of lens for those patients.

How successful are intraocular lenses?

More than 90% of the people who have cataracts removed see better after surgery than they did before. An important part of successful cataract surgery with an intraocular lens implant is following your doctor's instructions after surgery. Eye drops are prescribed after surgery to help the eye heal better and to prevent infection. Your doctor will have to examine your eye after surgery to make sure it is healing properly and to check your vision. It is important to keep these appointments with your doctor.

Does anyone need to wear eyeglasses or contact lenses after receiving an intraocular lens?

Most intraocular lenses are chosen to focus at what doctors call "distance" vision. By "distance," they mean anything farther than 2 or 3 feet away from the eye. If the lenses are focusing at distance, eyeglasses will be needed to see clearly close-up. Many people who have cataract surgery are already used to wearing bifocals, so they are familiar with this type of vision.

Section 23.2

The C-Flex™ Intraocular Lens

"New Device Approval—C-flex™ intraocular lens—P060011" is from the Centers for Devices and Radiological Health, U.S. Food and Drug Administration (FDA, www.fda.gov), June 1, 2007.

What is it?

C-flex™ (Product name: C-flex™ intraocular lens model 570C) is a plastic lens used to restore vision and replace the natural lens of the eye after it is removed during cataract surgery. A cataract is a gradual thickening, hardening, and clouding of the eye's lens, resulting in loss of vision. Cataracts are often the result of aging, but can have other causes.

How does it work?

C-flex™ acts as a healthy eye lens to correctly focuses light on the retina and restore vision.

When is it used?

C-flex™ is used to restore vision in adult patients who have had a cataractous lens removed.

What will it accomplish?

C-flex™ restores vision by acting as a substitute for the removed natural lens.

When should it not be used?

C-flex™ should not be implanted in patients who:

- are younger than 21 years;
- have extremely small eyes;
- have chronic or active ocular disease excluding cataracts; and
- are pregnant or nursing.

For additional information, see The Summary of Safety and Effectiveness and labeling at: http://www.fda.gov/cdrh/pdf6/p060011.html

Are there other considerations?

The patient and surgeon should consider the potential risks and benefits in deciding whether or not to implant this device. A surgeon may choose not to use this device if:

- there is inflammation/infection in the eye,
- removing the cataract was especially difficult, or
- there is a defect in the eye that would not allow normal placement of the lens.

Part Four

Glaucoma

Chapter 24

Glaucoma: A Leading Cause of Blindness

Glaucoma: How Much Do You Know?

Fifty million Americans are at risk for vision loss from glaucoma, a leading cause of blindness in the United States. Are you one of them? If you are, do you know how to reduce your risk of blindness? To determine how high your Eye-Q is, answer the following questions about glaucoma.

Glaucoma is more common in African Americans than in Whites.

True. In a study funded by the National Eye Institute, researchers at Johns Hopkins University reported that glaucoma is three to four times more likely to occur in African Americans than in Whites. In addition, glaucoma is six times more likely to cause blindness in African Americans than in Whites.

Glaucoma tends to run in families.

True. Although glaucoma tends to run in families, a hereditary

The quiz, "Glaucoma: How Much Do You Know?" is from the National Eye Institute (NEI, www.nei.nih.gov), part of the National Institutes of Health, December 2006. The text following the heading "Glaucoma Defined" is from "Glaucoma: What You Should Know," a booklet by the National Eye Institute (NEI, www.nei.nih.gov), part of the National Institutes of Health, April 2006.

basis has not been established. If someone in your immediate family has glaucoma, you should have a comprehensive dilated eye examination every one to two years.

A *person can have glaucoma and not know it.*

True. The early stages of open-angle glaucoma, the most common form, usually have no warning signs. However, as the disease progresses, a person with glaucoma may notice his or her side vision gradually failing.

People over age 60 are more likely to get glaucoma.

True. Everyone over age 60 is at an increased risk for glaucoma, especially Mexican Americans. Other groups at increased risk include African Americans over age 40 and people with a family history of glaucoma.

Eye pain is often a symptom of glaucoma.

False. People with glaucoma usually do not experience pain from the disease.

Glaucoma can be controlled.

True. Although glaucoma cannot be cured, it usually can be controlled by eyedrops or pills, conventional surgery, or laser surgery. Sometimes eye care professionals will recommend a combination of surgery and medication.

Glaucoma is caused by increased eye pressure.

False. Increased eye pressure means you are at increased risk for glaucoma, but does not mean you have the disease. A person has glaucoma only if the optic nerve is damaged. If you have increased eye pressure but no damage to the optic nerve, you do not have glaucoma. Follow the advice of your doctor.

Vision lost from glaucoma can be restored.

False. Vision loss from glaucoma is permanent. However, with early detection and treatment, the progression of visual loss can be slowed, or halted, and the risk of blindness reduced.

A complete glaucoma exam consists only of measuring eye pressure.

False. A measurement of eye pressure by tonometry, though an important part of a comprehensive eye exam, is, by itself, not sufficient for the detection of glaucoma. Glaucoma is detected most often during an eye examination through dilated pupils. Drops are put into the eyes during the exam to enlarge the pupils, which allows the eye care professional to see more of the inside of the eye to check for signs of glaucoma. When indicated, a visual field test should also be performed.

People at risk for glaucoma should have an eye examination through dilated pupils.

True. An eye examination through dilated pupils is the best way to diagnose glaucoma. Individuals at increased risk for the disease should have their eyes examined through dilated pupils every one to two years by an eye care professional.

Glaucoma Defined

What is glaucoma?

Glaucoma is a group of diseases that can damage the eye's optic nerve and result in vision loss and blindness. Glaucoma occurs when the normal fluid pressure inside the eyes slowly rises. However, with early treatment, you can often protect your eyes against serious vision loss.

What is the optic nerve?

The optic nerve is a bundle of more than 1 million nerve fibers. It connects the retina to the brain. The retina is the light-sensitive tissue at the back of the eye. A healthy optic nerve is necessary for good vision.

What are some other forms of glaucoma?

Open-angle glaucoma is the most common form. Some people have other types of the disease.

Low-tension or normal-tension glaucoma: Optic nerve damage and narrowed side vision occur in people with normal eye pressure. Lowering eye pressure at least 30 percent through medicines slows the disease in some people. Glaucoma may worsen in others despite low pressures.

A comprehensive medical history is important in identifying other potential risk factors, such as low blood pressure, that contribute to low-tension glaucoma. If no risk factors are identified, the treatment options for low-tension glaucoma are the same as for open-angle glaucoma.

Angle-closure glaucoma: The fluid at the front of the eye cannot reach the angle and leave the eye. The angle gets blocked by part of the iris. People with this type of glaucoma have a sudden increase in eye pressure. Symptoms include severe pain and nausea, as well as redness of the eye and blurred vision. If you have these symptoms, you need to seek treatment immediately.

This is a medical emergency. If your doctor is unavailable, go to the nearest hospital or clinic. Without treatment to improve the flow of fluid, the eye can become blind in as few as one or two days. Usually, prompt laser surgery and medicines can clear the blockage and protect sight.

Congenital glaucoma: Children are born with a defect in the angle of the eye that slows the normal drainage of fluid. These children usually have obvious symptoms, such as cloudy eyes, sensitivity to light, and excessive tearing. Conventional surgery typically is the suggested treatment, because medicines may have unknown effects in infants and be difficult to administer. Surgery is safe and effective. If surgery is done promptly, these children usually have an excellent chance of having good vision.

Secondary glaucomas: These can develop as complications of other medical conditions. These types of glaucomas are sometimes associated with eye surgery or advanced cataracts, eye injuries, certain eye tumors, or uveitis (eye inflammation). Pigmentary glaucoma occurs when pigment from the iris flakes off and blocks the meshwork, slowing fluid drainage. A severe form, called neovascular glaucoma, is linked to diabetes. Corticosteroid drugs used to treat eye inflammations and other diseases can trigger glaucoma in some people. Treatment includes medicines, laser surgery, or conventional surgery.

Causes and Risk Factors

How does open-angle glaucoma damage the optic nerve?

In the front of the eye is a space called the anterior chamber. A clear fluid flows continuously in and out of the chamber and nourishes nearby tissues. The fluid leaves the chamber at the open angle where the cornea and iris meet. When the fluid reaches the angle, it flows through a spongy meshwork, like a drain, and leaves the eye.

Sometimes, when the fluid reaches the angle, it passes too slowly through the meshwork drain. As the fluid builds up, the pressure inside the eye rises to a level that may damage the optic nerve. When the optic nerve is damaged from increased pressure, open-angle glaucoma—and vision loss—may result. That's why controlling pressure inside the eye is important.

Does increased eye pressure mean that I have glaucoma?

Not necessarily. Increased eye pressure means you are at risk for glaucoma, but does not mean you have the disease. A person has glaucoma only if the optic nerve is damaged. If you have increased eye pressure

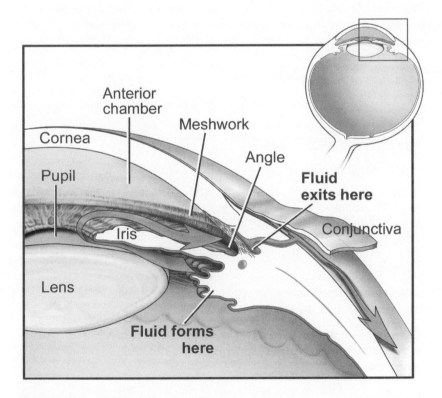

Figure 24.1. Fluid pathway in the eye.

but no damage to the optic nerve, you do not have glaucoma. However, you are at risk. Follow the advice of your eye care professional.

Can I develop glaucoma if I have increased eye pressure?

Not necessarily. Not every person with increased eye pressure will develop glaucoma. Some people can tolerate higher eye pressure better than others. Also, a certain level of eye pressure may be high for one person but normal for another.

Whether you develop glaucoma depends on the level of pressure your optic nerve can tolerate without being damaged. This level is different for each person. That's why a comprehensive dilated eye exam is very important. It can help your eye care professional determine what level of eye pressure is normal for you.

Can I develop glaucoma without an increase in my eye pressure?

Yes. Glaucoma can develop without increased eye pressure. This form of glaucoma is called low-tension or normal-tension glaucoma. It is not as common as open-angle glaucoma.

Who is at risk for glaucoma?

Anyone can develop glaucoma. Some people are at higher risk than others. They include:

- African Americans over age 40;
- everyone over age 60, especially Mexican Americans; and
- people with a family history of glaucoma.

Among African Americans, studies show that glaucoma is:

- five times more likely to occur in African Americans than in Caucasians;
- about four times more likely to cause blindness in African Americans than in Caucasians; and
- fifteen times more likely to cause blindness in African Americans between the ages of 45 to 64 than in Caucasians of the same age group.

A comprehensive dilated eye exam can reveal more risk factors, such as high eye pressure, thinness of the cornea, and abnormal optic nerve anatomy. In some people with certain combinations of these high-risk factors, medicines in the form of eyedrops reduce the risk of developing glaucoma by about half.

Medicare covers an annual comprehensive dilated eye exam for some people at high risk for glaucoma.

What can I do to protect my vision?

Studies have shown that the early detection and treatment of glaucoma, before it causes major vision loss, is the best way to control the disease. So, if you fall into one of the high-risk groups for the disease, make sure to have your eyes examined through dilated pupils every one to two years by an eye care professional.

If you are being treated for glaucoma, be sure to take your glaucoma medicine every day. See your eye care professional regularly.

You also can help protect the vision of family members and friends who may be at high risk for glaucoma—African Americans over age 40; everyone over age 60, especially Mexican Americans; and people with a family history of the disease. Encourage them to have a comprehensive dilated eye exam at least once every two years. Remember: Lowering eye pressure in glaucoma's early stages slows progression of the disease and helps save vision.

Symptoms and Detection

What are the symptoms of glaucoma?

At first, there are no symptoms. Vision stays normal, and there is no pain. However, as the disease progresses, a person with glaucoma may notice his or her side vision gradually failing. That is, objects in front may still be seen clearly, but objects to the side may be missed.

As glaucoma remains untreated, people may miss objects to the side and out of the corner of their eye. Without treatment, people with glaucoma will slowly lose their peripheral (side) vision. They seem to be looking through a tunnel. Over time, straight-ahead vision may decrease until no vision remains.

Glaucoma can develop in one or both eyes.

How is glaucoma detected?

Glaucoma is detected through a comprehensive eye exam that includes:

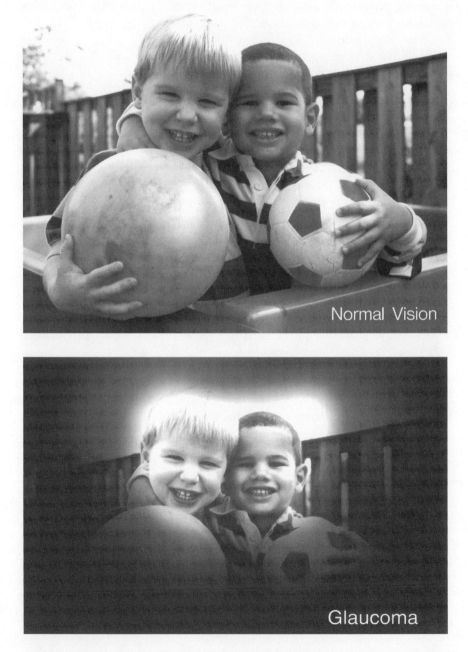

Figure 24.2. *Normal vision and same scene as viewed by a person with glaucoma.*

- **Visual acuity test:** This eye chart test measures how well you see at various distances. A tonometer measures pressure inside the eye to detect glaucoma.

- **Visual field test:** This test measures your side (peripheral) vision. It helps your eye care professional tell if you have lost side vision, a sign of glaucoma.

- **Dilated eye exam:** Drops are placed in your eyes to widen, or dilate, the pupils. Your eye care professional uses a special magnifying lens to examine your retina and optic nerve for signs of damage and other eye problems. After the exam, your close-up vision may remain blurred for several hours.

- **Tonometry:** An instrument (right) measures the pressure inside the eye. Numbing drops may be applied to your eye for this test.

- **Pachymetry:** A numbing drop is applied to your eye. Your eye care professional uses an ultrasonic wave instrument to measure the thickness of your cornea.

Treatment

Can glaucoma be treated?

Yes. Immediate treatment for early stage, open-angle glaucoma can delay progression of the disease. That's why early diagnosis is very important.

Glaucoma treatments include medicines, laser trabeculoplasty, conventional surgery, or a combination of any of these. While these treatments may save remaining vision, they do not improve sight already lost from glaucoma.

Medicines: Medicines, in the form of eyedrops or pills, are the most common early treatment for glaucoma. Some medicines cause the eye to make less fluid. Others lower pressure by helping fluid drain from the eye.

Before you begin glaucoma treatment, tell your eye care professional about other medicines you may be taking. Sometimes the drops can interfere with the way other medicines work.

Glaucoma medicines may be taken several times a day. Most people have no problems. However, some medicines can cause headaches or other side effects. For example, drops may cause stinging, burning, and redness in the eyes. Many drugs are available to treat glaucoma. If you have problems with one medicine, tell your eye care professional. Treatment with a different dose or a new drug may be possible.

Because glaucoma often has no symptoms, people may be tempted to stop taking, or may forget to take, their medicine. You need to use the drops or pills as long as they help control your eye pressure. Regular use is very important. Make sure your eye care professional shows you how to put the drops into your eye.

Laser trabeculoplasty: Laser trabeculoplasty helps fluid drain out of the eye. Your doctor may suggest this step at any time. In many cases, you need to keep taking glaucoma drugs after this procedure.

Laser trabeculoplasty is performed in your doctor's office or eye clinic. Before the surgery, numbing drops will be applied to your eye. As you sit facing the laser machine, your doctor will hold a special lens to your eye. A high-intensity beam of light is aimed at the lens and reflected onto the meshwork inside your eye. You may see flashes of bright green or red light. The laser makes several evenly spaced burns that stretch the drainage holes in the meshwork. This allows the fluid to drain better.

Like any surgery, laser surgery can cause side effects, such as inflammation.

Your doctor may give you some drops to take home for any soreness or inflammation inside the eye. You need to make several follow-up visits to have your eye pressure monitored.

If you have glaucoma in both eyes, only one eye will be treated at a time. Laser treatments for each eye will be scheduled several days to several weeks apart.

Studies show that laser surgery is very good at reducing the pressure in some patients. However, its effects can wear off over time. Your doctor may suggest further treatment.

Conventional surgery: Conventional surgery makes a new opening for the fluid to leave the eye. Your doctor may suggest this treatment at any time. Conventional surgery often is done after medicines and laser surgery have failed to control pressure.

Conventional surgery is performed in an eye clinic or hospital. Before the surgery, you will be given medicine to help you relax. Your doctor will make small injections around the eye to numb it. A small piece of tissue is removed to create a new channel for the fluid to drain from the eye.

For several weeks after the surgery, you must put drops in the eye to fight infection and inflammation. These drops will be different from those you may have been using before surgery.

As with laser surgery, conventional surgery is performed on one eye at a time. Usually the operations are four to six weeks apart. Conventional surgery is about 60 to 80 percent effective at lowering eye pressure. If the new drainage opening narrows, a second operation may be needed. Conventional surgery works best if you have not had previous eye surgery, such as a cataract operation. In some instances, your vision may not be as good as it was before conventional surgery. Conventional surgery can cause side effects, including cataract, problems with the cornea, and inflammation or infection inside the eye. The buildup of fluid in the back of the eye may cause some patients to see shadows in their vision. If you have any of these problems, tell your doctor so a treatment plan can be developed.

Conventional surgery makes a new opening for the fluid to leave the eye.

How should I use my glaucoma eyedrops?

If eyedrops have been prescribed for treating your glaucoma, you need to use them properly and as instructed by your eye care professional. Proper use of your glaucoma medication can improve the medicine's effectiveness and reduce your risk of side effects. To properly apply your eyedrops, follow these steps:

- First, wash your hands.
- Hold the bottle upside down.
- Tilt your head back.
- Hold the bottle in one hand and place it as close as possible to the eye.
- With the other hand, pull down your lower eyelid. This forms a pocket.
- Place the prescribed number of drops into the lower eyelid pocket. If you are using more than one eyedrop, be sure to wait at least five minutes before applying the second eyedrop.
- Close your eye or press the lower lid lightly with your finger for at least one minute. Either of these steps keeps the drops in the eye and helps prevent the drops from draining into the tear duct, which can increase your risk of side effects

What can I do if I already have lost some vision from glaucoma?

If you have lost some sight from glaucoma, ask your eye care professional about low vision services and devices that may help you make the most of your remaining vision. Ask for a referral to a specialist in low vision.

Many community organizations and agencies offer information about low vision counseling, training, and other special services for people with visual impairments. A nearby school of medicine or optometry may provide low vision services.

Current Research

A large amount of research is being done in the United States to learn what causes glaucoma and to improve its diagnosis and treatment. For instance, the National Eye Institute (NEI) is funding a number of studies to find out what causes fluid pressure to increase in the eye. By learning more about this process, doctors may be able to find the exact cause of the disease and learn better how to prevent and treat it. The NEI also supports clinical trials of new drugs and surgical techniques that show promise against glaucoma.

Chapter 25

Types of Glaucoma

Chapter Contents

Section 25.1

Signs and Symptoms of Different Types of Glaucoma

"Types of Glaucoma," © 2005 Glaucoma Research Foundation
(www.glaucoma.org). Reprinted with permission.

The two main types of glaucoma are primary open angle glaucoma (POAG), and angle closure glaucoma. These are marked by an increase of intraocular pressure (IOP), or pressure inside the eye. When optic nerve damage has occurred despite a normal IOP, this is called normal tension glaucoma. Secondary glaucoma refers to any case in which another disease causes or contributes to increased eye pressure, resulting in optic nerve damage and vision loss.

Angle Closure Glaucoma

This type of glaucoma is also known as acute glaucoma or narrow angle glaucoma. It is much more rare and is very different from open angle glaucoma in that the eye pressure usually rises very quickly.

This happens when the drainage canals get blocked or covered over, like a sink with something covering the drain.

With angle closure glaucoma, the iris is not as wide and open as it should be. The outer edge of the iris bunches up over the drainage canals, when the pupil enlarges too much or too quickly. This can happen when entering a dark room.

A simple test can be used to see if your angle is normal and wide or abnormal and narrow. Treatment of angle closure glaucoma usually involves surgery to remove a small portion of the outer edge of the iris. This helps unblock the drainage canals so that the extra fluid can drain. Usually surgery is successful and long lasting. However, you should still receive regular checkups.

Symptoms of angle closure glaucoma may include headaches, eye pain, nausea, rainbows around lights at night, and very blurred vision.

Normal Tension Glaucoma (NTG)

Normal tension glaucoma is also known as low-tension glaucoma or normal pressure glaucoma. In this type of glaucoma, the optic nerve is damaged even though intraocular pressure (IOP) is not very high. Doctors do not know why some people's optic nerves suffer damage even though pressure levels are in the "normal" range (between 12-22 mm Hg).

Those at higher risk for this form of glaucoma are people with a family history of normal tension glaucoma, people of Japanese ancestry, and people with a history of systemic heart disease, such as irregular heart rhythm. Normal tension glaucoma is usually detected after an examination of the optic nerve.

The Glaucoma Research Foundation sponsored a collaborative international study to help determine the best treatment for this type of glaucoma. The study concluded that eye drops used to lower intraocular pressure were effective even in cases of normal tension glaucoma. Currently, most doctors treat normal tension glaucoma by keeping normal eye pressures as low as possible with medicines, laser surgery, or filtering surgery.

Pediatric Glaucoma

The pediatric glaucomas consist of congenital glaucoma (present at birth), infantile glaucoma (appears during the first three years), juvenile glaucoma (age three through the teenage or young adult years), and all the secondary glaucomas occurring in the pediatric age group.

Congenital glaucoma is present at birth and most cases are diagnosed during the first year of life. Sometimes symptoms are not recognized until later in infancy or early childhood.

The range of treatment is very different from that for adult glaucoma. It is very important to catch pediatric glaucoma early in order to prevent blindness.

Primary Open Angle Glaucoma

This is the most common form of glaucoma, affecting about three million Americans. It happens when the eye's drainage canals become clogged over time. The inner eye pressure (also called intraocular pressure or IOP) rises because the correct amount of fluid can't drain out of the eye. With open angle glaucoma, the entrances to the drainage canals are clear and should be working correctly. The clogging problem occurs further inside the drainage canals, similar to a clogged pipe below the drain in a sink.

Most people have no symptoms and no early warning signs. If open angle glaucoma is not diagnosed and treated, it can cause a gradual loss of vision. This type of glaucoma develops slowly and sometimes without noticeable sight loss for many years. It usually responds well to medication, especially if caught early and treated.

Secondary Glaucoma

Glaucoma can occur as the result of an eye injury, inflammation, tumor or in advanced cases of cataract or diabetes. It can also be caused by certain drugs such as steroids. This form of glaucoma may be mild or severe. The type of treatment will depend on whether it is open angle or angle closure glaucoma.

Pseudoexfoliative Glaucoma

This form of secondary open angle glaucoma occurs when a flaky, dandruff-like material peels off the outer layer of the lens within the eye. The material collects in the angle between the cornea and iris and can clog the drainage system of the eye, causing eye pressure to rise.

Pseudoexfoliative glaucoma is common in those of Scandinavian descent. Treatment usually includes medications or surgery.

Pigmentary Glaucoma

A form of secondary open angle glaucoma, this occurs when the pigment granules in the back of the iris (the colored part of the eye) break into the clear fluid produced inside the eye. These tiny pigment granules flow toward the drainage canals in the eye and slowly clog them, causing eye pressure to rise. Treatment usually includes medications or surgery.

Traumatic Glaucoma

Injury to the eye may cause secondary open angle glaucoma. This type of glaucoma can occur immediately after the injury or years later.

It can be caused by blunt injuries that "bruise" the eye (called blunt trauma) or by injuries that penetrate the eye.

In addition, conditions such as severe nearsightedness, previous injury, infection, or prior surgery may make the eye more vulnerable to a serious eye injury.

Neovascular Glaucoma

The abnormal formation of new blood vessels on the iris and over the eye's drainage channels can cause a form of secondary open angle glaucoma.

Neovascular glaucoma is always associated with other abnormalities, most often diabetes. It never occurs on its own. The new blood vessels block the eye's fluid from exiting through the trabecular meshwork (the eye's drainage canals), causing an increase in eye pressure. This type of glaucoma is very difficult to treat.

Iridocorneal Endothelial Syndrome (ICE)

This rare form of glaucoma usually appears in only one eye, rather than both. Cells on the back surface of the cornea spread over the eye's drainage tissue and across the surface of the iris, increasing eye pressure and damaging the optic nerve. These corneal cells also form adhesions that bind the iris to the cornea, further blocking the drainage channels.

Iridocorneal endothelial syndrome occurs more frequently in light-skinned females. Symptoms can include hazy vision upon awakening and the appearance of halos around lights. Treatment can include medications and filtering surgery. Laser therapy is not effective in these cases.

Section 25.2

Childhood Glaucoma

Childhood glaucoma—also referred to as congenital glaucoma, pediatric, or infantile glaucoma—occurs in babies and young children. It is usually diagnosed within the first year of life.

This is a rare condition that may be inherited, caused by incorrect development of the eye's drainage system before birth. This leads to increased intraocular pressure, which in turn damages the optic nerve.

Symptoms of childhood glaucoma include enlarged eyes, cloudiness of the cornea, and photosensitivity (sensitivity to light).

How Is It Treated?

In an uncomplicated case, surgery can often correct such structural defects. Both medication and surgery are required in some cases.

Medical treatments may involve the use of topical eye drops and oral medications. These treatments help to either increase the exit of fluid from the eye or decrease the production of fluid inside the eye. Each results in lower eye pressure.

There are two main types of surgical treatments: filtering surgery and laser surgery. Filtering surgery (also known as micro surgery) involves the use of small surgical tools to create a drainage canal in the eye. In contrast, laser surgery uses a small but powerful beam of light to make a small opening in the eye tissue.

What to Expect

Thousands of children with glaucoma can live full lives. This is the ultimate goal of glaucoma management. Although lost vision cannot be restored, it is possible to optimize each child's remaining vision. Equally important is to encourage your child's independence and participation in his or her own self-care.

Signs of Childhood Glaucoma

- Unusually large eyes
- Excessive tearing
- Cloudy eyes
- Light sensitivity

Chapter 26

Glaucoma Risk Factors and Prevention

Chapter Contents

Section 26.1

Ocular Hypertension Increases Risk of Glaucoma

"Ocular Hypertension," © 2007 American Optometric Association (www.aoa.org). Reprinted with permission.

Ocular hypertension has no noticeable signs or symptoms. Ocular hypertension is an increase in the pressure in your eyes that is above the range considered normal with no detectable changes in vision or damage to the structure of your eyes. The term is used to distinguish people with elevated pressure from those with glaucoma, a serious eye disease that causes damage to the optic nerve and vision loss.

Ocular hypertension can occur in people of all ages, but it occurs more frequently in African Americans, those over age 40, and those with family histories of ocular hypertension and/or glaucoma. It is also more common in those who are very nearsighted or who have diabetes.

Ocular hypertension has no noticeable signs or symptoms. Your doctor of optometry can check the pressure in your eyes with an instrument called a tonometer and can examine the inner structures of your eyes to assess your overall eye health.

Not all people with ocular hypertension will develop glaucoma. However, there is an increased risk of glaucoma among those with ocular hypertension, so regular comprehensive optometric examinations are essential to your overall eye health.

There is no cure for ocular hypertension, however, careful monitoring and treatment, when indicated, can decrease the risk of damage to your eyes.

Section 26.2

Preventing or Delaying Glaucoma with Eyedrops

From "Eyedrops May Delay or Prevent Glaucoma in African Americans at Higher Risk," a press release by the National Eye Institute (NEI, www.nei.nih.gov), part of the National Institutes of Health, June 14, 2004.

Eyedrops that reduce elevated pressure inside the eye can delay or possibly prevent the onset of glaucoma in African Americans at higher risk for developing the disease, researchers have found. This makes it more important to identify African Americans at higher risk for developing glaucoma so they can receive prompt evaluation for possible medical treatment. These results are reported in the June 2004 issue of *Archives of Ophthalmology*.

Scientists found that daily pressure-lowering eyedrops reduced the development of primary open-angle glaucoma in African Americans by almost 50 percent. Primary open-angle glaucoma is the most common form of glaucoma and one of the nation's leading causes of vision loss. Of the African American study participants who received the eyedrops, 8.4 percent developed glaucoma. By comparison, 16.1 percent of the African American study participants who did not receive the eyedrops developed glaucoma. The study was funded by the National Eye Institute (NEI) and the National Center on Minority Health and Health Disparities (NCMHD), two components of the federal government's National Institutes of Health.

The results of this study, called the Ocular Hypertension Treatment Study (OHTS), are a followup to initial results released two years ago. In those findings, researchers discovered that treating people with elevated eye pressure could delay or prevent the onset of glaucoma. At that time, results for the subgroup of African Americans trended in the same direction, but were not conclusive.

Primary open-angle glaucoma affects about 2.2 million Americans age 40 and over, half of whom are not aware they have the disease. Vision loss from glaucoma occurs when the optic nerve is damaged. In most cases, elevated eye pressure, also called ocular hypertension, contributes to this damage. This causes gradual loss of peripheral (side) vision. As the disease progresses, the field of vision gradually narrows and blindness can result. Glaucoma has no early symptoms, and by the time people experience problems with their vision, they usually have a significant amount of optic nerve damage. However, if detected early, glaucoma can usually be controlled and serious vision loss prevented. Comprehensive dilated eye examinations are recommended at least once every two years for African Americans over age 40 and all people over age 60.

"This is the first study to recruit large numbers of African Americans to examine the benefit of pressure-lowering eyedrops to prevent or delay the onset of glaucoma," said Paul A. Sieving, M.D., Ph.D., director of the NEI. "The results underscore that African Americans over age 40 should receive a comprehensive dilated eye exam at least once every two years to see if they are at higher risk for glaucoma."

These results do not imply that every African American with high eye pressure requires treatment, according to Eve Higginbotham, M.D., chair of the Department of Ophthalmology at the University of Maryland Medical Center and first author of the journal article. "When determining treatment, doctors should take into account several risk factors, including specific anatomical characteristics of the optic nerve and the cornea," Dr. Higginbotham said. "While African Americans participating in the study were more likely than others to have these specific physical characteristics, the study results underscore the importance of measuring these ocular risk factors rather than relying solely on the race or ethnicity of the individual."

Dr. Higginbotham suggested that before determining treatment, the doctor and patient should also discuss the patient's health status and life expectancy, and the burden of daily treatment, including cost, inconvenience, and possible side effects.

Elevated eye pressure results when the fluid that flows in and out of the eye drains too slowly, gradually increasing pressure inside the eye. It is estimated that between three and six million people in the United States are at increased risk for developing primary open-angle glaucoma, representing between four and seven percent of the population above age 40. In this study, ocular hypertension was defined as pressure of 24 mm Hg or greater in at least one eye.

The OHTS studied more than 1,600 people, including 408 African Americans, 40 to 80 years of age, who had elevated eye pressure but no signs of glaucoma. Half were assigned daily pressure-lowering eyedrops, and the other half were assigned to observation (no medication). In the medication group, the number of African Americans participants developing glaucoma was significantly lower (8.4 percent) compared to the observation group (16.1 percent).

"The study also confirms that the risk for developing glaucoma is higher among African Americans compared with others," said Michael Kass, M.D., of the Washington University Department of Ophthalmology and Visual Sciences and chair of the study. "A number of risk factors may be contributing to the increased prevalence of visual impairment from glaucoma in African Americans. These include a family history of glaucoma; earlier onset of the disease compared to other races; later detection of the disease; and economic and social barriers to treatment."

Glaucoma is a leading cause of blindness in African Americans, said John Ruffin Ph.D., director of the NCMHD. "Glaucoma is almost three times as common in African Americans than Whites," Dr. Ruffin said. "However, if glaucoma is detected and treated early in its progression, it can usually be slowed and serious vision loss can be delayed."

Dr. Ruffin said Medicare covers an annual dilated eye examination for people at higher risk for glaucoma. This important preventive benefit defines higher risk as people with diabetes; those with a family history of glaucoma; and African Americans aged 50 and older.

In addition to support from the NEI and NCMHD, the Ocular Hypertension Treatment Study was supported by Research to Prevent Blindness and Merck Research Laboratories. The study was conducted at 22 clinical centers across the country.

Chapter 27

Diagnosing Glaucoma

Chapter Contents

Section 27.1

Working with Your Doctor If You've Been Diagnosed with Glaucoma

"Working With Your Doctor," © 2005 Glaucoma Research Foundation (www.glaucoma.org). Reprinted with permission.

If you have been diagnosed with glaucoma, obtaining treatment and following your treatment regimen are essential to preserving your eyesight. A good relationship with your eye doctor is the foundation of effective treatment.

The most recent diagnostic and treatment advances won't help if you don't obtain and follow the instructions from your doctor. Don't be afraid to ask questions!

Ask questions about the medications, results, and possible side effects. If side effects are intolerable, let your doctor(s) know as soon as possible so they can work on finding a more suitable medication.

Here are some specific questions you can ask to help you gather all of the information you need.

The Basics

- What type of glaucoma do I have?

- Did something cause my condition? And if so, what?

- How will my vision be affected now and in the future?

- Is it hereditary? What should I tell my family about my condition?

- What is my expected prognosis?

Treatment

- What are my treatment options?

- Which ones are most appropriate for me? Why?

- What are the possible risks and side effects of this treatment?

- What could happen without treatment?
- What medications do you recommend? Will they interact with any other medications or dietary supplements I am taking?
- How long will this treatment last?
- How will I know if the treatment is working?
- How often will I need checkups?

Lifestyle Changes

- Should I follow a special diet?
- What type of exercise could help my condition?
- What special precautions should I take when working or driving?
- Which activities should I avoid?

Support

- Can you recommend any glaucoma support groups?

More Tips for Working with Your Doctor

- **Make sure you have the information you need:** Detailed regimens can be hard to remember. Ask the doctor to write out the treatment plan in large clear letters, and if necessary, color-code the medications and instructions.

- **Bring a friend to your appointment:** Ask a friend or family member to come with you to your appointment and help you capture all the details. This can be especially helpful if your diagnosis is recent, since the diagnosis may create a shock-like state that makes it hard to absorb all the information the doctor provides.

- **Write things down:** In addition to taking your own notes at the doctor's office, keep a journal of drug reactions, their timing, etc. so you won't have to rely on memory at your next appointment.

- **Utilize the medical support team:** Trained staff at your doctor's office, such as nurses and technicians, can be an enormous support to helping you manage your disease. These knowledgeable professionals can often give you the information, time, and attention that can make a big difference.

Section 27.2

Discovery of Glaucoma Gene Will Improve Early Diagnosis

"Health Center Research Team Discovers New Glaucoma Gene,"
April 20, 2005. Reprinted with permission from University of
Connecticut Health Center Office of Communications.

Researchers at the University of Connecticut Health Center have
discovered a gene that causes late-onset primary open-angle glaucoma.

The discovery was made by Mansoor Sarfarazi, Ph.D., director,
Molecular Ophthalmic Genetics Laboratory and professor of human
molecular genetics, Surgical Research Center, Department of Surgery,
and his graduate assistant and doctoral candidate Sharareh Monemi,
M.D.

The gene is the third glaucoma-causing gene discovered by the
Molecular Ophthalmic Genetics Laboratory. The newly identified gene
is WDR36 and maps to the GLC1G locus on chromosome 5q22.1.

The discovery will enhance screening for the late-onset form of
glaucoma. It will improve early diagnosis of glaucoma, which allows
earlier and better treatment, and the discovery also advances the likelihood of gene-targeted therapies.

"Finding this gene was gratifying," Sarfarazi said. "This discovery
will improve screening of at-high-risk individuals and help to identify those who could develop glaucoma decades later. It will also help
in designing more effective treatments for them."

"But the real work has just begun," he said. "There's always more
to learn."

Peter J. Deckers, M.D., dean of the School of Medicine and executive vice president, said Sarfarazi's discovery was the latest example
of the high quality scientific research now being conducted at the
Health Center.

"This laboratory continues to work at the cutting edge of gene definition as causative factors in serious ocular problems," he said, "and
as a result of their seminal research contributions have established

for themselves, and the Health Center, an international reputation in the new biology of this decade—specifically molecular diagnosis, and in time, molecular treatment."

Glaucoma affects more than 2 million Americans and more than 33 million people worldwide. After cataracts, it is the second largest cause of blindness. Although there is no cure, medication or surgery can be effective treatments.

The numbers involved in the discovery were daunting: the researchers were originally faced with a universe of three billion base pairs of DNA material. That number was winnowed to 35 million pairs by locating the region of the chromosome where the gene was thought to reside. Additional study further narrowed the number to 7 million and colleagues working on a similar problem in Oregon helped narrow it further to 2 million base pairs of DNA.

In the end, Sarfarazi and Monemi investigated over 34,000 base pairs of DNA before the one mutation they were searching for turned up.

"This was like hunting," Sarfarazi said. "Of the original 35 million base pairs, only one change eventually proved to be significant. But this was like searching for the proverbial needle in a haystack."

The WDR36 gene is conserved—nearly the same—along the evolutionary path from the mouse to rat, dog, chimp and human, Sarfarazi said. Essential genes, vital to an important biological function such as vision, change less through evolution than other non-essential genes, he said.

Monemi was thrilled with the work.

"With my background as a physician, I understand the importance of helping patients," she said. "Not having your vision from birth is one thing, but losing it to glaucoma decades later would be terrible. This work can help make that loss less common."

The research should help Monemi's career too: it's the subject of her doctoral thesis.

Sarfarazi's Molecular Ophthalmic Genetics Laboratory also discovered another gene known as Optineurin that causes adult-onset primary open angle glaucoma in 2002. In 1997, he further identified and published information on the CYP1B1 gene that causes primary congenital glaucoma.

The current work was published in the March [2005] issue of the journal *Human Molecular Genetics*.

Chapter 28

Treating Glaucoma

Chapter Contents

Section 28.1

Surgical Treatment for Glaucoma

Surgery involves either laser treatment or making a cut in the eye to reduce the intraocular pressure (IOP). The type of surgery your doctor recommends will depend on the type and severity of your glaucoma and the general health of your eye. Surgery can help lower pressure when medication is not sufficient, however it cannot reverse vision loss.

Doctors often recommend laser surgery before filtering microsurgery, unless the eye pressure is very high or the optic nerve is badly damaged. During laser surgery, a tiny but powerful beam of light is used to make several small scars in the eye's trabecular meshwork (the eye's drainage system). The scars help increase the flow of fluid out of the eye.

In contrast, filtering microsurgery involves creating a drainage hole with the use of a small surgical tool. When laser surgery does not successfully lower eye pressure, or the pressure begins to rise again, the doctor may recommend filtering microsurgery.

Filtering Microsurgery

When medicines and laser surgeries do not lower eye pressure adequately, doctors may recommend a procedure called filtering microsurgery (sometimes called conventional or cutting surgery).

In filtering microsurgery, a tiny drainage hole is made in the sclera (the white part of the eye) in a procedure called a trabeculectomy or a sclerostomy. The new drainage hole allows fluid to flow out of the eye and helps lower eye pressure. This prevents or reduces damage to the optic nerve.

Pain during the Microsurgery

In most cases, there is no pain involved. The surgery is usually done with a local anesthetic and relaxing medications. Often a limited type of anesthesia, called intravenous (IV) sedation, is used.

In addition, an injection is given around or behind the eye to prevent eye movement. This injection is not painful when IV sedation is used first. The patient will be relaxed and drowsy and will not experience any pain during surgery.

Success Rate

Most of the related studies document follow-up for a one-year period. In those reports, it shows that in older patients, glaucoma filtering surgery is successful in about 70% to 90% of cases, for at least one year.

Occasionally, the surgically created drainage hole begins to close and the pressure rises again. This happens because the body tries to heal the new opening in the eye, as if the opening were an injury. This rapid healing occurs most often in younger people, because they have a stronger healing system. Anti-wound healing drugs, such as mitomycin-C and 5-FU, help slow down the healing of the opening. If needed, glaucoma filtering surgery can be done a number of times in the same eye.

Outpatient Procedure

Usually, filtering surgery is an outpatient procedure, requiring no overnight hospital stay. Within a few days after surgery, the eye doctor will need to check on the eye pressure. The doctor will also look for any signs of infection or increase in inflammation.

Recovery Time

For at least one week after surgery, patients are advised to keep water out of the eye. Most daily activities can be done, however, it is important to avoid driving, reading, bending, and doing any heavy lifting.

Each case is different, so check with your doctor for specific advice.

Appearance of the Eye after Surgery

The eye will be red and irritated shortly after surgery, and there may be increased eye tearing or watering. The inner eye fluid flows through the surgically created hole and forms a small blister-like bump called a bleb. The bleb, usually located on the upper surface of the eye, is covered by the eyelid, and is usually not visible.

243

Changes in Vision and Medication

There may be some vision changes, such as blurred vision, for about six weeks after the surgery. After that time, vision will usually return to the same level it was before surgery.

Vision can sometimes improve after surgery in patients who had been using pilocarpine. After stopping pilocarpine drops, the pupil returns to normal size, allowing more light to enter the eye.

In a few cases, the vision may be worse due to very low pressure. Cataracts or wrinkle in the macula area of the eye may develop.

After surgery, you may need to change your contact lenses or glasses. Gas permeable or soft contact lenses may be worn. However, the bleb may cause fitting problems, and special care will be needed to avoid infection of the bleb. Contact lens users should discuss these problems with their eye doctor following surgery.

Laser Surgery

Laser surgeries have become important in the treatment of different eye problems and diseases.

During the laser surgery, the eye is numbed so that there is little or no pain. The eye doctor then holds a special lens to the eye. The laser beam is aimed into the eye, and there is a bright light, like a camera flash.

Risks of Laser Surgery

Laser surgery is still surgery, and can carry some risks. Some people experience a short-term increase in their intraocular pressure (IOP) soon after surgery. In others who require YAG CP (cyclophotocoagulation) surgery, there is a risk of the IOP dropping too low to maintain the eye's normal metabolism and shape. The use of antiglaucoma medication before and after surgery can help to reduce this risk.

The following are the most common laser surgeries to treat glaucoma.

- **Laser Peripheral Iridotomy (LPI):** For the treatment of narrow angles and narrow-angle glaucoma. Narrow-angle glaucoma occurs when the angle between the iris and the cornea in the eye is too small. This causes the iris to block fluid drainage, increasing inner eye pressure. LPI makes a small hole in the iris, allowing it to fall back from the fluid channel and helping the fluid drain.

244

- **Argon Laser Trabeculoplasty (ALT):** For the treatment of primary open angle glaucoma (POAG). The laser beam opens the fluid channels of the eye, helping the drainage system work better. In many cases, medication will still be needed. Usually, half the fluid channels are treated first. If necessary, the other fluid channels can be treated in a separate session another time. This method prevents over-correction and lowers the risk of increased pressure following surgery. Argon laser trabeculoplasty has successfully lowered eye pressure in up to 75% of patients treated.

- **Selective Laser Trabeculoplasty (SLT):** For the treatment of primary open angle glaucoma (POAG). SLT uses a combination of frequencies that allow the laser to work at very low levels. It treats specific cells "selectively," leaving untreated portions of the trabecular meshwork intact. For this reason, it is believed that SLT, unlike other types of laser surgery, may be safely repeated many times.

- **Neodymium: YAG laser cyclophotocoagulation (YAG CP):** An alternative to filtering microsurgery that is typically used later in the treatment algorithm. This surgery destroys part of the ciliary body, the part of the eye that produces intraocular fluid. The procedure may need to be repeated in order to permanently control glaucoma.

Pain or Discomfort from Glaucoma Laser Surgery

There is a slight stinging sensation associated with LPI and ALT. In YAG CP laser surgery, a local anesthetic is used to numb the eye. Once the eye has been numbed, there should be little or no pain and discomfort.

Long-Term Benefits of Glaucoma Laser Surgery

Glaucoma laser surgeries help to lower the intraocular pressure (IOP) in the eye. The length of time the IOP remains lower depends on the type of laser surgery, the type of glaucoma, age, race, and many other factors. Some people may need the surgery repeated to better control the pressure IOP.

Medication Following Laser Surgery

In most cases, medications are still necessary to control and maintain eye pressure. However, surgery may lessen the amount of medication needed.

Recovery Time

In general, patients can resume normal daily activities the next day after laser surgery.

The procedure is usually performed in an eye doctor's office or eye clinic. Before the surgery, your eye will be numbed with medicine. Your eye may be a bit irritated and your vision slightly blurry after the surgery. You should arrange a ride home after your surgery.

Increased Risk of Cataracts

There is a small risk of developing cataracts after some types of laser surgery for glaucoma. However, the potential benefits of the surgery usually outweigh any risks.

There is a common myth that lasers can be used to remove cataracts; this is not the case except in experimental studies. After a cataract has been taken out with conventional cutting surgery, there often remains an outer membrane lens capsule. This membrane can slowly thicken and cloud vision, just as the cataract did. Laser surgery can open this membrane, helping to clear vision without an operation. This laser procedure is called a capsulotomy.

It is important to discuss all of your questions or concerns about laser surgery with your eye doctor.

Section 28.2

Eyedrops: An Important Part of Glaucoma Treatment

"Eyedrop Tips," © 2005–2007 Glaucoma Research Foundation (www.glaucoma.org). Reprinted with permission.

Prescription eye drops for glaucoma help maintain the pressure in your eye at a healthy level and are an important part of the treatment routine for many people. Always check with your doctor if you are having difficulty.

Remember:

- Follow your doctor's orders.

- Be sure your doctor knows about any other drugs you may be taking (including over-the-counter items like vitamins, aspirin, and herbal supplements) and about any allergies you may have.

- Wash your hands before putting in your eye drops.

- Be careful not to let the tip of the dropper touch any part of your eye.

- Make sure the dropper stays clean.

- If you are putting in more than one drop or more than one type of eye drop, wait five minutes before putting the next drop in. This will keep the first drop from being washed out by the second before it has had time to work.

- Store eye drops and all medicines out of the reach of children.

Steps for Putting in Eye Drops

1. Start by tilting your head backward while sitting, standing, or lying down. With your index finger placed on the soft spot just below the lower lid, gently pull down to form a pocket.

2. Let a drop fall into the pocket.

3. Slowly let go of the lower lid. Close your eyes but try not to shut them tight or squint. This may push the drops out of your eye.

4. Gently press on the inside corner of your closed eyes with your index finger and thumb for two to three minutes. This will help keep any drops from getting into your system and keep them in your eye, where they are needed.

5. Blot around your eyes to remove any excess.

If you are still having trouble putting eye drops in, here are some tips that may help.

If Your Hands Are Shaking

Try approaching your eye from the side so you can rest your hand on your face to help steady your hand.

If shaky hands are still a problem, you might try using a 1- or 2-pound wrist weight (you can get these at any sporting goods store). The extra weight around the wrist of the hand you're using can decrease mild shaking.

If You Are Having Trouble Getting the Drop into Your Eye

Try this: With your head turned to the side or lying on your side, close your eyes. Place a drop in the inner corner of your eyelid (the side closest to the bridge of your nose). By opening your eyes slowly, the drop should fall right into your eye.

If you are still not sure the drop actually got in your eye, put in another drop. The eyelids can hold only about one drop, so any excess will just run out of the eye. It is better to have excess run out than to not have enough medication in your eye.

Having Trouble Holding onto the Bottle?

If the eye drop bottle feels too small to hold (in cases where a dropper isn't used and the drop comes directly from the bottle), try wrapping something (like a paper towel) around the bottle.

You can use anything that will make the bottle wider. This may be helpful in some mild cases of arthritis in the hands.

Assistive devices are available to help you put in your eye drops.

Section 28.3

Alternative Medicine Treatments for Glaucoma

Homeopathic Remedies: Herbs

Proponents of homeopathic medicine believe that symptoms represent the body's attack against disease, and that substances which induce the symptoms of a particular disease or diseases can help the body ward off illness.

Holistic Treatments

Holistic medicine is a system of health care designed to assist individuals in harmonizing mind, body, and spirit. Some of the more popular therapies include good nutrition, physical exercise, and self-regulation techniques including meditation, biofeedback, and relaxation training. While holistic treatments can be part of a good physical regimen, there is no proof of their usefulness in glaucoma therapy.

Eating and Drinking

No conclusive studies prove a connection between specific foods and glaucoma, but it is reasonable to assume that what you eat and drink and your general health have an effect on the disease.

Some studies have shown that significant caffeine intake over a short time can slightly elevate intraocular eye pressure (IOP) for one to three hours. However, other studies indicate that caffeine has no meaningful impact on IOP. To be safe, people with glaucoma are advised to limit their caffeine intake to moderate levels.

Studies have also shown that as many as 80% of people with glaucoma who consume an entire quart of water over the course of twenty minutes experience elevated IOP, as compared to only 20% of people who don't have glaucoma. Since many commercial diet programs stress the importance of drinking at least eight glasses of water each day, to be safe, people with glaucoma are encouraged to consume water in small amounts throughout the day.

Good Nutrition

The ideal way to ensure a proper supply of essential vitamins and minerals is by eating a balanced diet. If you are concerned about your own diet, you may want to consult with your doctor about taking a multivitamin or multimineral nutritional supplement.

Some of the vitamins and minerals important to the eye include zinc and copper, antioxidant vitamins C, E, and A (as beta carotene), and selenium, an antioxidant mineral.

Bilberry

An extract of the European blueberry, bilberry is available through the mail and in some health food stores. It is most often advertised as an antioxidant eye health supplement that advocates claim can protect and strengthen the capillary walls of the eyes, and thus is especially effective in protecting against glaucoma, cataracts, and macular degeneration. There is some data indicating that bilberry may improve night vision and recovery time from glare, but there is no evidence that it is effective in the treatment or prevention of glaucoma.

Remember that the Food and Drug Administration (FDA) has not tested homeopathic remedies for safety or effectiveness. There is no guarantee that they contain consistent ingredients, or that dosage recommendations are accurate. It would be a serious mistake to use homeopathic remedies and dismiss valid therapies, delaying proven treatment for serious conditions.

Physical Exercise

There is some evidence suggesting that regular exercise can reduce eye pressure on its own, and can also have a positive impact on other glaucoma risk factors including diabetes and high blood pressure.

In a recent study, people with glaucoma who exercised regularly for three months reduced their IOPs an average of 20%. These people rode stationary bikes 4 times per week for 40 minutes. Measurable improvements in eye pressure and physical conditioning were seen at the end of three months. These beneficial effects were maintained by continuing to exercise at least three times per week; lowered IOP was lost if exercise was stopped for more than two weeks.

In an ongoing study, glaucoma patients who walked briskly 4 times per week for 40 minutes were able to lower their IOP enough to eliminate the need for beta blockers. Final results are not available, but there is hope that glaucoma patients with extremely high IOP who maintain an exercise schedule and continue beta-blocker therapy could significantly reduce their IOP.

Regular exercise may be a useful addition to the prevention of visual loss from glaucoma, but only your eye doctor can assess the effects of exercise on your eye pressure. Some forms of glaucoma (such as closed-angle) are not responsive to the effects of exercise, and other forms of glaucoma (for example, pigmentary glaucoma) may actually develop a temporary increase in IOP after vigorous exercise. And remember—exercise cannot replace medications or doctor visits!

Yoga and Recreational Body Inversion

The long-term effects of repeatedly assuming a head-down or inverted position on the optic nerve head (the nerve that carries visual images to the brain) have not been adequately demonstrated, but due to the potential for increased IOP, people with glaucoma should be careful about these kinds of exercises.

Glaucoma patients should let their doctors know if yoga shoulder and headstands or any other recreational body inversion exercises that result in head-down or inverted postures over extended periods of time are part of their exercise routines.

Self-Regulation Techniques

The results of studies regarding changes in IOP following relaxation and biofeedback sessions have generated some optimism in controlling selected cases of open-angle glaucoma, but further research is needed.

However, findings that reduced blood pressure and heart rate can be achieved with relaxation and biofeedback techniques show promise that non-medicinal and non-surgical techniques may be effective methods of treating and controlling open-angle glaucoma.

Section 28.4

Medical Marijuana for Glaucoma

Advocates of medicinal marijuana cite evidence that hemp products can lower intraocular pressure (IOP) in people with glaucoma. However, these products are less effective than safer and more available medicines. Most research regarding marijuana use took place before some current medications with fewer side effects were available.

The high dose of marijuana necessary to produce a clinically relevant effect on IOP in the short term requires constant inhalation, as much as every three hours.

The number of significant side effects generated by long-term oral use of marijuana or long-term inhalation of marijuana smoke make marijuana a poor choice in the treatment of glaucoma, a chronic disease requiring proven and effective treatment.

Currently, marijuana is designated as a Schedule I drug (drugs which have a high potential for abuse and no medical application or proven therapeutic value).

The only marijuana currently approved at the Federal level for medical use is Marinol, a synthetic form of tetrahydrocannabinol (THC), the most active component of marijuana. It was developed as an antiemetic (an agent that reduces nausea used in chemotherapy treatments), which can be taken orally in capsule form. The effects of Marinol on glaucoma are not impressive.

To date, no studies have shown that marijuana—or any of its approximately 400 chemical components—can safely and effectively lower intraocular pressure better than the variety of drugs currently on the market.

Currently, there are no National Eye Institute studies in the United States concerning the use of marijuana to treat glaucoma.

The Glaucoma Research Foundation will continue to monitor the research community for any new and well-designed studies regarding the use of marijuana to effectively treat glaucoma.

Chapter 29

Living with Glaucoma

Chapter Contents

Section 29.1

Adjusting to Daily Life If You Have Glaucoma

"Daily Life," © 2005 Glaucoma Research Foundation
(www.glaucoma.org). Reprinted with permission. This article
appeared in the January 2005 issue of *Gleams*.

You will probably need to make just a few changes to your lifestyle in order to manage your glaucoma effectively. As long as you are diagnosed early, visit your doctor regularly, and follow your recommended course of treatment, you can continue to live your life fully.

Try to schedule time for taking medication around daily routines such as waking, mealtimes, and bedtime. In this way, your medications will become a natural part of your day.

In addition to taking care of your physical health, it's equally important to pay attention to the other side of glaucoma—the emotional and psychological aspects of having this disease.

Be sure to share your feelings. Especially in the beginning, it can be helpful to talk about your fears. Confide in your spouse, a relative, a close friend, or a member of the clergy. You may also want to talk with other people who have glaucoma. Sharing ideas and feelings about living with a chronic health condition can be useful and comforting.

Don't let glaucoma limit your life. You can continue with what you were doing before glaucoma was diagnosed. You can make new plans and start new ventures. The eye care community, including the Glaucoma Research Foundation, will keep looking for better methods to treat glaucoma and will eventually find a cure.

Some daily activities such as driving or playing certain sports may become more challenging. Loss of contrast sensitivity, problems with glare, and light sensitivity are some of the possible effects of glaucoma that may interfere with your activities.

The key issue is to trust your judgment. If you are having trouble seeing at night, you may want to consider not driving at night. Stay safe by adjusting your schedule so that you do most of your travel during the day.

Sunglasses or tinted lenses can help with glare and contrast. Yellow, amber, and brown are the best tints to block out glare from fluorescent lights. On a bright day, try using brown lenses for your glasses. For overcast days or at night, try using the lighter tints of yellow and amber.

Experiment to see what works best for you under different circumstances.

Section 29.2

Questions and Answers about Living with Glaucoma

How often should I see my eye doctor?

As a newly diagnosed person with glaucoma, you may need to have your eye pressure checked every week or month until it is under control. Even when your eye pressure is at a safe level, you may need to see your doctor several times a year for checkups.

It is important that your doctor listens and responds to your concerns and questions, is willing to explain your treatment options, and is available for calls and checkups. If you do not feel confident and comfortable with your doctor, remember, you always have the right to seek a second opinion.

A good working relationship with your eye doctor is the key to effective glaucoma care.

Will a diagnosis of glaucoma limit my life?

We are limited only by what we think we can or cannot do. You can continue with what you were doing before glaucoma was diagnosed. You can make new plans and start new ventures. And you can trust the eye care community to keep looking for better treatment methods for glaucoma. Take good care of yourself and your eyes, and get on with enjoying your life.

What can I do to help others?

As a glaucoma patient, you have the opportunity to teach your friends and relatives about this disease. Many people are unaware of the importance of eye checkups and do not know that individuals with glaucoma may have no symptoms. You can help protect their eye health by encouraging them to have their eye pressure and optic nerves checked regularly.

Source: *Understanding And Living With Glaucoma.*

Part Five

Macular Degeneration

Chapter 30

Juvenile Macular Degeneration: Stargardt Disease

What Is Stargardt Disease?

Stargardt disease is the most common form of inherited juvenile macular degeneration. It is characterized by a reduction of central vision with a preservation of peripheral (side) vision.

Clinical Description

Stargardt disease, also known as fundus flavimaculatus, is usually diagnosed in individuals under the age of 20 when decreased central vision is first noticed. On examination, the retina of an affected individual shows a macular lesion surrounded by yellow-white flecks, or spots, with irregular shapes. The retina consists of layers of light-sensing cells that line the inner back wall of the eye and are important in normal vision. The macula is found in the center of the retina and is responsible for the fine, detailed central vision used in reading and color vision.

The progression of visual loss is variable. One study of 95 individuals with Stargardt disease showed that once a visual acuity of 20/40 was reached, there was often rapid progression of additional visual loss until acuity was reduced to 20/200 (legal blindness). By age 50, approximately 50 percent of all those studied had visual acuities of 20/200 or worse. Eventually, almost all individuals with Stargardt disease are expected to have visual acuities in the range of 20/200 to 20/400. The reduced visual acuity due to Stargardt disease cannot be corrected with prescription eyeglasses or contact lenses. In late stages of the disease, there may also be noticeable impairment of color vision.

What Causes Stargardt Disease?

In 1997, Foundation Fighting Blindness researchers isolated the gene for Stargardt disease. The ABCR gene produces a protein involved in energy transport to and from photoreceptor cells in the retina. Mutations in the ABCR gene, which cause Stargardt disease, produce a dysfunctional protein that cannot perform its transport function. As a result, photoreceptor cells degenerate and vision loss occurs.

Symptoms

- Bilateral, decreased central vision in childhood or young adulthood
- Visual acuity may start at the 20/40 level and later decline to 20/200 or slightly worse
- Central scotoma (blind spot in central vision)
- Abnormal color vision
- Photophobia—an abnormal visual intolerance of light
- Night blindness

Diagnosis

At the beginning stage of the disease, the retina may appear normal upon routine examination. As the disease progresses, clinical signs of the condition can be viewed with ophthalmoscopy. Your ophthalmologist or retinal specialist may perform additional common diagnostic procedures—visual acuity tests, color vision testing, the Amsler grid test or an automated macular field test to assess vision. Other tests may also be ordered, such as an electrodiagnostic test to examine macular function.

As with macular degeneration patients, fluorescein angiography may be necessary to document the pattern of blood vessels and determine whether dye leaks from the vessels. A doctor can determine which areas of the macula are damaged and whether there are abnormal blood vessels to be treated.

Risk Factors

Stargardt disease, an early-onset form of macular degeneration, is an inherited disease. The condition is programmed into your cells at conception. It is not caused by injury, infection or exposure to a toxic agent. Because Stargardt disease is an inherited condition, there is nothing that can be done to reduce the risk of developing the disease.

However, recent findings in rodent models of Stargardt disease find that unprotected, prolonged exposure to light can accelerate vision loss. Therefore, The Foundation Fighting Blindness strongly recommends that patients with Stargardt disease wear brimmed hats or visors and sunglasses when outdoors.

Stargardt disease is an autosomal recessive disease. In autosomal recessive diseases, unaffected parents, who are carriers, have one gene with a disease-causing mutation paired with one normal gene. Each of their children then has a 25 percent chance (or one chance in four) of inheriting the two diseased genes (one from each parent) needed to cause the disorder. Carriers are unaffected because they have only one copy of the gene.

What You Can Do to Reduce Risk

Unfortunately, there is no treatment that has been proven to improve the visual loss or to retard the progressing of the disease.

Treatment

The discovery of the ABCR gene now allows researchers to study the underlying biochemical interactions that result from mutations in this gene. Understanding how genetic mutations lead to retinal degeneration is critical for the development of experimental therapies. Although there is currently no treatment for Stargardt disease, individuals benefit from the use of low vision aids and orientation and mobility training.

Sources: The Foundation Fighting Blindness (FFB) http://www.blindness .org; Lighthouse International

Chapter 31

Understanding Age-Related Macular Degeneration (ARMD)

What is age-related macular degeneration?

Age-related macular degeneration (AMD) is a disease associated with aging that gradually destroys sharp, central vision. Central vision is needed for seeing objects clearly and for common daily tasks such as reading and driving. AMD affects the macula, the part of the eye that allows you to see fine detail. AMD causes no pain.

In some cases, AMD advances so slowly that people notice little change in their vision. In others, the disease progresses faster and may lead to a loss of vision in both eyes. AMD is a leading cause of vision loss in Americans 60 years of age and older.

AMD occurs in two forms: wet and dry.

Where is the macula?

The macula is located in the center of the retina, the light-sensitive tissue at the back of the eye. The retina instantly converts light, or an image, into electrical impulses. The retina then sends these impulses, or nerve signals, to the brain.

What is wet AMD?

Wet AMD occurs when abnormal blood vessels behind the retina start to grow under the macula. These new blood vessels tend to be very

Excerpted from "Age-Related Macular Degeneration" is from the National Eye Institute (NEI, www.nei.nih.gov), part of the National Institutes of Health, April 2006.

fragile and often leak blood and fluid. The blood and fluid raise the macula from its normal place at the back of the eye. Damage to the macula occurs rapidly.

With wet AMD, loss of central vision can occur quickly. Wet AMD is also known as advanced AMD. It does not have stages like dry AMD.

An early symptom of wet AMD is that straight lines appear wavy. If you notice this condition or other changes to your vision, contact your eye care professional at once. You need a comprehensive dilated eye exam.

What is dry AMD?

Dry AMD occurs when the light-sensitive cells in the macula slowly break down, gradually blurring central vision in the affected eye. As dry AMD gets worse, you may see a blurred spot in the center of your vision. Over time, as less of the macula functions, central vision is gradually lost in the affected eye.

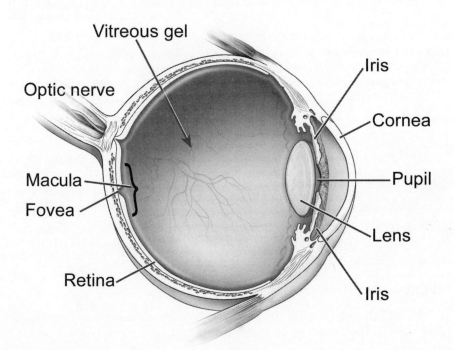

Figure 31.1. The location of the macula and retina in the eye.

The most common symptom of dry AMD is slightly blurred vision. You may have difficulty recognizing faces. You may need more light for reading and other tasks. Dry AMD generally affects both eyes, but vision can be lost in one eye while the other eye seems unaffected.

One of the most common early signs of dry AMD is drusen.

What are drusen?

Drusen are yellow deposits under the retina. They often are found in people over age 60. Your eye care professional can detect drusen during a comprehensive dilated eye exam.

Drusen alone do not usually cause vision loss. In fact, scientists are unclear about the connection between drusen and AMD. They do know that an increase in the size or number of drusen raises a person's risk of developing either advanced dry AMD or wet AMD. These changes can cause serious vision loss.

Dry AMD has three stages, all of which may occur in one or both eyes:

1. **Early AMD:** People with early AMD have either several small drusen or a few medium-sized drusen. At this stage, there are no symptoms and no vision loss.

2. **Intermediate AMD:** People with intermediate AMD have either many medium-sized drusen or one or more large drusen. Some people see a blurred spot in the center of their vision. More light may be needed for reading and other tasks.

3. **Advanced Dry AMD:** In addition to drusen, people with advanced dry AMD have a breakdown of light-sensitive cells and supporting tissue in the central retinal area. This breakdown can cause a blurred spot in the center of your vision. Over time, the blurred spot may get bigger and darker, taking more of your central vision. You may have difficulty reading or recognizing faces until they are very close to you.

If you have vision loss from dry AMD in one eye only, you may not notice any changes in your overall vision. With the other eye seeing clearly, you still can drive, read, and see fine details. You may notice changes in your vision only if AMD affects both eyes. If blurriness occurs in your vision, see an eye care professional for a comprehensive dilated eye exam.

Ninety percent of all people with AMD have this type. Scientists are still not sure what causes dry AMD.

Frequently Asked Questions about Wet and Dry AMD

Which is more common—the dry form or the wet form?

The dry form is much more common. More than 85 percent of all people with intermediate and advanced AMD combined have the dry form.

However, if only advanced AMD is considered, about two thirds of patients have the wet form. Because almost all vision loss comes from advanced AMD, the wet form leads to significantly more vision loss than the dry form.

Can the dry form turn into the wet form?

Yes. All people who have the wet form had the dry form first.

The dry form can advance and cause vision loss without turning into the wet form. The dry form also can suddenly turn into the wet form, even during early stage AMD. There is no way to tell if or when the dry form will turn into the wet form.

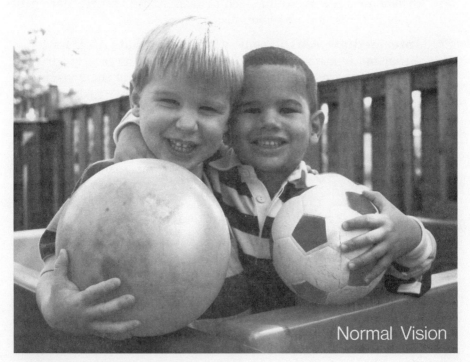

Normal Vision

Figure 31.2. *Normal vision.*

The dry form has early and intermediate stages. Does the wet form have similar stages?

No. The wet form is considered advanced AMD.

Can advanced AMD be either the dry form or the wet form?

Yes. Both the wet form and the advanced dry form are considered advanced AMD. Vision loss occurs with either form. In most cases, only advanced AMD can cause vision loss.

People who have advanced AMD in one eye are at especially high risk of developing advanced AMD in the other eye.

Causes and Risk Factors

Who is at risk for AMD?

The greatest risk factor is age. Although AMD may occur during middle age, studies show that people over age 60 are clearly at greater risk than other age groups. For instance, a large study found that people in middle-age have about a 2 percent risk of getting AMD, but this risk increased to nearly 30 percent in those over age 75.

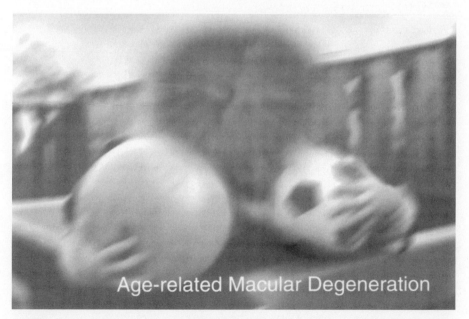

Figure 31.3. Vision of someone with age-related macular degeneration.

Other risk factors include:

- **Smoking:** Smoking may increase the risk of AMD.

- **Obesity:** Research studies suggest a link between obesity and the progression of early and intermediate stage AMD to advanced AMD.

- **Race:** Whites are much more likely to lose vision from AMD than African Americans.

- **Family history:** Those with immediate family members who have AMD are at a higher risk of developing the disease.

- **Gender:** Women appear to be at greater risk than men.

Can my lifestyle make a difference?

Your lifestyle can play a role in reducing your risk of developing AMD.

- Eat a healthy diet high in green leafy vegetables and fish.
- Don't smoke.
- Maintain normal blood pressure.
- Watch your weight.
- Exercise.

Symptoms and Detection

What are the symptoms?

Both dry and wet AMD cause no pain.

For dry AMD: the most common early sign is blurred vision. As fewer cells in the macula are able to function, people will see details less clearly in front of them, such as faces or words in a book. Often this blurred vision will go away in brighter light. If the loss of these light-sensing cells becomes great, people may see a small—but growing—blind spot in the middle of their field of vision.

For wet AMD: the classic early symptom is that straight lines appear crooked. This results when fluid from the leaking blood vessels gathers and lifts the macula, distorting vision. A small blind spot may also appear in wet AMD, resulting in loss of one's central vision.

How is AMD detected?

Your eye care professional may suspect AMD if you are over age 60 and have had recent changes in your central vision. To look for signs of the disease, he or she will use eye drops to dilate, or enlarge, your pupils. Dilating the pupils allows your eye care professional to view the back of the eye better.

AMD is detected during a comprehensive eye exam that includes:

1. **Visual acuity test:** This eye chart test measures how well you see at various distances.

2. **Dilated eye exam:** Drops are placed in your eyes to widen, or dilate, the pupils. Your eye care professional uses a special magnifying lens to examine your retina and optic nerve for signs of AMD and other eye problems. After the exam, your close-up vision may remain blurred for several hours.

3. **Tonometry:** An instrument measures the pressure inside the eye. Numbing drops may be applied to your eye for this test.

Your eye care professional also may do other tests to learn more about the structure and health of your eye.

During an eye exam, you may be asked to look at an Amsler grid. The pattern of the grid resembles a checkerboard. You will cover one eye and stare at a black dot in the center of the grid. While staring at the dot, you may notice that the straight lines in the pattern appear wavy. You may notice that some of the lines are missing. These may be signs of AMD.

Do **not** depend on the grid displayed in Figure 31.4 for any diagnoses—check with your eye care professional.

If your eye care professional believes you need treatment for wet AMD, he or she may suggest a fluorescein angiogram. In this test, a special dye is injected into your arm. Pictures are taken as the dye passes through the blood vessels in your retina. The test allows your eye care professional to identify any leaking blood vessels and recommend treatment.

Treatment

How is wet AMD treated?

Wet AMD can be treated with laser surgery, photodynamic therapy, and injections into the eye. None of these treatments is a cure for wet AMD. The disease and loss of vision may progress despite treatment.

Laser surgery: This procedure uses a laser to destroy the fragile, leaky blood vessels. A high energy beam of light is aimed directly onto the new blood vessels and destroys them, preventing further loss of vision. However, laser treatment may also destroy some surrounding healthy tissue and some vision. Only a small percentage of people with wet AMD can be treated with laser surgery. Laser surgery is more effective if the leaky blood vessels have developed away from the fovea, the central part of the macula. Laser surgery is performed in a doctor's office or eye clinic.

The risk of new blood vessels developing after laser treatment is high. Repeated treatments may be necessary. In some cases, vision loss may progress despite repeated treatments.

Photodynamic therapy: A drug called verteporfin is injected into your arm. It travels throughout the body, including the new blood vessels in your eye. The drug tends to "stick" to the surface of new blood vessels. Next, a light is shined into your eye for about 90 seconds. The light activates the drug. The activated drug destroys the

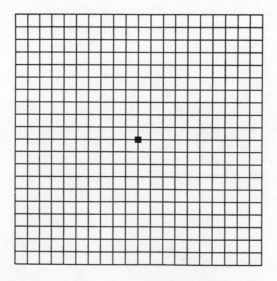

Figure 31.4. The Amsler grid is used to detect age-related macular degeneration.

new blood vessels and leads to a slower rate of vision decline. Unlike laser surgery, this drug does not destroy surrounding healthy tissue. Because the drug is activated by light, you must avoid exposing your skin or eyes to direct sunlight or bright indoor light for five days after treatment.

Photodynamic therapy is relatively painless. It takes about 20 minutes and can be performed in a doctor's office.

Photodynamic therapy slows the rate of vision loss. It does not stop vision loss or restore vision in eyes already damaged by advanced AMD. Treatment results often are temporary. You may need to be treated again.

Injections: Wet AMD can now be treated with new drugs that are injected into the eye (anti-VEGF therapy). Abnormally high levels of a specific growth factor occur in eyes with wet AMD and promote the growth of abnormal new blood vessels. This drug treatment blocks the effects of the growth factor.

You will need multiple injections that may be given as often as monthly. The eye is numbed before each injection. After the injection, you will remain in the doctor's office for a while and your eye will be monitored. This drug treatment can help slow down vision loss from AMD and in some cases improve sight.

How is dry AMD treated?

Once dry AMD reaches the advanced stage, no form of treatment can prevent vision loss. However, treatment can delay and possibly prevent intermediate AMD from progressing to the advanced stage, in which vision loss occurs.

The National Eye Institute's Age-Related Eye Disease Study (AREDS) found that taking a specific high-dose formulation of antioxidants and zinc significantly reduces the risk of advanced AMD and its associated vision loss. Slowing AMD's progression from the intermediate stage to the advanced stage will save the vision of many people.

Age-Related Eye Disease Study (AREDS)

What is the dosage of the AREDS formulation?

The specific daily amounts of antioxidants and zinc used by the study researchers were 500 milligrams of vitamin C, 400 International

Units of vitamin E, 15 milligrams of beta carotene (often labeled as equivalent to 25,000 International Units of vitamin A), 80 milligrams of zinc as zinc oxide, and two milligrams of copper as cupric oxide. Copper was added to the AREDS formulation containing zinc to prevent copper deficiency anemia, a condition associated with high levels of zinc intake.

Who should take the AREDS formulation?

People who are at high risk for developing advanced AMD should consider taking the formulation. You are at high risk for developing advanced AMD if you have either:

1. Intermediate AMD in one or both eyes.

    or

2. Advanced AMD (dry or wet) in one eye but not the other eye.

Your eye care professional can tell you if you have AMD, its stage, and your risk for developing the advanced form.

The AREDS formulation is not a cure for AMD. It will not restore vision already lost from the disease. However, it may delay the onset of advanced AMD. It may help people who are at high risk for developing advanced AMD keep their vision.

Can people with early stage AMD take the AREDS formulation to help prevent the disease from progressing to the intermediate stage?

There is no apparent need for those diagnosed with early stage AMD to take the AREDS formulation. The study did not find that the formulation provided a benefit to those with early stage AMD. If you have early stage AMD, a comprehensive dilated eye exam every year can help determine if the disease is progressing. If early stage AMD progresses to the intermediate stage, discuss taking the formulation with your doctor.

Can diet alone provide the same high levels of antioxidants and zinc as the AREDS formulation?

No. The high levels of vitamins and minerals are difficult to achieve from diet alone. However, previous studies have suggested that people who have diets rich in green leafy vegetables have a lower risk of developing AMD.

Can a daily multivitamin alone provide the same high levels of antioxidants and zinc as the AREDS formulation?

No. The formulation's levels of antioxidants and zinc are considerably higher than the amounts in any daily multivitamin.

If you are already taking daily multivitamins and your doctor suggests you take the high-dose AREDS formulation, be sure to review all your vitamin supplements with your doctor before you begin. Because multivitamins contain many important vitamins not found in the AREDS formulation, you may want to take a multivitamin along with the AREDS formulation. For example, people with osteoporosis need to be particularly concerned about taking vitamin D, which is not in the AREDS formulation.

How can I take care of my vision now that I have AMD?

Dry AMD: If you have dry AMD, you should have a comprehensive dilated eye exam at least once a year. Your eye care professional can monitor your condition and check for other eye diseases. Also, if you have intermediate AMD in one or both eyes, or advanced AMD in one eye only, your doctor may suggest that you take the AREDS formulation containing the high levels of antioxidants and zinc.

Because dry AMD can turn into wet AMD at any time, you should get an Amsler grid from your eye care professional. Use the grid every day to evaluate your vision for signs of wet AMD. This quick test works best for people who still have good central vision. Check each eye separately. Cover one eye and look at the grid. Then cover your other eye and look at the grid. If you detect any changes in the appearance of this grid or in your everyday vision while reading the newspaper or watching television, get a comprehensive dilated eye exam.

Wet AMD: If you have wet AMD and your doctor advises treatment, do not wait. After laser surgery or photodynamic therapy, you will need frequent eye exams to detect any recurrence of leaking blood vessels. Studies show that people who smoke have a greater risk of recurrence than those who don't. In addition, check your vision at home with the Amsler grid. If you detect any changes, schedule an eye exam immediately.

What can I do if I have already lost some vision from AMD?

If you have lost some sight from AMD, don't be afraid to use your eyes for reading, watching TV, and other routine activities. Normal use of your eyes will not cause further damage to your vision.

If you have lost some sight from AMD, ask your eye care professional about low vision services and devices that may help you make the most of your remaining vision. Ask for a referral to a specialist in low vision. Many community organizations and agencies offer information about low vision counseling, training, and other special services for people with visual impairments. A nearby school of medicine or optometry may provide low vision services.

Chapter 32

Frequently Asked Questions about ARMD

How do I know if I have age-related macular degeneration (AMD)?

Your ophthalmologist or optometrist can give you a definite diagnosis after a dilated retinal examination. To a trained professional, the signs of macular degeneration are apparent when the eye is dilated and a special lens is used to see the retina. These may include the presence of protein deposits in the retina, growth of new blood vessels, leaking blood vessels, or swelling of the retina.

To the patient, the first symptom of AMD is often that straight lines (telephone wires or door frames) look wavy. There may be blurring or loss of central vision, especially in the case of wet AMD. Remember to check each eye separately for vision changes. Your eyes work together to help each other out. You may have a problem in one eye but not notice it because the other eye is "masking" it.

Will I go blind? Will I eventually see nothing but blackness?

It is very important to understand that macular degeneration does **not** cause blindness. AMD affects the central vision only. Your peripheral vision will remain and you will always be able to see out of the

"Frequently Asked Questions," © 2007 The Macular Degeneration Partnership. For additional information, call toll-free 888-430-9898 or visit www.amd.org. Reprinted with permission.

corner of your eye. If you have other eye problems like cataracts or glaucoma, these may affect your peripheral vision.

I have a cataract. Is it safe to have it removed or will it make my macular degeneration worse?

The decision to remove a cataract is always an individual one. Surgery is usually considered when the cataract interferes with daily activities. Removing the cataract can let more light into the eye, which may help someone with macular degeneration to see better. Recent research has concluded that cataract removal does not appear to contribute to worsening of age-related macular degeneration. Any surgery has risks. Your doctor will make a careful examination of your eye to determine if the benefits of surgery outweigh any risks.

I have had dry AMD for years. Does this mean I'm going to get wet AMD, too?

The course of development for macular degeneration is different in each person. Some people have only the dry form for decades and never develop the wet form. However, if you have the dry form, your risk of progressing to wet AMD is higher and increases each year. If you have AMD in one eye, your risk is of getting AMD in the other eye is also higher. This is why it is so important to use the Amsler Grid daily to check for any changes that may occur. There are now several good therapies for wet macular degeneration, but early detection and treatment are essential.

No one else in my family has AMD. Why did I get it?

Macular degeneration does tend to run in families—your risk of AMD is higher if there are other family members who have it. But we don't fully understand how this works. If there is a gene that determines AMD and multiple family members have it, why don't they all get the eye disease? Much of the research is focused on identifying the gene or genes of AMD and figuring out why some people get it and others don't. Other factors appear to contribute to the development of AMD. You may have developed it because of lifestyle factors such as diet, smoking, high blood pressure, or exposure to ultraviolet light. Unfortunately, we don't have all the answers to this question. We do know that if you have a particular gene (complement factor H) and you smoke, your risk of getting AMD is almost nine times greater than for a nonsmoker who has the gene. Smoking is the number one factor for AMD that is under your control.

I keep trying magnifiers to help me read, but they just don't work! What can I do?

Some people find immediate help in using common hand-held magnifying glasses. But for many people, this approach is not enough. Just as your eyeglasses are a different prescription from someone else, your magnifier may need to be professionally prescribed just for you. See a low vision specialist or visit a Low Vision Center in your area. You can also explore other devices such as closed circuit television, screen readers, or voice systems. Don't give up! There is a whole world of assistive devices available. Find the one that works for you.

I've heard that vitamins can help prevent macular degeneration. What's the story on that?

The National Eye Institute Age-Related Eye Disease Study (AREDS) showed that a combination of antioxidants and zinc could slow the progression of the disease and vision loss in people with intermediate AMD. The supplement, is marketed under many labels, including Bausch & Lomb Ocuvite PreserVision and I-Caps. Many other brands now include the AREDS formula: beta carotene, vitamin C, vitamin E, zinc and copper. Other ingredients may also be helpful, including lutein, zeaxanthin, and omega-3 fatty acids. A new clinical trial, AREDS-2, is just getting started to study these ingredients. Ask your doctor if these vitamins are appropriate for you.

Chapter 33

Risk Factors for ARMD

Chapter Contents

Section 33.1

Genes Can Influence Risk of ARMD

Excerpted from "Variations in Genes Can Influence the Risk of Developing Age-Related Macular Degeneration and Other Disease Such as Cancer," a press release by the National Eye Institute (NEI, www.nei.nih.gov), part of the National Institutes of Health, May 5, 2006.

A team of researchers has determined that variations in certain genes involved in fighting infection can successfully predict the risk of developing age-related macular degeneration (AMD), the leading cause of blindness in white Americans over the age of 60. The team, led by Bert Gold, Ph.D., and Michael Dean, Ph.D., of the National Cancer Institute (NCI), part of the National Institutes of Health (NIH), identified a genetic variant that is associated with an increased risk of developing AMD. They also found two genetic variants that protect against developing this disease. Study results appear online March 5, 2006 in *Nature Genetics*.

The genes analyzed in this study—Complement Factor B (BF) and Complement Component 2 (C2)—contain the instructions to make proteins that activate the body's immune defense against microbial infections. These defense responses are part of a system called the complement pathways. These pathways involve numerous proteins in the blood that work in association with the body's immune cells and antibodies to destroy bacteria, viruses, or fungi invading the body. Some complement proteins can stimulate inflammation, the redness and swelling that result in tissues when they are infected.

Previous studies have shown that genetic variations in complement pathway genes can cause a dysfunction in the inflammatory response that plays a central role in the pathology of AMD. Based on these findings, investigators initiated this study, which screened almost 900 patients with AMD and 400 unaffected individuals for genetic variants in the BF and C2 genes. Data analysis revealed that specific variants in each gene were associated with AMD. One genetic variant conferred an increased risk for AMD, while two genetic variants showed protection against developing this disease. These results, when analyzed in association with results linking AMD and genetic variants of Complement Factor H—a gene than contains the instructions to make a protein that inhibits the complement system—showed that 56 percent of the unaffected individuals had a variant that conferred protection to AMD while 74 percent of those with AMD had no protective variants.

"These studies confirm that AMD has a strong genetic component," said Paul Sieving, M.D., Ph.D., director, National Eye Institute, at NIH. "This may support the development of screening tests for risk of developing AMD, which would allow us to administer treatment early in the course of disease. Knowing the underlying genetic alterations for risk could also aid in developing preventive therapies tailored to an individual's genetic background."

AMD is a disease that blurs or destroys sharp, central vision. Approximately 7.3 million Americans have intermediate stages of AMD with a high risk of increasing vision loss, while 1.8 million are visually impaired due to this disease. There is no known cure for AMD.

"We were studying a very common disease, but no one knew its cause. It was unexpected to find that the immune system was involved in causing AMD," said Gold, Laboratory of Genomic Diversity at NCI and lead author of this study. "Understanding how genetic variations in complement pathway genes are causing this common, complex disease could be very helpful in understanding other complex diseases, such as cancer."

In the cancer field, there is increasing interest in how infection and chronic inflammation could promote tumor growth. Studies have shown that inflammatory cells can promote tumor growth by producing a favorable growth environment.

Complement proteins play an important role in inflammation. This discovery of a link between genetic variants in complement genes and AMD may be relevant to the role of complement in cancer progression.

Section 33.2

Laser Treatment Does Not Prevent ARMD

From "Laser Treatment Does Not Prevent Vision Loss for People with Early Age-Related Macular Degeneration," a press release by the National Eye Institute (NEI, www.nei.nih.gov), part of the National Institutes of Health, November 1, 2006.

An extensive government-supported study has found that low-intensity laser treatment, thought to be possibly beneficial in slowing or preventing the loss of vision from age-related macular degeneration (AMD), is ineffective in preventing complications of AMD or loss of vision. This is the major conclusion of the Complications of Age-Related Macular Degeneration Prevention Trial (CAPT), a research study of more than 1,000 people that will be published in the November 2006 issue of the journal *Ophthalmology*. The study was supported by grants from the National Eye Institute (NEI) of the National Institutes of Health (NIH).

The presence of yellowish deposits under the retina, called drusen, is the first sign of early AMD. Eyes with large drusen are at increased risk of progressing to advanced AMD, with accompanying loss of vision. First considered in the 1970s, low-intensity laser treatment has been shown to reduce the extent of drusen. However, the studies evaluating the impact of laser treatment on vision have been small, and the results inconsistent.

This study was designed to assess the safety and effectiveness of laser treatment in preventing vision loss among people with large drusen in both eyes. It found there was no difference in vision or in progression to advanced AMD between treated and untreated eyes, which were closely observed for the duration of the trial.

"AMD is the leading cause of vision loss in the United States for people over age 60," said NEI director Paul A. Sieving, M.D., Ph.D. "This is an important study because after 35 years of inconsistent results from preventive laser treatment trials, we now know that this approach does not seem to stop vision loss from AMD. Doctors using this technique should reconsider its use in patients with good vision, such as those studied in this trial."

"At present, the only established way to decrease the risk of vision loss in people with large drusen (early AMD) is to take daily supplements of vitamins and minerals as used in the NEI-supported Age-Related Eye Disease Study (AREDS)," Sieving continued. "This study found that high-dose antioxidant vitamins and minerals (vitamins C and E, beta-carotene, zinc, and copper), taken by mouth by people at risk of developing advanced AMD, reduced the risk of progression to advanced AMD by 25 percent and the risk of moderate vision loss by 19 percent. People at risk for AMD are advised not to smoke and to maintain a healthy lifestyle, with a diet including leafy green vegetables and fish."

A total of 1,052 participants over the age of 50 (average age of 71) who had 10 or more large drusen and a visual acuity of 20/40 or better in each eye were enrolled through 22 clinical centers. One eye of each participant was treated and the other eye was observed throughout the five years of the trial. After five years, 20.5 percent of the treated eyes and 20.5 percent of the untreated eyes had lost three or more lines of visual acuity on a standard eye chart. Likewise, 20 percent of treated and untreated eyes progressed to advanced AMD. Change in visual acuity was strongly associated with the development of advanced AMD, but not with the treatment group.

"Laser treatment applied to eyes with large drusen that are at high risk for vision loss from AMD had neither a clinically significant beneficial nor harmful effect," said Stuart L. Fine, M.D., professor of ophthalmology and director of the Scheie Eye Institute at the University of Pennsylvania, and CAPT chairman. "There is no evidence from this trial to suggest that people with large drusen should seek preventive laser treatment."

The NEI has just launched a nationwide study to see if a modified combination of vitamins, minerals, and fish oil can further slow the progression of vision loss from AMD. This new study, called the Age-Related Eye Disease Study 2 (AREDS2), will build upon results from the earlier AREDS study.

Section 33.3

Regular Exercise May Stave off Degenerative Eye Disease

Regular exercise can cut the likelihood of developing the degenerative eye disease age-related macular degeneration by 70%, suggests research published in the *British Journal of Ophthalmology*.

Age-related macular degeneration, or ARMD for short, refers to a condition in which the light sensitive cells in the macula at the back of the eye stop working. This affects central vision and therefore activities, such as driving.

It is usually divided into two types—"dry" or non-exudative ARMD—and "wet" or exudative AMRD. The authors base their findings on the number of cases of ARMD arising over 15 years among almost 4,000 U.S. men and women in Beaver Dam, Wisconsin.

Participants were aged between 43 and 86 at the start of the study in 1988-90, and were assessed at five yearly intervals. As well as detailed eye examinations, they were asked about their lifestyle and the amount of regular physical activity they took, including climbing flights of stairs, daily walks, and sessions of formal exercise.

One in four had an active lifestyle, and nearly one in four climbed more than six flights of stairs a day while around one in eight walked more than 12 blocks a day.

After taking account of other risk factors, such as weight, blood fat levels, and age, those with an active lifestyle were 70% less likely to develop "wet" AMRD than those who had a sedentary lifestyle.

Regular walkers were 30% less likely to develop this variant.

Other factors, such as diet, may explain the findings, caution the authors. But physical activity is known to reduce systemic inflammation and irregularities in cells lining the arteries, both of which are thought to have a role in the condition, they say.

Physically active people are also likely to be "biologically" younger than those with a sedentary lifestyle, which could also be important as ARMD is associated with aging, they add.

Chapter 34

Nutrition, Antioxidants, and ARMD

"I don't recognize people unless I'm almost nose to nose," says Mardella Richey. "When I go out to dinner, restaurants are so dark I wouldn't recognize my own mother." Even a daily task like cooking can be a problem. "I can't read what it says on the bottle—if it's curry powder or celery powder," says Richey, who recently confused one for the other when making tomato soup. (The curried soup wasn't bad!)

Richey is among some nine million Americans with age-related macular degeneration (AMD), the leading cause of vision loss for people over 60. AMD destroys sharp central vision, which is necessary for seeing objects clearly and for common daily tasks such as reading and driving.

Nearly two million people have the advanced form of the disease, called wet AMD, which can cause rapid vision loss in both eyes. An early symptom of wet AMD is that straight lines may appear wavy and distorted, and images on TV may appear blurry. It is caused when abnormal blood vessels grow beneath the retina and leak blood and fluid under the macula, the small area near the center of the retina responsible for central vision.

Initial Study Encouraging

Richey participated in the Age-Related Eye Disease Study (AREDS), a nationwide clinical trial launched by the National Eye Institute

From "Nutrition and the Aging Eye," in *NIH MedlinePlus,* a magazine published by the National Institutes of Health (www.fnlm.org), pp. 18–19, January 2007.

(NEI) in 1992, results from which were published in 2001. The AREDS study showed that an experimental combination of three antioxidant vitamins (C, E, and beta carotene) and the minerals zinc and copper reduced the risk of progressing to advanced AMD by 25 percent and the risk of moderate vision loss by 19 percent.

Says AREDS lead investigator Emily Chew, M.D., deputy director of NEI's Division of Epidemiology and Clinical Research, "The results were of public health significance. About seven million people are at risk of developing AMD in the next five years, so you could reduce the risk of developing advanced AMD and its accompanying vision loss by 300,000 people if all seven million took the AREDS supplement. That's pretty big savings in health care and productivity."

Foods Lower AMD Risk

As a follow-up to AREDS, last October, in partnership with nearly 100 clinical centers nationwide, NEI began AREDS2, a study to determine how high doses of antioxidant and fish oil supplements affect the risk of advanced AMD, the need for cataract surgery, and moderate vision loss. Four thousand participants between the ages of 50 and 85 who have AMD are being sought for the study. The trial is "double-masked," meaning neither investigators nor participants know who is getting which combinations of the antioxidants and supplements or a placebo.

From earlier studies, NEI researchers knew that adults eating kale, mustard greens, collard greens, and raw or cooked spinach (vegetables high in lutein and zeaxanthin, two antioxidants from the same family as beta carotene), were at considerably less risk of developing advanced AMD than those who didn't. And adults consuming more sources of the omega-3 fatty acids DHA and EPA (found in fish, especially salmon) also appeared to be at less risk.

Over the next five years, researchers will be testing the effects of the two kinds of nutrients—the vegetable-derived vitamins lutein and zeaxanthin, and the fatty acids DHA and EPA—in four participant groups. One group is to receive lutein and zeaxanthin supplements; one will get DHA and EPA; one will get both the vitamins and the fatty acids; and a fourth (control) group will get a placebo.

All participants will be given the choice of also taking the initial AREDS combination of vitamins (C, E, and beta carotene) and minerals (zinc and copper). They may also instead choose to participate in a second part of the study in which the original AREDS formulation will be further tested by eliminating beta carotene and/or reducing the amount of zinc.

What Is Macular Degeneration?

In "dry" macular degeneration, small yellowish deposits known as drusen form under the retina, affecting the macula, the small area near the center of the retina that helps produce the sharp central vision needed for reading or driving.

In "wet" macular degeneration, blood vessels growing up from below the retina leak blood under the retina. Pressure from these pockets of blood damage the light-sensing cells, destroying the ability to see straight ahead.

"Symptoms of AMD don't usually start until the 60s or later," says study chair Dr. Emily Chew of the National Eye Institute. "But you get signs in the 50s. In some cases, where it's genetic, you can get them younger than that."

Advances in Macular Degeneration Research

On June 30, [2006], the Food and Drug Administration (FDA) approved a promising new drug—ranibizumab (marketed as Lucentis)—for treatment of neovascular age-related macular degeneration (AMD). Though the neovascular form of AMD represents only about 10 percent of AMD cases, it is the form that causes most vision loss.

Now, a similar drug—bevacizumab (marketed as Avastin)—from the same manufacturer is also being used successfully by many ophthalmologists to treat AMD. This second drug is currently only FDA-approved for treatment of metastatic cancer, but ophthalmologists continue to use it "off-label" (not yet officially approved) for AMD treatment. The second drug is considerably cheaper for patients than ranibizumab.

"The good news for patients is that there are two new medications for neovascular age-related macular degeneration, both of which appear to work better than the alternatives," stated Robert Steinbrook, M.D., in the October 5, 2006, issue of *The New England Journal of Medicine.* "But since they have never been directly compared, physicians can only speculate about which drug is superior with regard to safety, efficacy, and frequency of administration."

Chapter 35

Are High Levels of Antioxidants and Zinc Right for You?

The Age-Related Eye Disease Study (AREDS)—sponsored by the federal government's National Eye Institute—has found that taking high levels of antioxidants and zinc can reduce the risk of developing advanced age-related macular degeneration (AMD) by about 25 percent.

This major clinical trial closely followed about 3,600 participants with varying stages of AMD. The results showed that the AREDS formulation, while not a cure for AMD, may play a key role in helping people at high risk for developing advanced AMD keep their remaining vision.

But is the AREDS formulation right for you? Here are some questions and answers that can help you make that decision.

Who should take the AREDS formulation?

People who are at high risk for developing advanced AMD should consider taking the combination of nutrients used in the study. Your eye care professional can tell you if you have AMD and are at risk for developing the advanced form of the disease. The doctor should give you a dilated eye exam in which drops are placed in your eyes. This allows for a careful examination of the inside of the eye to look for signs of AMD.

"The AREDS Formulation and Age-Related Macular Degeneration," is from the National Eye Institute (NEI, www.nei.nih.gov), part of the National Institutes of Health, October 2003.

Before taking these high levels of vitamins and minerals, you should talk with your doctor about the risk of developing advanced AMD and whether taking the AREDS formulation is right for you.

What is the dosage of the AREDS formulation?

The specific daily amounts of antioxidants and zinc used by the study researchers were 500 milligrams of vitamin C; 400 International Units of vitamin E; 15 milligrams of beta-carotene (often labeled as equivalent to 25,000 International Units of vitamin A); 80 milligrams of zinc as zinc oxide; and two milligrams of copper as cupric oxide. Copper was added to the AREDS formulations containing zinc to prevent copper deficiency anemia, a condition associated with high levels of zinc intake.

Can I take a daily multivitamin if I am taking the AREDS formulation?

Yes. A daily multivitamin contains many important nutrients not found in the AREDS formulation. For example, elderly people with osteoporosis need to be particularly concerned about taking vitamin D, which is not in the AREDS formulation. The AREDS formulation is not a substitute for a multivitamin. In the Age-Related Eye Disease Study, two thirds of the study participants took multivitamins along with the AREDS formulation.

If you are already taking daily multivitamins and your doctor suggests you take the AREDS formulation, be sure to review all your vitamins with your doctor before you begin.

Can a daily multivitamin alone provide the same high levels of antioxidants and zinc as the AREDS formulation?

No. The AREDS formulation's levels of antioxidants and zinc are considerably higher than the amounts in any daily multivitamin.

Can diet alone provide the same high levels of antioxidants and zinc as the AREDS formulation?

No. The high levels of vitamins and minerals are difficult to achieve from diet alone. However, previous studies have suggested that people who have diets rich in green, leafy vegetables have a lower risk of developing AMD.

Will taking the AREDS formulation prevent a person from developing AMD?

No. There is no known treatment that can prevent the development of AMD. The study did not show that the AREDS formulation prevented people from developing early signs of AMD. No recommendation has been made for taking the AREDS formulation to prevent early AMD.

Taking the formulation reduced the rate of advanced AMD in people at high risk by about 25 percent over a 6-year period. We do not know if this treatment effect will persist over a longer period. However, by continuing to follow the AREDS participants, we hope to find out if the treatment effect will last longer than six years.

Where can I buy the AREDS formulation?

You can purchase the AREDS formulation at drug stores, supermarkets, health food stores, and other retail outlets that sell pharmaceutical products. The vitamins and minerals can also be purchased separately; be certain to include copper whenever taking high levels of zinc. Taking beta-carotene is not recommended for smokers.

Are there any side effects from the AREDS formulation?

Some AREDS participants reported minor side effects from the treatments. About 7.5 percent of participants assigned to the zinc treatments—compared with five percent who did not have zinc in their assigned treatment—had urinary tract problems that required hospitalization. Yellowing of the skin, a well-known side effect of large doses of beta-carotene, was reported slightly more often by participants taking antioxidants.

Are former smokers at an increased risk for developing lung cancer if they take high doses of beta-carotene?

Large clinical trials sponsored by the National Cancer Institute demonstrated that beta-carotene increases the risk of lung cancer in current smokers. In these trials, most of these smokers were heavy smokers. The only other large clinical trial evaluating beta-carotene was the Physicians Health Study (PHS). In the PHS, there was no evidence of increased cancer risk in those randomly assigned to beta-carotene, but few physicians were active smokers. There also was no evidence of an increased risk of lung cancer in former smokers. However, many studies suggest that former smokers maintain some increased risk of lung cancer for years after stopping smoking. Therefore, it is reasonable to expect that beta-carotene may also slightly increase their risk of cancer, at least for a period of several years.

In deciding whether to include beta-carotene in a formulation designed to slow the development of advanced AMD, you and your doctor should balance the apparent increase in the risk of lung cancer associated with beta-carotene with the risk of AMD progression.

What about other antioxidants such as bilberry and lutein?

The AREDS did not study bilberry, lutein, or other antioxidants, so we don't know how they may affect eye disease. Future clinical trials may eventually provide answers about these or other antioxidants.

Should young people with inherited macular degeneration take the AREDS formulation?

The AREDS only studied age-related macular degeneration. We have no recommendations for younger people with the inherited (juvenile) forms of macular degeneration.

Where can I obtain more information?

For more information, contact your eye care professional or the National Eye Institute at 301-496-5248 or visit the NEI website at www .nei.nih.gov/amd.

Chapter 36

Treatments for
Macular Degeneration

Chapter Contents

Section 36.1

Therapies to Treat Wet and Dry ARMD

Dry Age-Related Macular Degeneration

Although several new drugs are being investigated and approved by regulatory agencies around the world for the treatment of the exudative (wet) type of AMD [age-related macular degeneration], aside from cessation of smoking and a healthy diet of dark green leafy vegetables and fruits supplemented by zinc and antioxidant vitamins (Vitamins E, C, and beta carotene), very little is currently available to help patients with dry AMD to prevent progression to more serious stages of debilitating disease.

However, this is an area which has ignited research interest, and the longer term future may be somewhat brighter for those with dry AMD.

Several companies are conducting research to explore how, or why, early, dry AMD converts to wet AMD or progresses to the late stages of the dry form—usually referred to as "geographic atrophy." A few different pathways such as inflammation and/or oxidative damage have been considered, mostly involving drusen. Small drusen usually appear early in AMD and may not result in vision loss. However, the numbers and size of the drusen may increase along with concomitant other changes such as RPE [retinal pigment epithelium] cell pathology, causing AMD to progress with resulting vision loss. Linkage of these events to the appearance of wet AMD or progression to geographic atrophy is a key question and yet under investigation. One possibility is that the drusen debris buildup leads to a diminished blood supply to the RPE and photoreceptor cells, resulting in a diminished oxygen supply (hypoxia). In an attempt to compensate for this imbalance, new, abnormal blood vessels (neovascularization) could be formed, leading to wet AMD. Continuing research may lead to more effective antioxidants, anti-inflammatory agents, etc., which could halt or even reverse the progression of early, dry AMD to the more severe wet form or to the end stage dry form.

Researchers are also very interested in genetics as a link to AMD and as a factor in progression from dry to wet AMD. Researchers have now located particular genes whose mutations are associated with an increased risk for AMD. For example, one of these genes, known as Factor H, codes for a protein (complement factor H), which is a powerful inhibitor of inflammation. People who possess an alternate version of the gene produce an aberrant complement factor H, which fails to provide adequate suppression of the complement pathway of inflammation. This means that people with the defective gene are more vulnerable to certain inflammatory processes which can lead to the development of AMD.

Nutritional Supplementation

The Age-Related Eye Disease Study (AREDS) group is hoping to demonstrate that modifications to the original vitamin formulation, shown to reduce the risk of advanced age-related macular degeneration (AMD) by 25% over seven years, will further reduce the risk of progression in patients at high risk for developing advanced disease.

The vitamin formulation used in the original AREDS protocol consisted of:

- 500 mg of vitamin C;

- 400 IU of vitamin E;

- 15 mg of beta-carotene (smokers excepted);

- 80 mg of zinc, and

- 2 mg of cupric oxide.

In AREDS2, patients with either bilateral large drusen or large drusen in one eye and advanced AMD in the other will be given either high doses of lutein and zeaxanthin, both carotenoids, or omega-3 fatty acids or both, plus the original AREDS formulation, for a total of six years.

- The AREDS2 investigation will also compare the original AREDS formulation by comparing low zinc (25 mg) vs. high zinc (80 mg), and will also compare formulations with and without beta-carotene. As investigators note, the rational for adding lutein and zeaxanthin to the new formulation was based on observations that subjects in the original AREDS trial were less likely to progress to advanced AMD when they had high dietary levels of the two carotenoids.

- Those who consumed at least two servings of fish a week in the original study were less likely to develop advanced AMD as well. Omega-3 fatty acids in the AREDS2 formulation will include both DHA [docosahexaenoic acid] and EPA [eicosapentaenoic acid], naturally found in fish oils.

Lasering of Drusen

Prophylactic laser treatment of drusen does not apparently affect the rate of vision loss over a five-year interval according to recently reported findings from the Complications of Age-Related Macular Degeneration Prevention Trial (CAPT). CAPT was designed to assess the safety and effectiveness of low-intensity laser treatment in preventing vision loss in patients with at least 10 large drusen in both eyes at study entry. During the study, patients received treatment in one eye only; the other eye was not treated. At the end of five years, 20.5 percent of both treated and observed eyes had visual acuity scores three lines worse than at study entry.

Another study (Laser to Drusen trial) confirmed that prophylactic laser of the fellow eye of patients with neovascular AMD is not beneficial. As a result of these findings, vitamin supplementation remains essentially the only prevention therapy for either atrophic or neovascular AMD. Nevertheless, 90 percent of all AMD is dry AMD, not wet, and novel approaches aimed at inhibiting destructive processes within the eye that give rise to dry AMD are now under exploration.

They include:

- **Anecortave Acetate:** Anecortave acetate, from Alcon Laboratories, attenuates new blood vessel growth. A Phase III trial is currently evaluating the safety and efficacy of the new agent in patients with dry AMD at risk for progressing to wet AMD. The trial will also assess a novel delivery system that allows for slow, sustained delivery of the drug behind the eye.

- **NT-501, Encapsulated Cell Technology (ECT) Based Intraocular Delivery of Ciliary Neurotrophic Factor (CNTF):** Neurotrophic factors are believed to retard progression of neurodegenerative diseases in general. In a Phase II study, CNTF will be delivered via Encapsulated Cell technology (ECT). In ECT, genetically engineered cells that overproduce CNTF are placed in a tiny capsule in the vitreous cavity of the eye. This design bypasses the blood-retinal barrier, facilitating drug delivery to the back of the eye. The drug is being tested in atrophic macular degeneration as well as early and late stages of retinitis pigmentosa. Neurotech USA has developed this research in collaboration with the Foundation Fighting Blindness and the National Eye Institute, and in licensing agreement with Amgen, Inc.

- **Fenretinide (ST-602):** Sirion Therapeutics is sponsoring this Phase II trial, enrolling up to 225 patients at 20 sites throughout the United States. The study will assess the ability of fenretinide to slow progression of geographic atrophy in AMD patients. Fenretinide is an oral agent felt to reduce the accumulation of lipofuscin in the eye by lowering the body's serum retinol (vitamin A). Lipofuscin is a waste product which gradually accumulates in all aging cells. In the retinal pigment epithelial cells, however, it can become a noxious substance. When oxidized by free radicals, lipofuscin becomes cytotoxic, damaging the RPE cells and initiating macular degeneration.

- **OT-551:** Othera Pharmaceuticals is working on OT-551, a proprietary small molecule, delivered topically by eyedrop, which acts in a novel way on several eye conditions, including AMD. OT-551 acts via multiple pathways to down-regulate the over expression of NF-kB (nuclear factor kappa B) in various disease states. The pathways affected by OT-551 include direct activity against oxidative stress and indirect activity against cytokine-induced inflammation and angiogenesis. A growing body of scientific literature points to oxidative stress, inflammation, and angiogenesis as the key targets for treating age-related macular degeneration (AMD). Othera has initiated a dry AMD study of patients with geographic atrophy, who will test the new eyedrops, used three times a day, over a period of up to two years. Othera has previously shown in a study soon to be published in *Investigative Ophthalmology and Vision Science*, that in an animal model of dry AMD, OT-551 is effective at protecting retinal cells from photo oxidative damage.

- **Anti-Inflammatory Compounds:** On March 20, 2007 Potentia Pharma (USA) announced Phase I clinical trials with a compound they believe will be effective for both wet and dry AMD. The working name for this compound is Proteus or POT-4, a complement inhibitor which shuts down the complement activation

299

system that could lead to local inflammation, tissue damage and up-regulation of angiogenic factors such as vascular endothelial growth factor (VEGF). According to Potentia, this is the first ever testing of a so-called complement inhibitor compound intended to interfere with complement activation. Several other companies, including Jerini (Germany and USA) and Peptech (Australia) are also working on the development of complement inhibitors. Jerini and Peptech are reportedly exploring how drugs developed to control inflammatory diseases, such as rheumatoid arthritis, might have applications in age-related macular degeneration. The theory is that, upon activation of the complement system, the extremely potent pro-inflammatory complement components C3 and C5a can be generated. Researchers looking at these compounds have reported positive preclinical results in several applications including age-related macular degeneration. The Jerini and Peptech research is in exploratory phases with no announcement of trials as of March 29, 2007.

Wet AMD

Essentially, persons with macular degeneration have, at present, three possible treatment options: thermal (heat laser); photodynamic therapy; or anti-VEFG drugs. Information on each of these is described below. Further information about experimental therapies is covered in the section on Clinical Trials at http://www.amdalliance.org/information/treatments/clinicaltrials.php.

Laser Photocoagulation

Laser photocoagulation is a surgical procedure involving the application of a hot laser to seal and halt or slow the progression of abnormal blood vessels. In the 1990s laser treatment was the only therapy available for AMD.

Through the use of a high-energy light that turns to heat when it hits the parts of the retina to be treated, laser photocoagulation seals the choroidal neovascularization (CNV) and inhibits the leaky blood vessels' growth, preventing further vision deterioration. A scar forms as a result of the treatment, and this scar creates a permanent blind spot in the field of vision. Vision does not usually improve after laser treatment and may even be somewhat worse. However, loss of vision following laser treatment, though immediate, is generally less severe than the eventual loss of vision that usually occurs if laser treatment is not done. In many cases, some visual distortion will disappear after laser treatment.

Photodynamic Therapy (PDT)

Photodynamic therapy (PDT) (trade name Visudyne) uses a non-thermal (or cold) laser with an intravenous light-sensitive drug to seal and halt or slow the progression of abnormal retina blood vessels. This treatment does not produce a blind spot on the retina. The light is shone directly at the targeted tissue and the drug accumulates in these cells. It therefore reduces damage to normal surrounding tissue and allows the treatment to be given again as needed.

However, early diagnosis of AMD is key, because once vision is lost due to the growth of abnormal blood vessels, it cannot be reclaimed by either treatment.

Anti-Angiogenesis Therapies

As of February 2006, pegaptanib sodium (trade name Macugen) is approved for use in Canada, the United States, and Europe. The United States Food and Drug Administration (FDA) approved Macugen for treatment of neovascular (wet) age-related macular degeneration. FDA approval came following successful clinical trials demonstrating that the drug reduced vision loss in 70 percent of clinical trial patients. It is also very encouraging that the drug is effective for all kinds of wet AMD, whether in the early or late stages.

Pegaptanib sodium (trade name Macugen) is what researchers call an anti-VEGF drug, or in other words, a drug which works by targeting the proteins which act to trigger abnormal blood vessel growth and leakage. Anti-VEGF drugs are delivered directly to the eye by an injection, which is repeated every four to six weeks.

Other anti-VEFG drugs on the horizon include ranibizumab (trade name Lucentis), from Genentech and Novartis. On June 30, 2006, the U.S. Food and Drug Administration (FDA) announced approval of Lucentis (ranibizumab). AMD Alliance International (AMDAI) loudly applauded the decision, which effectively makes available in the United States a groundbreaking treatment for wet age-related macular degeneration. This approval is based on the evidence presented from several years of rigorous clinical trials, in which Lucentis was shown to maintain vision in 95 percent of trial participants, and improve vision in approximately 30 to 40 percent of trial participants. This decision means that treatment with Lucentis will now be widely available in the United States through retinal specialists. The FDA approval of course only covers the United States. Introduction of Lucentis in other countries is expected to follow in the coming year. AMD Alliance International applauds the introduction of new treatments, which bring hope and help to those with macular degeneration.

Angiostatic Therapies

In other research developments, a completely different class of AMD drugs, called angiostatic therapies, is showing promise. This class of drugs proposed yet another approach to treatment of AMD, in this case by administering a type of steroid to stop the abnormal growth of blood vessels in the eye. Unlike the anti-VEGF treatments, angiostatic drugs are delivered through a canula, to the back of the eye.

One possible angiostatic treatment is anecortave acetate (Retaane), from Alcon Laboratories. Although early clinical results were not as stellar as hoped, scientists working on the treatment believe this may be a result of drug delivery problems, not the drug itself and are making adjustments. On May 24, 2005, the Food and Drug Administration released what is called an "approvable" letter, basically meaning that the drug is approvable but some further study is required. Alcon recently reported that their researchers and officials will "meet with the FDA to discuss the approvable letter, the clinical studies submitted with the NDA and other ongoing clinical studies for Retaane suspension to determine the steps necessary to gain final approval for the wet AMD indication." Retaane has received market approval for use in Australia. In early March 2006, a request for market approval in Europe was withdrawn, by Alcon, from regulatory consideration.

Combination Therapies

Other investigations are also showing promise, including combination therapies, which combine traditional PDT therapy with new drugs to increase the effectiveness of PDT. Combination treatments pair one or more existing or new AMD treatments to see if the end result might be greater than what could be achieved individually. More and more medical practitioners believe that combination methods are the way of the future for wet AMD treatment. Usually the idea is that one kind of treatment will take care of existing AMD in the patient, and the other will help to prevent any future developments.

Statement on Bevacizumab: Position Statement Released by AMD Alliance International, April 28, 2006

The role, efficacy, and safety of antivascular endothelial growth factor (VEGF) therapies for use in the treatment of age-related macular degeneration (AMD) were first established by clinical trials of pegaptanib sodium, (Macugen, [OSI] Eyetech/Pfizer) and later by clinical trials for ranibizumab (Lucentis, Genentech, Inc.).

Pegaptanib sodium: Phase III clinical trials for pegaptanib sodium demonstrated that after 1 year of treatment, individuals who were treated with 0.3 mg and 1 mg pegaptanib sodium experienced less vision loss than those who were treated with a placebo. Individuals who were treated with pegaptanib sodium experienced lasting results for 2 years. The most common side effect (occurring in approximately 1.3 percent of cases) was endophthalmitis, which was caused by the injection.

Ranibizumab: Phase III clinical trials for ranibizumab demonstrated superior results after 1 year of treatment, and showed that the majority of individuals who were treated with ranibizumab improved or maintained vision 2 years later. The improvement in visual acuity endpoints in the ranibizumab-treated groups (0.3 mg and 0.5 mg) was maintained at year 2, while individuals in the control group continued to experience vision deterioration. At 2 years, at least 90 percent of individuals who were treated with ranibizumab maintained or improved vision compared to approximately 53 percent of individuals who were treated with sham injections. Treatment side effects were mild to moderate, affected less than 3 percent of individuals, and included conjunctival hemorrhage, increased IOP [intraocular pressure], vitreous floaters, and endophthalmitis.

Broadening the anti-VEGF theory: Ranibizumab was developed by Genentech, Inc. The company had previously developed bevacizumab (Avastin, Genentech, Inc.), an anti-VEGF drug that is currently approved by the Food and Drug Administration (FDA) as an intravenous therapy for metastatic colorectal cancer patients. Bevacizumab for use in cancer therapy is currently being investigated. Ranibizumab is a molecular fragment of an antibody, and bevacizumab is a full-length antibody. They are both thought to work by a similar principle—the drug blocks the production of VEGF. VEGF, which is also produced by cancer cells, prompts the abnormal growth of blood vessels, also known as angiogenesis. Bevacizumab binds with VEGF and interferes with its ability to stimulate blood vessel growth.

In early 2004, Philip Rosenfeld, M.D., Ph.D., and colleagues at the Bascom Palmer Eye Institute in Miami, Florida, initiated the use of bevacizumab in the treatment of AMD. Their first study was called Systemic Avastin for Neovascular AMD (SANA). In this and subsequent studies, which consisted of intravitreal injections of bevacizumab, individuals who were clinically followed reported improvements in visual acuity comparable to ranibizumab with no serious adverse events. It is important to note that these clinical studies were not conducted as randomized clinical trials. Based on these results, the use of bevacizumab for the treatment of AMD appears to have been broadly accepted by retinal specialists around the world.

The use of bevacizumab in the eyes, an indication for which it is not approved, is called off-label use. It is reasoned conjecture on the part of the AMD Alliance International that the off-label use of bevacizumab was first suggested for reasons of economy and availability in the face of a significant unmet need. Treatment with ranibizumab is not yet available unless an individual is registered in a clinical trial, or, as is possible in some European countries, receives the treatment on what is called a 'named-patient' basis. The FDA is expected to respond to Genentech's application for the approval of ranibizumab in the United States by June 30, 2006.

Safety and efficacy of bevacizumab: There is growing anecdotal evidence about the efficacy of the off-label use of bevacizumab. However, at this time, published reports on bevacizumab are limited to a number of human clinical case series in and a few animal studies on intravitreal injection. Most notable among the animal studies is one conducted by Anat Lowenstein, M.D., who reported no safety issues in rabbit testing. Published human research on the safety and efficacy of bevacizumab is limited to the previously mentioned small human study at Bascom Palmer Eye Institute.

There have, however, been reports of serious life-threatening adverse events that can be attributed to bevacizumab when it is used in clinical trials on cancer patients. Most notably, a 4.4 percent risk of thromboembolic events has been referenced. It is noted that when used as a cancer treatment, bevacizumab is administered systemically rather than locally.

Our position on bevacizumab: The off-label use of drugs is legal in North America, Europe, and Asia, and is a practice that is accepted by physicians, health care providers and institutions, and some insurers. As stated earlier, there is growing anecdotal evidence about the efficacy of the off-label use of bevacizumab. However, there have been no randomized controlled clinical trials, nor are there any broad, scientifically accepted published reports in this regard. In fact, due to the fact that bevacizumab is a full-length antibody, some researchers assert that it will not be as effective in the long term because it cannot penetrate all layers of the eye as well as the fragment antibody ranibizumab. Answers to all of the questions about bevacizumab will only be known following the completion of clinical trials and publication of the results. Genentech, Inc., has stated that it is not planning to conduct any clinical trials involving the medication.

On April 20, 2006, the American Academy of Ophthalmology (AAO) issued a statement declaring their support for Medicare reimbursement consideration for the cost of bevacizumab usage in cases where individuals who are deemed by their treating physician to have failed FDA-approved therapies and/or are likely to have greater benefit from the use of intravitreal bevacizumab.

Individuals also have access to a clinical trial of ranibizumab, sponsored by Genentech, Inc., the makers of bevacizumab. The trial, known as Safety Assessment of Intravitreal Lucentis for AMD (SAILOR), is a 1-year, Phase IIIb study that is designed to evaluate the safety of ranibizumab, the VEGF inhibitor, which, as discussed above, has not yet been approved by the FDA. The trial provides access to the drug for eligible individuals in advance of the FDA's response and is open to individuals with all subtypes of new or recurrent active subfoveal wet AMD. For more information, see www.clinicaltrials.gov or www.amdalliance.org. Eligible patients are not able access these clinical trials outside the United States.

Meanwhile, until options such as ranibizumab become widely available, individuals are desperately seeking options and answers. Our position is that individuals must make an informed decision about treatment in consultation with their own retinal specialist. According to the American Medical Association, informed consent refers to significantly more than the process of signing a consent to treat form. Rather, informed consent refers to the communication that takes place between individuals and their physician.

The process of arriving at an informed decision includes questions such as:

1. What is my exact diagnosis?

2. What is the typical progression for an individual with my eye condition?

3. What treatment options and/or care do you recommend?

4. How will each of these treatments and/or care options help me?

5. What are the risks and side effects for my unique eye condition?

6. What are the proven and unproven benefits of treatment for my unique eye condition?

7. Are the differences in the evidence gathered through randomized clinical trials versus clinical studies significant for me?

8. Regardless of cost or coverage by my insurance, what are some alternative treatments?

Section 36.2

Macular Translocation: Experimental Treatment for Wet ARMD

"Macular Translocation," © 2006 The Cleveland Clinic Cole Eye Institute, 9500 Euclid Avenue Mail Stop W14, Cleveland, OH 44195, www.clevelandclinic.org/eye. Additional information is available from the Cleveland Clinic Health Information Center, 216-444-3771, toll-free 800-223-2273 extension 43771, or at http://www.clevelandclinic.org/health.

What is macular translocation?

The eye is often compared to a camera. The front of the eye contains a lens that focuses images on the inside of the back of the eye. The back of the eye, called the retina, is covered with special nerve cells that react to light. These nerve cells are very close together in the middle of the retina where the eye focuses the images that we see. This small middle section, called the macula, is essential to clarity and sharpness of vision. Sometimes the retina is damaged by unwanted new blood vessels growing on it. This damages the macula and causes vision loss.

In macular translocation, the macula is moved away from abnormal new blood vessel growth (choroidal neovascular membrane) to an area of healthier retinal tissue to preserve as much vision as possible.

Can this procedure be performed if the patient has either the dry (atrophic) or the wet (exudative) form of age-related macular degeneration?

This procedure is only for patients who have the wet (exudative) form of age-related macular degeneration. It is used only for patients whose abnormal blood vessels are located in the very center of the macula and are not associated with a scar. Better results are achieved in patients who have small abnormal blood vessels of more recent onset.

Will the patient need tests before the procedure?

The patient will require a comprehensive ophthalmological evaluation as well as fluorescein angiogram. Sometimes an indocyanine green angiogram is also needed.

How is the procedure performed?

This is a vitreoretinal surgical procedure—a bubble of air is placed in the eye and the patient is required to maintain a sitting up or leaning to one side position for a few days following the surgery.

Is more than one treatment needed?

In about 10% of the cases, a secondary treatment is required.

What results can the patient expect?

The treatment is still experimental. So far, about 20% of the patients treated have had improvement in the vision. There continues to be improvement up to six months after the procedure.

Is age a factor for macular translocation surgery?

No.

If the patient has been diagnosed as legally blind, can this procedure still be performed?

Yes.

If a doctor told a patient that nothing else can be done for them, can macular translocation surgery still be performed?

The patient needs to be evaluated to determine whether they are eligible to undergo the procedure.

If lasers were used as a prior treatment, can this procedure still be performed?

Yes.

Are there any risks or side effects the patient should be concerned about?

The risks will be discussed when the patient is evaluated.

If the patient has other medical disorders, can this procedure still be performed?

Yes.

Section 36.3

Rehabilitation for Degeneration

Currently, there are no treatment options available that restore lost vision; and for most AMD [age-related macular degeneration] patients there are not even treatments that prevent further vision loss. For many AMD patients, the hardest challenge is adapting to life with impaired vision. However, by retraining existing peripheral vision, modifying the patient's environment, and using available low vision devices and aids, AMD patients can continue to maintain their lifestyle and independence.

Also known as "sight enhancement" services, low vision rehabilitation services are available in most countries but systems of delivery and the range of services available vary considerably. Public health care funding for low vision rehabilitation services and devices, as detailed in the 2003 AMD Alliance International Global Campaign Report, also varies significantly. Please contact your local Alliance member for advice, information and referral, or ask your eye doctor for a referral to a low vision specialist near you. You can find contact details of member organizations at the AMD Alliance International website at www.amdalliance.org. Alternatively, contact any reputable visual impairment organization in your own country. Learning about vision rehabilitation services early, and understanding how they can actually improve everyday functioning, can greatly help you deal with AMD and your changing vision. Rehabilitation includes low vision assessment, adaptive living, low vision devices, vision training, counseling support, and benefits advice as well as orientation and mobility training.

It is important that you seek assistance from low vision specialists and vision rehabilitation experts. These experts can help you use your remaining sight to its fullest and teach you new ways to accomplish everyday tasks—whether it's traveling safely, taking care of your home, preparing meals, cooking safely, managing your medications, reading a book, writing a letter, shopping, or watching television. Low vision rehabilitation is a team effort often involving the low vision specialist (an optometrist or ophthalmologist skilled in the examination, treatment, and management of patients with visual impairments), rehabilitation teachers, mobility and orientation specialists, occupational therapists, technicians, and other professions as needed.

Critical to the success of vision rehabilitation is the low vision assessment. This is different from a regular eye exam which determines how well you can see the eye chart. The low vision assessment is designed to accurately measure how your vision functions in day-to-day living—being able to see faces, street signs, newspaper print, stove dials, etc. Not only does the assessment measure how well you see at a distance and up close, additional tests evaluate contrast sensitivity and locate blurry or distorted areas in the visual field. The vision specialist is interested in knowing if your vision is affected by glare and different lighting conditions; do you see better when you look slightly away from the object? In addition, the low vision specialist wants to determine how your vision impairment impacts your life. Do you travel independently? Can you safely prepare your own meals? What about grocery shopping, making phone calls or taking medications? Can you write checks and manage other financial tasks? This information allows the creation of a vision rehabilitation program that is right for you.

Part Six

Disorders of the Cornea, Retina, and Lacrimal Glands (Tear Ducts)

Chapter 37

Facts about the Cornea, Corneal Diseases, and Their Treatment

What Is the Cornea?

The cornea is the eye's outermost layer. It is the clear, dome-shaped surface that covers the front of the eye.

Structure of the Cornea

Although the cornea is clear and seems to lack substance, it is actually a highly organized group of cells and proteins. Unlike most tissues in the body, the cornea contains no blood vessels to nourish or protect it against infection. Instead, the cornea receives its nourishment from the tears and aqueous humor that fills the chamber behind it. The cornea must remain transparent to refract light properly, and the presence of even the tiniest blood vessels can interfere with this process. To see well, all layers of the cornea must be free of any cloudy or opaque areas.

The corneal tissue is arranged in five basic layers, each having an important function.

Epithelium: The epithelium is the cornea's outermost region, comprising about 10 percent of the tissue's thickness. The epithelium functions primarily to: (1) Block the passage of foreign material, such as

From "Facts About the Cornea and Corneal Disease," by the National Eye Institute (NEI, www.nei.nih.gov), part of the National Institutes of Health, January 2007.

dust, water, and bacteria, into the eye and other layers of the cornea; and (2) Provide a smooth surface that absorbs oxygen and cell nutrients from tears, then distributes these nutrients to the rest of the cornea. The epithelium is filled with thousands of tiny nerve endings that make the cornea extremely sensitive to pain when rubbed or scratched. The part of the epithelium that serves as the foundation on which the epithelial cells anchor and organize themselves is called the basement membrane.

Bowman Layer: Lying directly below the basement membrane of the epithelium is a transparent sheet of tissue known as the Bowman layer. It is composed of strong layered protein fibers called collagen. Once injured, the Bowman layer can form a scar as it heals. If these scars are large and centrally located, some vision loss can occur.

Stroma: Beneath the Bowman layer is the stroma, which comprises about 90 percent of the cornea's thickness. It consists primarily of water (78 percent) and collagen (16 percent), and does not contain any blood vessels. Collagen gives the cornea its strength, elasticity, and form. The collagen's unique shape, arrangement, and spacing are essential in producing the cornea's light-conducting transparency.

Descemet Membrane: Under the stroma is the Descemet membrane, a thin but strong sheet of tissue that serves as a protective barrier against infection and injuries. The Descemet membrane is composed of collagen fibers (different from those of the stroma) and is made by the endothelial cells that lie below it. The Descemet membrane is regenerated readily after injury.

Endothelium: The endothelium is the extremely thin, innermost layer of the cornea. Endothelial cells are essential in keeping the cornea clear. Normally, fluid leaks slowly from inside the eye into the middle corneal layer (stroma). The endothelium's primary task is to pump this excess fluid out of the stroma. Without this pumping action, the stroma would swell with water, become hazy, and ultimately opaque. In a healthy eye, a perfect balance is maintained between the fluid moving into the cornea and fluid being pumped out of the cornea. Once endothelium cells are destroyed by disease or trauma, they are lost forever. If too many endothelial cells are destroyed, corneal edema and blindness ensue, with corneal transplantation the only available therapy.

Refractive Errors

About 120 million people in the United States wear eyeglasses or contact lenses to correct nearsightedness, farsightedness, or astigmatism. These vision disorders—called refractive errors—affect the cornea and are the most common of all vision problems in this country.

Refractive errors occur when the curve of the cornea is irregularly shaped (too steep or too flat). When the cornea is of normal shape and curvature, it bends, or refracts, light on the retina with precision. However, when the curve of the cornea is irregularly shaped, the cornea bends light imperfectly on the retina. This affects good vision. The refractive process is similar to the way a camera takes a picture. The cornea and lens in your eye act as the camera lens. The retina is similar to the film. If the image is not focused properly, the film (or retina) receives a blurry image. The image that your retina "sees" then goes to your brain, which tells you what the image is.

When the cornea is curved too much, or if the eye is too long, faraway objects will appear blurry because they are focused in front of the retina. This is called myopia, or nearsightedness. Myopia affects over 25 percent of all adult Americans.

Hyperopia, or farsightedness, is the opposite of myopia. Distant objects are clear, and close-up objects appear blurry. With hyperopia, images focus on a point beyond the retina. Hyperopia results from an eye that is too short.

Astigmatism is a condition in which the uneven curvature of the cornea blurs and distorts both distant and near objects. A normal cornea is round, with even curves from side to side and top to bottom. With astigmatism, the cornea is shaped more like the back of a spoon, curved more in one direction than in another. This causes light rays to have more than one focal point and focus on two separate areas of the retina, distorting the visual image. Two thirds of Americans with myopia also have astigmatism.

Refractive errors are usually corrected by eyeglasses or contact lenses. Although these are safe and effective methods for treating refractive err ors, refractive surgeries are becoming an increasingly popular option.

What Is the Function of the Cornea?

Because the cornea is as smooth and clear as glass but is strong and durable, it helps the eye in two ways:

1. It helps to shield the rest of the eye from germs, dust, and other harmful matter. The cornea shares this protective task with the eyelids, the eye socket, tears, and the sclera, or white part of the eye.

2. The cornea acts as the eye's outermost lens. It functions like a window that controls and focuses the entry of light into the eye. The cornea contributes between 65 percent to 75 percent of the eye's total focusing power.

When light strikes the cornea, it bends—or refracts—the incoming light onto the lens. The lens further refocuses that light onto the retina, a layer of light sensing cells lining the back of the eye that starts the translation of light into vision. For you to see clearly, light rays must be focused by the cornea and lens to fall precisely on the retina. The retina converts the light rays into impulses that are sent through the optic nerve to the brain, which interprets them as images.

The refractive process is similar to the way a camera takes a picture. The cornea and lens in the eye act as the camera lens. The retina is similar to the film. If the image is not focused properly, the film (or retina) receives a blurry image.

The cornea also serves as a filter, screening out some of the most damaging ultraviolet (UV) wavelengths in sunlight. Without this protection, the lens and the retina would be highly susceptible to injury from UV radiation.

How Does the Cornea Respond to Injury?

The cornea copes very well with minor injuries or abrasions. If the highly sensitive cornea is scratched, healthy cells slide over quickly and patch the injury before infection occurs and vision is affected. If the scratch penetrates the cornea more deeply, however, the healing process will take longer, at times resulting in greater pain, blurred vision, tearing, redness, and extreme sensitivity to light. These symptoms require professional treatment. Deeper scratches can also cause corneal scarring, resulting in a haze on the cornea that can greatly impair vision. In this case, a corneal transplant may be needed.

What Are Some Diseases and Disorders Affecting the Cornea?

Some diseases and disorders of the cornea are:

Allergies: Allergies affecting the eye are fairly common. The most common allergies are those related to pollen, particularly when the weather is warm and dry. Symptoms can include redness, itching, tearing, burning, stinging, and watery discharge, although they are not usually severe enough to require medical attention. Antihistamine decongestant eyedrops can effectively reduce these symptoms, as does rain and cooler weather, which decreases the amount of pollen in the air.

An increasing number of eye allergy cases are related to medications and contact lens wear. Also, animal hair and certain cosmetics, such as mascara, face creams, and eyebrow pencil, can cause allergies that affect the eye. Touching or rubbing eyes after handling nail polish, soaps, or chemicals may cause an allergic reaction. Some people have sensitivity to lip gloss and eye makeup. Allergy symptoms are temporary and can be eliminated by not having contact with the offending cosmetic or detergent.

Conjunctivitis (Pinkeye): This term describes a group of diseases that cause swelling, itching, burning, and redness of the conjunctiva, the protective membrane that lines the eyelids and covers exposed areas of the sclera, or white of the eye. Conjunctivitis can spread from one person to another and affects millions of Americans at any given time. Conjunctivitis can be caused by a bacterial or viral infection, allergy, environmental irritants, a contact lens product, eyedrops, or eye ointments.

At its onset, conjunctivitis is usually painless and does not adversely affect vision. The infection will clear in most cases without requiring medical care. But for some forms of conjunctivitis, treatment will be needed. If treatment is delayed, the infection may worsen and cause corneal inflammation and a loss of vision.

Corneal Infections: Sometimes the cornea is damaged after a foreign object has penetrated the tissue, such as from a poke in the eye. At other times, bacteria or fungi from a contaminated contact lens can pass into the cornea. Situations like these can cause painful inflammation and corneal infections called keratitis. These infections can reduce visual clarity, produce corneal discharges, and perhaps erode the cornea. Corneal infections can also lead to corneal scarring, which can impair vision and may require a corneal transplant.

As a general rule, the deeper the corneal infection, the more severe the symptoms and complications. It should be noted that corneal infections, although relatively infrequent, are the most serious complication of contact lens wear.

Minor corneal infections are commonly treated with antibacterial eye drops. If the problem is severe, it may require more intensive antibiotic or antifungal treatment to eliminate the infection, as well as steroid eye drops to reduce inflammation. Frequent visits to an eye care professional may be necessary for several months to eliminate the problem.

Dry Eye: The continuous production and drainage of tears is important to the eye's health. Tears keep the eye moist, help wounds heal, and protect against eye infection. In people with dry eye, the eye produces fewer or less quality tears and is unable to keep its surface lubricated and comfortable.

The tear film consists of three layers—an outer, oily (lipid) layer that keeps tears from evaporating too quickly and helps tears remain on the eye; a middle (aqueous) layer that nourishes the cornea and conjunctiva; and a bottom (mucin) layer that helps to spread the aqueous layer across the eye to ensure that the eye remains wet. As we age, the eyes usually produce fewer tears. Also, in some cases, the lipid and mucin layers produced by the eye are of such poor quality that tears cannot remain in the eye long enough to keep the eye sufficiently lubricated.

The main symptom of dry eye is usually a scratchy or sandy feeling as if something is in the eye. Other symptoms may include stinging or burning of the eye; episodes of excess tearing that follow periods of very dry sensation; a stringy discharge from the eye; and pain and redness of the eye. Sometimes people with dry eye experience heaviness of the eyelids or blurred, changing, or decreased vision, although loss of vision is uncommon.

Dry eye is more common in women, especially after menopause. Surprisingly, some people with dry eye may have tears that run down their cheeks. This is because the eye may be producing less of the lipid and mucin layers of the tear film, which help keep tears in the eye. When this happens, tears do not stay in the eye long enough to thoroughly moisten it.

Dry eye can occur in climates with dry air, as well as with the use of some drugs, including antihistamines, nasal decongestants, tranquilizers, and antidepressant drugs. People with dry eye should let their health care providers know all the medications they are taking because some of them may intensify dry eye symptoms.

People with connective tissue diseases, such as rheumatoid arthritis, can also develop dry eye. It is important to note that dry eye is sometimes a symptom of Sjögren syndrome, a disease that attacks the body's lubricating glands, such as the tear and salivary glands. A complete physical examination may diagnose any underlying diseases.

Artificial tears, which lubricate the eye, are the principal treatment for dry eye. They are available over-the-counter as eyedrops. Sterile ointments are sometimes used at night to help prevent the eye from drying. Using humidifiers, wearing wrap-around glasses when outside, and avoiding outside windy and dry conditions may bring relief. For people with severe cases of dry eye, temporary or permanent closure of the tear drain (small openings at the inner corner of the eyelids where tears drain from the eye) may be helpful.

Corneal Dystrophies: A corneal dystrophy is a condition in which one or more parts of the cornea lose their normal clarity due to a buildup of cloudy material. There are over 20 corneal dystrophies that affect all parts of the cornea. These diseases share many traits:

- They are usually inherited.

- They affect the right and left eyes equally.

- They are not caused by outside factors, such as injury or diet.

- Most progress gradually.

- Most usually begin in one of the five corneal layers and may later spread to nearby layers.

- Most do not affect other parts of the body, nor are they related to diseases affecting other parts of the eye or body.

- Most can occur in otherwise totally healthy people, male or female.

Corneal dystrophies affect vision in widely differing ways. Some cause severe visual impairment, while a few cause no vision problems and are discovered during a routine eye examination. Other dystrophies may cause repeated episodes of pain without leading to permanent loss of vision.

Some of the most common corneal dystrophies include Fuchs dystrophy, keratoconus, lattice dystrophy, and map-dot-fingerprint dystrophy.

Fuchs Dystrophy: Fuchs dystrophy is a slowly progressing disease that usually affects both eyes and is slightly more common in women than in men. Although doctors can often see early signs of

Fuchs dystrophy in people in their 30s and 40s, the disease rarely affects vision until people reach their 50s and 60s.

Fuchs dystrophy occurs when endothelial cells gradually deteriorate without any apparent reason. As more endothelial cells are lost over the years, the endothelium becomes less efficient at pumping water out of the stroma. This causes the cornea to swell and distort vision. Eventually, the epithelium also takes on water, resulting in pain and severe visual impairment.

Epithelial swelling damages vision by changing the cornea's normal curvature, and causing a sight-impairing haze to appear in the tissue. Epithelial swelling will also produce tiny blisters on the corneal surface. When these blisters burst, they are extremely painful.

At first, a person with Fuchs dystrophy will awaken with blurred vision that will gradually clear during the day. This occurs because the cornea is normally thicker in the morning; it retains fluids during sleep that evaporate in the tear film while we are awake. As the disease worsens, this swelling will remain constant and reduce vision throughout the day.

When treating the disease, doctors will try first to reduce the swelling with drops, ointments, or soft contact lenses. They also may instruct a person to use a hair dryer, held at arm's length or directed across the face, to dry out the epithelial blisters. This can be done two or three times a day.

When the disease interferes with daily activities, a person may need to consider having a corneal transplant to restore sight. The short-term success rate of corneal transplantation is quite good for people with Fuchs dystrophy. However, some studies suggest that the long-term survival of the new cornea can be a problem.

Herpes Zoster (Shingles): This infection is produced by the varicella-zoster virus, the same virus that causes chickenpox. After an initial outbreak of chickenpox (often during childhood), the virus remains inactive within the nerve cells of the central nervous system. But in some people, the varicella-zoster virus will reactivate at another time in their lives. When this occurs, the virus travels down long nerve fibers and infects some part of the body, producing a blistering rash (shingles), fever, painful inflammations of the affected nerve fibers, and a general feeling of sluggishness.

Varicella-zoster virus may travel to the head and neck, perhaps involving an eye, part of the nose, cheek, and forehead. In about 40 percent of those with shingles in these areas, the virus infects the cornea. Doctors will often prescribe oral antiviral treatment to reduce the risk of the virus infecting cells deep within the tissue, which could inflame and scar the cornea. The disease may also cause decreased corneal sensitivity, meaning that foreign matter, such as eyelashes, in the eye are not felt as keenly. For many, this decreased sensitivity will be permanent.

Although shingles can occur in anyone exposed to the varicella-zoster virus, research has established two general risk factors for the disease: (1) Advanced age; and (2) A weakened immune system. Studies show that people over age 80 have a five times greater chance of having shingles than adults between the ages of 20 and 40. Unlike herpes simplex I, the varicella-zoster virus does not usually flare up more than once in adults with normally functioning immune systems.

Be aware that corneal problems may arise months after the shingles are gone. For this reason, it is important that people who have had facial shingles schedule follow-up eye examinations.

Iridocorneal Endothelial Syndrome: More common in women and usually diagnosed between ages 30-50, iridocorneal endothelial (ICE) syndrome has three main features: (1) Visible changes in the iris, the colored part of the eye that regulates the amount of light entering the eye; (2) Swelling of the cornea; and (3) The development of glaucoma, a disease that can cause severe vision loss when normal fluid inside the eye cannot drain properly. ICE is usually present in only one eye.

ICE syndrome is actually a grouping of three closely linked conditions: iris nevus (or Cogan-Reese) syndrome; Chandler syndrome; and essential (progressive) iris atrophy (hence the acronym ICE). The most common feature of this group of diseases is the movement of endothelial cells off the cornea onto the iris. This loss of cells from the cornea often leads to corneal swelling, distortion of the iris, and variable degrees of distortion of the pupil, the adjustable opening at the center of the iris that allows varying amounts of light to enter the eye. This cell movement also plugs the fluid outflow channels of the eye, causing glaucoma.

The cause of this disease is unknown. While we do not yet know how to keep ICE syndrome from progressing, the glaucoma associated with the disease can be treated with medication, and a corneal transplant can treat the corneal swelling.

Keratoconus: This disorder—a progressive thinning of the cornea—is the most common corneal dystrophy in the United States, affecting one in every 2,000 Americans. It is more prevalent in teenagers and adults in their 20s. Keratoconus arises when the middle of the cornea thins and gradually bulges outward, forming a rounded cone shape. This abnormal curvature changes the cornea's refractive power, producing moderate to severe distortion (astigmatism) and blurriness (nearsightedness) of vision. Keratoconus may also cause swelling and a sight-impairing scarring of the tissue.

Studies indicate that keratoconus stems from one of several possible causes:

- An inherited corneal abnormality. About seven percent of those with the condition have a family history of keratoconus.

- An eye injury, i.e., excessive eye rubbing or wearing hard contact lenses for many years.

- Certain eye diseases, such as retinitis pigmentosa, retinopathy of prematurity, and vernal keratoconjunctivitis.

- Systemic diseases, such as Leber congenital amaurosis, Ehlers-Danlos syndrome, Down syndrome, and osteogenesis imperfecta.

Keratoconus usually affects both eyes. At first, people can correct their vision with eyeglasses. But as the astigmatism worsens, they must rely on specially fitted contact lenses to reduce the distortion and provide better vision. Although finding a comfortable contact lens can be an extremely frustrating and difficult process, it is crucial because a poorly fitting lens could further damage the cornea and make wearing a contact lens intolerable.

In most cases, the cornea will stabilize after a few years without ever causing severe vision problems. But in about 10 to 20 percent of people with keratoconus, the cornea will eventually become too scarred or will not tolerate a contact lens. If either of these problems occur, a corneal transplant may be needed. This operation is successful in more than 90 percent of those with advanced keratoconus. Several studies have also reported that 80 percent or more of these patients have 20/40 vision or better after the operation.

The National Eye Institute is conducting a natural history study—called the Collaborative Longitudinal Evaluation of Keratoconus Study—to identify factors that influence the severity and progression of keratoconus.

Lattice Dystrophy: Lattice dystrophy gets its name from an accumulation of amyloid deposits, or abnormal protein fibers, throughout the middle and anterior stroma. During an eye examination, the doctor sees these deposits in the stroma as clear, comma-shaped over-lapping dots and branching filaments, creating a lattice effect. Over time, the lattice lines will grow opaque and involve more of the stroma. They will also gradually converge, giving the cornea a cloudiness that may also reduce vision.

In some people, these abnormal protein fibers can accumulate under the cornea's outer layer—the epithelium. This can cause erosion of the epithelium. This condition is known as recurrent epithelial erosion. These erosions: (1) Alter the cornea's normal curvature, resulting in temporary vision problems; and (2) Expose the nerves that line the cornea, causing severe pain. Even the involuntary act of blinking can be painful.

To ease this pain, a doctor may prescribe eyedrops and ointments to reduce the friction on the eroded cornea. In some cases, an eye patch may be used to immobilize the eyelids. With effective care, these erosions usually heal within three days, although occasional sensations of pain may occur for the next six to eight weeks.

By about age 40, some people with lattice dystrophy will have scarring under the epithelium, resulting in a haze on the cornea that can greatly obscure vision. In this case, a corneal transplant may be needed. Although people with lattice dystrophy have an excellent chance for a successful transplant, the disease may also arise in the donor cornea in as little as three years. In one study, about half of the transplant patients with lattice dystrophy had a recurrence of the disease from between two to 26 years after the operation. Of these, 15 percent required a second corneal transplant. Early lattice and recurrent lattice arising in the donor cornea responds well to treatment with the excimer laser.

Although lattice dystrophy can occur at any time in life, the condition usually arises in children between the ages of two and seven.

Map-Dot-Fingerprint Dystrophy: This dystrophy occurs when the epithelium's basement membrane develops abnormally (the basement membrane serves as the foundation on which the epithelial cells, which absorb nutrients from tears, anchor and organize themselves). When the basement membrane develops abnormally, the epithelial cells cannot properly adhere to it. This, in turn, causes recurrent epithelial erosions, in which the epithelium's outermost layer rises slightly, exposing a small gap between the outermost layer and the rest of the cornea.

Epithelial erosions can be a chronic problem. They may alter the cornea's normal curvature, causing periodic blurred vision. They may also expose the nerve endings that line the tissue, resulting in moderate to severe pain lasting as long as several days. Generally, the pain will be worse on awakening in the morning. Other symptoms include sensitivity to light, excessive tearing, and foreign body sensation in the eye.

Map-dot-fingerprint dystrophy, which tends to occur in both eyes, usually affects adults between the ages of 40 and 70, although it can develop earlier in life. Also known as epithelial basement membrane dystrophy, map-dot-fingerprint dystrophy gets its name from the unusual appearance of the cornea during an eye examination. Most often, the affected epithelium will have a map-like appearance, i.e., large, slightly gray outlines that look like a continent on a map. There may also be clusters of opaque dots underneath or close to the map-like patches. Less frequently, the irregular basement membrane will form concentric lines in the central cornea that resemble small fingerprints.

Typically, map-dot-fingerprint dystrophy will flare up occasionally for a few years and then go away on its own, with no lasting loss of vision. Most people never know that they have map-dot-fingerprint dystrophy, since they do not have any pain or vision loss. However, if treatment is needed, doctors will try to control the pain associated with the epithelial erosions. They may patch the eye to immobilize it, or prescribe lubricating eyedrops and ointments. With treatment, these erosions usually heal within three days, although periodic flashes of pain may occur for several weeks thereafter. Other treatments include anterior corneal punctures to allow better adherence of cells; corneal scraping to remove eroded areas of the cornea and allow regeneration of healthy epithelial tissue; and use of the excimer laser to remove surface irregularities.

Ocular Herpes: Herpes of the eye, or ocular herpes, is a recurrent viral infection that is caused by the herpes simplex virus and is the most common infectious cause of corneal blindness in the United States. Previous studies show that once people develop ocular herpes, they have up to a 50 percent chance of having a recurrence. This second flare-up could come weeks or even years after the initial occurrence.

Ocular herpes can produce a painful sore on the eyelid or surface of the eye and cause inflammation of the cornea. Prompt treatment with antiviral drugs helps to stop the herpes virus from multiplying and destroying epithelial cells. However, the infection may spread deeper into the cornea and develop into a more severe infection called stromal keratitis, which causes the body's immune system to attack and destroy stromal cells. Stromal keratitis is more difficult to treat than less severe ocular herpes infections. Recurrent episodes of stromal keratitis can cause scarring of the cornea, which can lead to loss of vision and possibly blindness.

Like other herpetic infections, herpes of the eye can be controlled. An estimated 400,000 Americans have had some form of ocular herpes. Each year, nearly 50,000 new and recurring cases are diagnosed in the United States, with the more serious stromal keratitis accounting for about 25 percent. In one large study, researchers found that recurrence rate of ocular herpes was 10 percent within one year, 23 percent within two years, and 63 percent within 20 years. Some factors believed to be associated with recurrence include fever, stress, sunlight, and eye injury.

Pterygium: A pterygium is a pinkish, triangular-shaped tissue growth on the cornea. Some pterygia grow slowly throughout a person's life, while others stop growing after a certain point. A pterygium rarely grows so large that it begins to cover the pupil of the eye.

Pterygia are more common in sunny climates and in the 20- to 40-year age group. Scientists do not know what causes pterygia to develop. However, since people who have pterygia usually have spent a significant time outdoors, many doctors believe ultraviolet (UV) light from the sun may be a factor. In areas where sunlight is strong, wearing protective eyeglasses, sunglasses, and/or hats with brims are suggested. While some studies report a higher prevalence of pterygia in men than in women, this may reflect different rates of exposure to UV light.

Because a pterygium is visible, many people want to have it removed for cosmetic reasons. It is usually not too noticeable unless it becomes red and swollen from dust or air pollutants. Surgery to remove a pterygium is not recommended unless it affects vision. If a pterygium is surgically removed, it may grow back, particularly if the patient is less than 40 years of age. Lubricants can reduce the redness and provide relief from the chronic irritation.

Stevens-Johnson Syndrome: Stevens-Johnson Syndrome (SJS), also called erythema multiforme major, is a disorder of the skin that can also affect the eyes. SJS is characterized by painful, blistery lesions on the skin and the mucous membranes (the thin, moist tissues that line body cavities) of the mouth, throat, genital region, and eyelids. SJS can cause serious eye problems, such as severe conjunctivitis; iritis, an inflammation inside the eye; corneal blisters and erosions; and corneal holes. In some cases, the ocular complications from SJS can be disabling and lead to severe vision loss.

Scientists are not certain why SJS develops. The most commonly cited cause of SJS is an adverse allergic drug reaction. Almost any drug—but most particularly sulfa drugs—can cause SJS. The allergic reaction to the drug may not occur until 7 to 14 days after first using it. SJS can also be preceded by a viral infection, such as herpes or the mumps, and its accompanying fever, sore throat, and sluggishness. Treatment for the eye may include artificial tears, antibiotics, or corticosteroids. About one third of all patients diagnosed with SJS have recurrences of the disease.

SJS occurs twice as often in men as women, and most cases appear in children and young adults under 30, although it can develop in people at any age.

What Is a Corneal Transplant? Is It Safe?

A corneal transplant involves replacing a diseased or scarred cornea with a new one. When the cornea becomes cloudy, light cannot penetrate the eye to reach the light-sensitive retina. Poor vision or blindness may result.

In corneal transplant surgery, the surgeon removes the central portion of the cloudy cornea and replaces it with a clear cornea, usually donated through an eye bank. A trephine, an instrument like a cookie cutter, is used to remove the cloudy cornea. The surgeon places the new cornea in the opening and sews it with a very fine thread. The thread stays in for months or even years until the eye heals properly (removing the thread is quite simple and can easily be done in an ophthalmologist's office). Following surgery, eye drops to help promote healing will be needed for several months.

Corneal transplants are very common in the United States; about 40,000 are performed each year. The chances of success of this operation have risen dramatically because of technological advances, such as less irritating sutures, or threads, which are often finer than a human hair; and the surgical microscope. Corneal transplantation has restored sight to many, who a generation ago would have been blinded permanently by corneal injury, infection, or inherited corneal disease or degeneration.

What Problems Can Develop from a Corneal Transplant?

Even with a fairly high success rate, some problems can develop, such as rejection of the new cornea. Warning signs for rejection are decreased vision, increased redness of the eye, increased pain, and increased sensitivity to light. If any of these last for more than six hours, you should immediately call your ophthalmologist. Rejection can be successfully treated if medication is administered at the first sign of symptoms.

A study supported by the National Eye Institute (NEI) suggests that matching the blood type, but not tissue type, of the recipient with that of the cornea donor may improve the success rate of corneal transplants in people at high risk for graft failure. Approximately 20 percent of corneal transplant patients—between 6,000 to 8,000 a year—reject their donor corneas. The NEI-supported study, called the Collaborative Corneal Transplantation Study, found that high-risk patients may reduce the likelihood of corneal rejection if their blood types match those of the cornea donors. The study also concluded that intensive steroid treatment after transplant surgery improves the chances for a successful transplant.

Are There Alternatives to a Corneal Transplant?

Phototherapeutic keratectomy (PTK) is one of the latest advances in eye care for the treatment of corneal dystrophies, corneal scars, and certain corneal infections. Only a short time ago, people with these disorders would most likely have needed a corneal transplant. By combining the precision of the excimer laser with the control of a computer, doctors can vaporize microscopically thin layers of diseased corneal tissue and etch away the surface irregularities associated with many corneal dystrophies and scars. Surrounding areas suffer relatively little trauma. New tissue can then grow over the now-smooth surface. Recovery from the procedure takes a matter of days, rather than months as with a transplant. The return of vision can occur rapidly, especially if the cause of the problem is confined to the top layer of the cornea. Studies have shown close to an 85 percent success rate in corneal repair using PTK for well-selected patients.

The PTK procedure is especially useful for people with inherited disorders, whose scars or other corneal opacities limit vision by blocking the way images form on the retina. PTK has been approved by the U.S. Food and Drug Administration.

Current Corneal Research

Vision research funded by the National Eye Institute (NEI) is leading to progress in understanding and treating corneal disease.

For example, scientists are learning how transplanting corneal cells from a patient's healthy eye to the diseased eye can treat certain conditions that previously caused blindness. Vision researchers continue to investigate ways to enhance corneal healing and eliminate the corneal scarring that can threaten sight. Also, understanding how genes produce and maintain a healthy cornea will help in treating corneal disease.

Genetic studies in families afflicted with corneal dystrophies have yielded new insight into 13 different corneal dystrophies, including keratoconus. To identify factors that influence the severity and progression of keratoconus, the NEI is conducting a natural history study—called the Collaborative Longitudinal Evaluation of Keratoconus (CLEK) Study—that is following more than 1,200 patients with the disease. Scientists are looking for answers to how rapidly their keratoconus will progress, how bad their vision will become, and whether they will need corneal surgery to treat it. Results from the CLEK Study will enable eye care practitioners to better manage this complex disease.

The NEI also supported the Herpetic Eye Disease Study (HEDS), a group of clinical trials that studied various treatments for severe ocular herpes. HEDS researchers reported that oral acyclovir reduced by 41 percent the chance that ocular herpes, a recurrent disease, would return. The study clearly showed that acyclovir therapy can benefit people with all forms of ocular herpes. Current HEDS research is examining the role of psychological stress and other factors as triggers of ocular herpes recurrences.

Chapter 38

Keratoconus

Keratoconus, often abbreviated to "KC," is a non-inflammatory eye condition in which the normally round dome-shaped cornea progressively thins causing a cone-like bulge to develop. This results in significant visual impairment. The cornea is the clear window of the eye and is responsible for refracting most of the light coming into the eye. Therefore, abnormalities of the cornea severely affect the way we see the world making simple tasks, like driving, watching TV, or reading a book difficult.

In its earliest stages, keratoconus causes slight blurring and distortion of vision and increased sensitivity to glare and light. These symptoms usually first appear in the late teens and early twenties. Keratoconus may progress for 10 to 20 years and then slow or stabilize. Each eye may be affected differently.

Eyeglasses or soft contact lenses may be used to correct the mild nearsightedness and astigmatism caused in the early stages of keratoconus. As the disorder progresses and the cornea continues to thin and change shape, rigid gas permeable contact lenses are generally prescribed to correct vision more adequately. The contact lenses must be carefully fitted, and frequent checkups and lens changes may be needed to achieve and maintain good vision.

"What Is Keratoconus?" © 2007 National Keratoconus Foundation. Reprinted with permission. For additional information, contact the National Keratoconus Foundation/Discovery Eye Foundation, 8733 Beverly Blvd., Ste 201, Los Angeles, CA 90048, 800-521-2524, 310-623-4466, www.nkcf.org.

In severe cases, a corneal transplant may be needed due to scarring, extreme thinning, or contact lens intolerance. This is a surgical procedure that replaces the keratoconus cornea with healthy donor tissue.

Who Gets Keratoconus?

The actual incidence of KC is not known. It is not a common eye disease, but it is by no means rare. It has been estimated to occur in 1 out of every 2,000 persons in the general population. Keratoconus is generally first diagnosed in young people at puberty or in their late teens. It is found in all parts of the United States and the rest of the world. It has no known significant geographic, cultural, or social pattern.

Living with Keratoconus

People react differently to the news that they have KC. Lack of knowledge often creates fear, so learn all that you can about this condition. Ask questions and discuss your concerns with your doctor and others who have keratoconus. This will be both enlightening and reassuring.

From a medical standpoint, the most important thing you can do is to keep in touch with your eye care practitioner and follow his/her instructions.

From an emotional and psychological standpoint, it is important to understand the nature of keratoconus and to talk freely about it with family and friends to be sure that they understand it. If at all possible, talk with other keratoconus patients. The mutual sharing of common experiences is both rewarding and reassuring.

Perhaps there is no better therapy than sharing your experiences with others in similar circumstances. Self-help groups can be extremely helpful. Support group meetings arranged for this purpose, with the help of the National Keratoconus Foundation, are extremely helpful. For more information about support groups in your area, e-mail the NKCF at: info@nkcf.org.

If none are available near you, another resource is Keratoconus-link (KC-link). This is a free, interactive forum for people with keratoconus—a worldwide support group! KC-link offers those with keratoconus a unique opportunity to share their KC experiences and concerns with others who can truly understand the daily frustrations of this condition. The camaraderie shared and support offered is invaluable. For more information go to www.nkcf.org/kclink.htm.

Those who participate in NKCF self-help groups are, almost without exception, successful in their chosen fields despite this disorder. They empathize that KC should not stop you from accomplishing your goals and might even serve as a motivation. People from all walks of life have experienced this disorder, including many individuals in the entertainment industry, medicine, sports, and business.

Those who handle their KC problems successfully develop their own coping mechanisms. These include wearing sunglasses for driving, carrying extra contact lenses, and planning ahead for local trips, and using a map because reading street signs is often difficult.

While it is important that you accept keratoconus as a fact in your life and realize that you have to adapt to it, it is essential for you to understand that adapting is not surrendering. You control your life; keratoconus does not.

Chapter 39

Retinal and Vitreous Detachment

Chapter Contents

Section 39.1

Retinal Detachment

From "Retinal Detachment Resource Guide," by the
National Eye Institute (NEI, www.nei.nih.gov), part of the
National Institutes of Health, December 2006.

What is retinal detachment?

The retina is the light-sensitive layer of tissue that lines the inside of the eye and sends visual messages through the optic nerve to the brain. When the retina detaches, it is lifted or pulled from its normal position. If not promptly treated, retinal detachment can cause permanent vision loss.

In some cases there may be small areas of the retina that are torn. These areas, called retinal tears or retinal breaks, can lead to retinal detachment.

What are the symptoms of retinal detachment?

Symptoms include a sudden or gradual increase in either the number of floaters, which are little "cobwebs" or specks that float about in your field of vision, and/or light flashes in the eye. Another symptom is the appearance of a curtain over the field of vision. A retinal detachment is a medical emergency. Anyone experiencing the symptoms of a retinal detachment should see an eye care professional immediately.

What are the different types of retinal detachment?

There are three different types of retinal detachment:

- **Rhegmatogenous:** A tear or break in the retina allows fluid to get under the retina and separate it from the retinal pigment epithelium (RPE), the pigmented cell layer that nourishes the retina. These types of retinal detachments are the most common.

- **Tractional:** In this type of detachment, scar tissue on the retina's surface contracts and causes the retina to separate from the RPE. This type of detachment is less common.

- **Exudative:** Frequently caused by retinal diseases, including inflammatory disorders and injury/trauma to the eye. In this type, fluid leaks into the area underneath the retina, but there are no tears or breaks in the retina.

Who is at risk for retinal detachment?

A retinal detachment can occur at any age, but it is more common in people over age 40. It affects men more than women, and Whites more than African Americans.

A retinal detachment is also more likely to occur in people who:

- are extremely nearsighted;

- have had a retinal detachment in the other eye;

- have a family history of retinal detachment;

- have had cataract surgery;

- have other eye diseases or disorders, such as retinoschisis, uveitis, degenerative myopia, or lattice degeneration; or

- have had an eye injury.

How is retinal detachment treated?

Small holes and tears are treated with laser surgery or a freeze treatment called cryopexy. These procedures are usually performed in the doctor's office. During laser surgery tiny burns are made around the hole to "weld" the retina back into place. Cryopexy freezes the area around the hole and helps reattach the retina.

Retinal detachments are treated with surgery that may require the patient to stay in the hospital. In some cases a scleral buckle, a tiny synthetic band, is attached to the outside of the eyeball to gently push the wall of the eye against the detached retina. If necessary, a vitrectomy may also be performed. During a vitrectomy, the doctor makes a tiny incision in the sclera (white of the eye). Next, a small instrument is placed into the eye to remove the vitreous, a gel-like substance that fills the center of the eye and helps the eye maintain a round shape. Gas is often injected to into the eye to replace the vitreous and reattach the retina; the gas pushes the retina back against the wall of the eye. During the healing process, the eye makes fluid that gradually replaces the gas and fills the eye. With all of these procedures, either laser or cryopexy is used to "weld" the retina back in place.

With modern therapy, over 90 percent of those with a retinal detachment can be successfully treated, although sometimes a second treatment is needed. However, the visual outcome is not always predictable. The final visual result may not be known for up to several months following surgery. Even under the best of circumstances, and even after multiple attempts at repair, treatment sometimes fails and vision may eventually be lost. Visual results are best if the retinal detachment is repaired before the macula (the center region of the retina responsible for fine, detailed vision) detaches. That is why it is important to contact an eye care professional immediately if you see a sudden or gradual increase in the number of floaters and/or light flashes, or a dark curtain over the field of vision.

National Eye Institute-Supported Research

The NEI supported The Silicone Study, a nationwide clinical trial that compared the use of silicone oil with long-acting intraocular gas for repairing a retinal detachment caused by proliferative vitreoretinopathy (PVR). With PVR, cells grow on the surface of the retina causing it to detach. This is a serious complication that sometimes follows retinal detachment surgery and is difficult to treat. The results indicate that both treatments are effective and give the surgeons more options for treating these difficult cases. More information on The Silicone Study is available at http://www.nei.nih.gov/neitrials/static/study39.asp.

Section 39.2

Vitreous Detachment

From "Facts About Vitreous Detachment," by the
National Eye Institute (NEI, www.nei.nih.gov), part of the
National Institutes of Health, December 2006.

Most of the eye's interior is filled with vitreous, a gel-like substance that helps the eye maintain a round shape. There are millions of fine fibers intertwined within the vitreous that are attached to the surface of the retina, the eye's light-sensitive tissue. As we age, the vitreous slowly shrinks, and these fine fibers pull on the retinal surface. Usually the fibers break, allowing the vitreous to separate and shrink from the retina. This is a vitreous detachment. In most cases, a vitreous detachment is not sight-threatening and requires no treatment.

As the vitreous shrinks, it becomes somewhat stringy, and the strands can cast tiny shadows on the retina that you may notice as floaters, which appear as little "cobwebs" or specks that seem to float about in your field of vision. If you try to look at these shadows they appear to quickly dart out of the way. One symptom of a vitreous detachment is a small but sudden increase in the number of new floaters. This increase in floaters may be accompanied by flashes of light (lightning streaks) in your peripheral, or side, vision. In most cases, either you will not notice a vitreous detachment, or you will find it merely annoying because of the increase in floaters.

A vitreous detachment is a common condition that usually affects people over age 50, and is very common after age 80. People who are nearsighted are also at increased risk. Those who have a vitreous detachment in one eye are likely to have one in the other, although it may not happen until years later.

Although a vitreous detachment does not threaten sight, once in a while some of the vitreous fibers pull so hard on the retina that they create a macular hole or lead to a retinal detachment. Both of these conditions are sight-threatening and should be treated immediately. If left untreated, a macular hole or detached retina can lead to permanent vision loss in the affected eye. Those who experience a sudden increase in floaters or an increase in flashes of light in peripheral

337

vision should have an eye care professional examine their eyes as soon as possible. The only way to diagnose the cause of the problem is by a comprehensive dilated eye examination. If the vitreous detachment has led to a macular hole or detached retina, early treatment can help prevent loss of vision.

Chapter 40

Macular Hole

What is a macular hole?

A macular hole is a small break in the macula, located in the center of the eye's light-sensitive tissue called the retina. The macula provides the sharp, central vision we need for reading, driving, and seeing fine detail.

A macular hole can cause blurred and distorted central vision. Macular holes are related to aging and usually occur in people over age 60.

Is a macular hole the same as age-related macular degeneration?

No. Macular holes and age-related macular degeneration are two separate and distinct conditions, although the symptoms for each are similar. Both conditions are common in people 60 and over. An eye care professional will know the difference.

What causes a macular hole?

Most of the eye's interior is filled with vitreous, a gel-like substance that fills about 80 percent of the eye and helps it maintain a round shape. The vitreous contains millions of fine fibers that are attached

From "Macular Hole Resource Guide," by the National Eye Institute (NEI, www.nei.nih.gov), part of the National Institutes of Health, December 2006.

to the surface of the retina. As we age, the vitreous slowly shrinks and pulls away from the retinal surface. Natural fluids fill the area where the vitreous has contracted. This is normal. In most cases, there are no adverse effects. Some patients may experience a small increase in floaters, which are little "cobwebs" or specks that seem to float about in your field of vision.

However, if the vitreous is firmly attached to the retina when it pulls away, it can tear the retina and create a macular hole. Also, once the vitreous has pulled away from the surface of the retina, some of the fibers can remain on the retinal surface and can contract. This increases tension on the retina and can lead to a macular hole. In either case, the fluid that has replaced the shrunken vitreous can then seep through the hole onto the macula, blurring and distorting central vision.

Macular holes can also occur from eye disorders, such as high myopia (nearsightedness), macular pucker, and retinal detachment; eye disease, such diabetic retinopathy and Best disease; and injury to the eye.

What are the symptoms of a macular hole?

Macular holes often begin gradually. In the early stage of a macular hole, people may notice a slight distortion or blurriness in their straight-ahead vision. Straight lines or objects can begin to look bent or wavy. Reading and performing other routine tasks with the affected eye become difficult.

Are there different types of a macular hole?

Yes. There are three stages to a macular hole:

- Foveal detachments (Stage I). Without treatment, about half of Stage I macular holes will progress.

- Partial-thickness holes (Stage II). Without treatment, about 70 percent of Stage II macular holes will progress.

- Full-thickness holes (Stage III).

The size of the hole and its location on the retina determine how much it will affect a person's vision. When a Stage III macular hole develops, most central and detailed vision can be lost. If left untreated, a macular hole can lead to a detached retina, a sight-threatening condition that should receive immediate medical attention.

How is a macular hole treated?

Although some macular holes can seal themselves and require no treatment, surgery is necessary in many cases to help improve vision. In this surgical procedure—called a vitrectomy—the vitreous gel is removed to prevent it from pulling on the retina and replaced with a bubble containing a mixture of air and gas. The bubble acts as an internal, temporary bandage that holds the edge of the macular hole in place as it heals. Surgery is performed under local anesthesia and often on an outpatient basis.

Following surgery, patients must remain in a face-down position, normally for a day or two but sometimes for as long as two to three weeks. This position allows the bubble to press against the macula and be gradually reabsorbed by the eye, sealing the hole. As the bubble is reabsorbed, the vitreous cavity refills with natural eye fluids.

Maintaining a face-down position is crucial to the success of the surgery. Because this position can be difficult for many people, it is important to discuss this with your doctor before surgery.

What are the risks of surgery?

The most common risk following macular hole surgery is an increase in the rate of cataract development. In most patients, a cataract can progress rapidly, and often becomes severe enough to require removal. Other less common complications include infection and retinal detachment either during surgery or afterward, both of which can be immediately treated.

For a few months after surgery, patients are not permitted to travel by air. Changes in air pressure may cause the bubble in the eye to expand, increasing pressure inside the eye.

How successful is this surgery?

Vision improvement varies from patient to patient. People that have had a macular hole for less than six months have a better chance of recovering vision than those who have had one for a longer period. Discuss vision recovery with your doctor before your surgery. Vision recovery can continue for as long as three months after surgery.

What if I cannot remain in a face-down position after the surgery?

If you cannot remain in a face-down position for the required period after surgery, vision recovery may not be successful. People who are unable to remain in a face-down position for this length of time may not be good candidates for a vitrectomy. However, there are a number of devices that can make the face-down recovery period easier on you. There are also some approaches that can decrease the amount of face-down time. Discuss these with your doctor.

Is my other eye at risk?

If a macular hole exists in one eye, there is a 10 percent to 15 percent chance that a macular hole will develop in your other eye over your lifetime. Your doctor can discuss this with you.

Chapter 41

Macular Pucker

What are other names for macular pucker?

Names for macular pucker include epiretinal membrane, preretinal membrane, cellophane maculopathy, retina wrinkle, surface wrinkling retinopathy, premacular fibrosis, and internal limiting membrane disease.

What is a macular pucker?

A macular pucker is scar tissue that has formed on the eye's macula, located in the center of the eye's light-sensitive tissue called the retina. The macula provides the sharp, central vision we need for reading, driving, and seeing fine detail. A macular pucker can cause blurred and distorted central vision.

Most of the eye's interior is filled with vitreous, a gel-like substance that fills about 80 percent of the eye and helps it maintain a round shape. The vitreous contains millions of fine fibers that are attached to the surface of the retina. As we age, the vitreous slowly shrinks and pulls away from the retinal surface. This is called a vitreous detachment, and is normal. In most cases, there are no adverse effects, except for a small increase in floaters, which are little "cobwebs" or specks that seem to float about in your field of vision.

From "Macular Pucker Resource Guide," by the National Eye Institute (NEI, www.nei.nih.gov), part of the National Institutes of Health, December 2006.

However, sometimes when the vitreous pulls away from the retina, there is microscopic damage to the retina's surface (Note: This is not a macular hole). When this happens, the retina begins a healing process to the damaged area and forms scar tissue, or an epiretinal membrane, on the surface of the retina. This scar tissue is firmly attached to the retina surface. When the scar tissue contracts, it causes the retina to wrinkle, or pucker, usually without any effect on central vision. However, if the scar tissue has formed over the macula, our sharp, central vision becomes blurred and distorted.

What causes a macular pucker?

Most macular puckers are related to vitreous detachment, which usually occurs in people over age 50. As you age, you are at increased risk for macular pucker.

A macular pucker can also be triggered by certain eye diseases and disorders, such as a detached retina and inflammation of the eye (uveitis). Also, people with diabetes sometimes develop an eye disease called diabetic retinopathy, which can cause a macular pucker. A macular pucker can also be caused by trauma from either surgery or an eye injury.

What are the symptoms of a macular pucker?

Vision loss from a macular pucker can vary from no loss to severe loss, although severe vision loss is uncommon. People with a macular pucker may notice that their vision is blurry or mildly distorted, and straight lines can appear wavy. They may have difficulty in seeing fine detail and reading small print. There may be a gray area in the center of your vision, or perhaps even a blind spot.

Is a macular pucker the same as age-related macular degeneration?

No. A macular pucker and age-related macular degeneration are two separate and distinct conditions, although the symptoms for each are similar. An eye care professional will know the difference.

Can macular pucker get worse?

For most people, vision remains stable and does not get progressively worse. Usually macular pucker affects one eye, although it may affect the other eye later.

Is a macular pucker similar to a macular hole?

A macular pucker and a macular hole are different conditions, although they both result from the same reason: The pulling on the retina from a shrinking vitreous. When the pulling causes microscopic damage, the retina can heal itself; scar tissue, or a macular pucker, can be the result. If the shrinking vitreous pulls too hard, it can tear the retina, creating a macular hole, which is more serious. Both conditions have similar symptoms—distorted and blurred vision. Also, a macular pucker will not develop into a macular hole. An eye care professional will know the difference.

How is a macular pucker treated?

A macular pucker usually requires no treatment. In many cases, the symptoms of vision distortion and blurriness are mild, and no treatment is necessary. People usually adjust to the mild visual distortion, since it does not affect activities of daily life, such as reading and driving. Neither eyedrops, medications, nor nutritional supplements will improve vision distorted from macular pucker. Sometimes the scar tissue—which causes a macular pucker—separates from the retina, and the macular pucker clears up.

Rarely, vision deteriorates to the point where it affects daily routine activities. However, when this happens, surgery may be recommended. This procedure is called a vitrectomy, in which the vitreous gel is removed to prevent it from pulling on the retina and replaced with a salt solution (Because the vitreous is mostly water, you will notice no change between the salt solution and the normal vitreous). Also, the scar tissue which causes the wrinkling is removed. A vitrectomy is usually performed under local anesthesia.

After the operation, you will need to wear an eye patch for a few days or weeks to protect the eye. You will also need to use medicated eyedrops to protect against infection.

How successful is this surgery?

Surgery to repair a macular pucker is very delicate, and while vision improves in most cases, it does not usually return to normal. On average, about half of the vision lost from a macular pucker is restored; some people have significantly more vision restored, some less. In most cases, vision distortion is significantly reduced. Recovery of vision can take up to three months. Patients should talk with their eye care professional about whether treatment is appropriate.

What are the risks of surgery?

The most common complication of a vitrectomy is an increase in the rate of cataract development. Cataract surgery may be needed within a few years after the vitrectomy. Other, less common complications are retinal detachment either during or after surgery, and infection after surgery. Also, the macular pucker may grow back, but this is rare.

What research is being done?

Research studies are being conducted to determine other treatments for macular pucker. Please note that both of the procedures described below need additional clinical testing. We suggest you share this information with your eye care professional.

Some physicians are researching the use of a surgical procedure in which scar tissue is peeled off without performing the vitrectomy.

Other doctors are researching a new surgical technique to remove the internal limiting membrane (a layer of the retina) for patients with both macular pucker and macular hole. This surgical technique is called Fluidic Internal Limiting Membrane Separation (FILMS). After a vitrectomy, fluid is injected between the membrane and the retina that causes the membrane, along with the scar tissue, to lift away. It is then removed with forceps.

Chapter 42

Retinal Vein Occlusion

What is retinal vein occlusion?

The eye is often compared to a camera. The front of the eye contains a lens that focuses images on the inside of the back of the eye. This area, called the retina, is covered with special nerve cells that react to light.

Nerve cells need a constant supply of blood to deliver oxygen and nutrients. Most people understand what happens in a "stroke." A small blood clot blocks the flow of blood through one of the arteries in the brain, and the area that is not getting blood becomes damaged. This same type of damage can happen to nerve cells anywhere in the body, not just the brain.

When the flow of blood through the retina is blocked, it is often because of a retinal vein occlusion. If this happens, the nerve cells of the retina can die and vision will be lost. Because all of the blood from the retina drains through one large vein, a blockage of that vein can affect all the vision in that eye.

Why do people get retinal vein occlusion?

Retinal vein occlusion happens when a blood clot or other substance in the blood, such as cholesterol, blocks the vein. Sometimes it happens

"Retinal Vein Occlusion," © 2006 The Cleveland Clinic Cole Eye Institute, 9500 Euclid Avenue Mail Stop W14, Cleveland, OH 44195, www.clevelandclinic .org/eye. Additional information is available from the Cleveland Clinic Health Information Center, 216-444-3771, toll-free 800-223-2273 extension 43771, or at http://www.clevelandclinic.org/health.

because the veins of the eye are too narrow. It is more likely to occur in people with diabetes, high blood pressure, high cholesterol levels, or other health problems that affect blood flow.

How does the doctor know whether someone has a retinal vein occlusion?

The symptoms of retinal vein occlusion are usually very obvious. There is a sudden, painless blurring or loss of vision. It almost always happens in just one eye. At first, the blurring or loss of vision might be slight, but it gets worse over the next few hours or days. Sometimes there is a complete loss of vision almost immediately.

If these symptoms occur, it is important to schedule an appointment with your doctor as soon as possible. Retinal vein occlusion often causes permanent damage to the retina and loss of vision. It can also lead to other eye problems.

How is retinal vein occlusion treated?

Unfortunately, there is no way to actually unblock retinal veins. However, the doctor can treat any health problems that seem to be related to the retinal vein occlusion.

Vision can rarely come back in some eyes that have had a retinal vein occlusion. In most eyes, the vision will not get better, but it will not get any worse either.

Sometimes the retinal vein occlusion will cause a dangerous condition called neovascular glaucoma. In neovascular glaucoma, abnormal blood vessels start growing inside the eye, and the pressure in the eye starts increasing. This can permanently destroy all vision in the eye. It can also cause great pain and cause the eye to deteriorate physically. If this condition seems likely to develop, your doctor might recommend a treatment called laser photocoagulation.

What happens in laser photocoagulation?

In laser photocoagulation, the surgeon focuses a laser beam onto multiple small spots on the retina where the abnormal blood vessels are growing. The laser beam heats up those spots, creating a tiny burn in the retina and stopping the growth.

This treatment is usually effective in stopping the growth of the blood vessels, but it will not bring back any vision that has been lost. Unfortunately, there is no known way to reverse the damage that is done by the more severe forms of retinal vein occlusion and neovascular glaucoma. The goal of treatment is to prevent further damage and possible loss of the eye itself.

Chapter 43

Disorders Linked to Retinal Degeneration

Chapter Contents

Section 43.1

Bardet-Biedl Syndrome

What is Bardet-Biedl syndrome?

Bardet-Biedl syndrome is a complex disorder that affects many parts of the body including the retina. Individuals with this syndrome have a retinal degeneration similar to retinitis pigmentosa (RP).

What are the symptoms?

The diagnosis of Bardet-Biedl syndrome is usually confirmed in childhood when visual problems due to RP are discovered. The first symptom of RP is night blindness. Night blindness makes it difficult to see in low light levels. RP then causes a progressive loss of peripheral (side) vision. Peripheral vision loss is often referred to as tunnel vision. Individuals with Bardet-Biedl also experience central vision loss during childhood or adolescence. RP symptoms progress rapidly and usually lead to severe visual impairment by early adulthood.

In addition to RP, polydactyly (extra fingers and/or toes) and obesity are defining characteristics of Bardet-Biedl syndrome. A diagnosis of Bardet-Biedl syndrome is usually first suspected when a child is born with polydactyly. Subsequent RP symptoms and obesity confirm the diagnosis. Extra fingers and toes are usually removed in infancy or early childhood. Slight webbing (extra skin) between fingers and between toes is also common. Most individuals have short, broad feet as well. Obesity may be present by childhood and is usually limited to the trunk of the body. Many individuals are also shorter than average.

Approximately half of all individuals with Bardet-Biedl syndrome experience developmental disabilities ranging from mild impairment or delayed emotional development to mental retardation. The degree of mental retardation can range from mild cognitive disability to severe mental retardation.

Individuals may also experience renal (kidney) disease. Renal abnormalities can affect the structure and the function of the kidneys and can lead to severe renal impairment.

Upon reaching adulthood, males with Bardet-Biedl syndrome can have small genitalia (testes and penis). Because female sexual organ size is more difficult to assess, it is not known how many women have this characteristic. Females with Bardet-Biedl can experience irregular menstrual cycles.

Is it an inherited disease?

Bardet-Biedl syndrome is genetically passed through families by the autosomal recessive pattern of inheritance.[1] In this type of inheritance both parents, called carriers, have one gene for the syndrome paired with one normal gene.[2] Each of their children then has a 25 percent chance (or 1 chance in 4) of inheriting the two Bardet-Biedl genes (one from each parent) needed to cause the disorder.[3] Carriers are unaffected because they have only one copy of the gene.[4] At this time, it is impossible to determine who is a carrier for Bardet-Biedl syndrome until after the birth of an affected child.

What treatment is available?

There are no treatments for all of the characteristics associated with Bardet-Biedl syndrome. As vision worsens, individuals will benefit from the use of low-vision aids and orientation as well as from mobility training. To manage the complications of renal disease associated with Bardet-Biedl syndrome, every individual with the disorder should be examined by a nephrologist, a physician who specializes in kidney diseases.

Are there other related syndromes?

Bardet-Biedl syndrome is often confused with Laurence-Moon syndrome. Individuals with Laurence-Moon syndrome almost always experience neurologic problems but rarely polydactyly. Polydactyly is a defining feature of Bardet-Biedl syndrome, while neurologic problems almost never occur. Laurence-Moon syndrome is extremely rare; only a few cases have been documented. Because of the similarity of these syndromes, Bardet-Biedl syndrome is often referred to as Laurence-Moon/Bardet-Biedl syndrome or Laurence-Moon/Biedl syndrome.

Health Reference Series *Medical Advisor's Notes and Updates*

1. At least eight different genes appear to be capable of causing Bardet-Biedl syndrome. There appear to be complex interactions among these genes, and this may account for the wide variation in features from patient to patient.

2. Carriers have at least one abnormal gene paired with normal genes.

3. The disorder is caused when children inherit a sufficient number of Bardet-Biedl genes (some coming from each parent).

4. Carriers are unaffected because they don't have enough abnormal copies of the genes to cause the disorder.

Section 43.2

Choroideremia

Reprinted with permission from "Choroideremia," © 2002 The Foundation Fighting Blindness (www.blindness.org). All rights reserved. The text that follows this document under the heading *"Health Reference Series* Medical Advisor's Notes and Updates" was provided to Omnigraphics by David A. Cooke, M.D., June 27, 2007. Dr. Cooke is not affiliated with the Foundation Fighting Blindness.

Choroideremia is a rare inherited disorder that causes progressive loss of vision due to degeneration of the choroid and retina.

What are the symptoms?

Choroideremia, formerly called tapetochoroidal dystrophy, occurs almost exclusively in males. In childhood, night blindness is the most common first symptom. As the disease progresses, there is loss of peripheral vision or "tunnel vision," and later a loss of central vision. Progression of the disease continues throughout the individual's life, although both the rate and the degree of visual loss can vary, even within the same family.

Vision loss due to choroideremia is caused by degeneration of several layers of cells that are essential to sight. These layers, which line the inside of the back of the eye, are called the choroids, the retinal pigment epithelium and the photoreceptors. The choroid consists of several blood vessel layers that are located between the retina and the sclera (the white of the eye). Choroidal vessels provide the retinal pigment epithelium and photoreceptors with oxygen and nutrients necessary for normal function. The retinal pigment epithelium and the photoreceptors are part of the retina. The epithelium is associated closely with the photoreceptors and is needed for normal function. The photoreceptors are responsible for converting light into the electrical impulses that transfer messages to the brain where "seeing" actually occurs.

The retinal pigment epithelium and the choroid initially deteriorate to cause choroideremia. Eventually, the photoreceptors break down as well. As the disease progresses, the clinical appearance of these cell layers changes in a characteristic manner and more vision is lost.

Is it an inherited disease?

Choroideremia is genetically passed through families by the X-linked pattern of inheritance. In this type of inheritance, the gene for the disease is located on the X chromosome. Females have two X chromosomes and can carry the disease gene on one of their X chromosomes. Because they have a healthy version of the gene on their other X chromosome, carrier females typically are not affected by X-linked diseases such as juvenile retinoschisis. Sometimes, however, when carrier females are examined, the retina shows minor signs of the disease.[1]

Males have only one X chromosome (paired with one Y chromosome) and are therefore genetically susceptible to X-linked diseases. Males cannot be carriers of X-linked diseases. Males affected with an X-linked disease always pass the gene on the X chromosome to their daughters, who then become carriers. Affected males never pass an X-linked disease gene to their sons because fathers pass the Y chromosome to their sons.

Female carriers have a 50 percent chance (or 1 chance in 2) of passing the X-linked disease gene to their daughters, who become carriers, and a 50 percent chance of passing the gene to their sons, who are then affected by the disease.

What treatment is available?

Recently, scientists discovered mutations on a gene on the X chromosome that causes choroideremia.[2] New research based on these findings now drives the search for a treatment. However, at present there is no effective treatment or cure.

Choroideremia is one of the few retinal degenerative diseases that might be detected prenatally in some cases; female carriers may want to seek information about this testing from a medical geneticist or a genetic counselor. All members of an affected family are encouraged to consult an ophthalmologist and to seek genetic counseling. These professionals can provide explanations of the disease and the recurrence risk for all family members and for future offspring.

Until a treatment is discovered, help is available through low vision aids, including optical, electronic, and computer-based devices. Personal, educational, and vocational counseling, as well as adaptive training skills, job placement, and income assistance, are available through community resources.

Are there any other related diseases?

Early in the course of the disease[3], choroideremia could be confused with X-linked retinitis pigmentosa. Both have symptoms of night blindness and tunnel vision. However, differences[4] are clear in a complete medical eye examination, especially as the disease progresses. The disease most similar clinically to choroideremia is gyrate atrophy. It too can be distinguished based on its inheritance, as an autosomal recessive disorder, and based on its cause, known to be a defect in an unrelated gene.

Health Reference Series *Medical Advisor's Notes and Updates*

1. Very rarely, a female carrier will have symptoms resembling affected males; this occurs when, by random chance, most of her retinal cells are utilizing the defective copy of the gene.

2. Choroideremia has been determined to be due to mutations in a gene on the X-chromosome that produces Rab escort protein

1 (REP-1). It is not completely understood how these mutations actually cause the retinal changes in choroideremia.

3. There are a number of diseases that cause degeneration of the retina, and in their earliest stages, it is sometimes difficult to tell them apart.

4. These differences involve the pattern of retinal involvement.

Section 43.3

Leber Congenital Amaurosis

What is Leber Congenital Amaurosis?

Leber congenital amaurosis (LCA) is an inherited retinal degenerative disease characterized by severe loss of vision at birth. A variety of other eye-related abnormalities including roving eye movements, deep-set eyes, and sensitivity to bright light also occur with this disease. Some patients with LCA also experience central nervous system abnormalities.

What are the symptoms?

Individuals with LCA have very reduced vision at birth. Within an infant's first few months of life, parents usually notice a lack of visual responsiveness and unusual roving eye movements, known as nystagmus. Eye examinations of infants with LCA reveal normal appearing retinas. However, electroretinography (ERG) tests, which measure visual function, detect little if any activity in the retina. A low level of retinal activity, measured by ERG, indicates very little visual function. ERG tests are key to establishing a diagnosis of LCA.

By early adolescence, various changes in the retinas of patients with LCA become readily apparent. Blood vessels often become narrow and constricted. A variety of pigmentary (color) changes can also occur in the retinal pigment epithelium (RPE), the supportive tissue underlying the retina. Sometimes, pigmentary changes are similar to another retinal degenerative disease known as retinitis pigmentosa.

Although the appearance of the retina undergoes marked changes with age, vision usually remains fairly stable through young adult life. Long-term visual prognosis remains to be defined. Visual acuity in patients with LCA is usually limited to the level of counting fingers or detecting hand motions or bright lights. Some patients are also extremely sensitive to light (photophobia). Patients with remaining vision are often extremely farsighted.

Many children with LCA habitually press on their eyes with their fists or fingers. This habitual pressing on the eyes is known clinically as oculodigital reflex. The eyes of individuals with LCA also usually appear sunken or deep set. Keratoconus (cone shape to the front of the eye) and cataracts (clouding of the lens, the clear, glass-like structure through which light passes) have also been reported with this disease.

In some cases, LCA is associated with central nervous system complications such as developmental delay, epilepsy, and motor skill impairment. Because LCA is relatively rare, the frequency of central nervous system complications is unknown.

Is it an inherited disease?

LCA is most typically passed through families by the autosomal recessive pattern of inheritance. In this type of inheritance, both parents, called carriers, have one gene for the disease paired with one normal gene. Each of their children has a 25 percent chance (or 1 chance in 4) of inheriting the two LCA genes (one from each parent) needed to cause the disorder. Carriers are unaffected because they have only one copy of the gene. At this time, it is impossible to determine who is a carrier for LCA until after the birth of an affected child.

Are there any other related diseases?

Initially, LCA can be confused with early onset retinitis pigmentosa (RP), congenital and hereditary optic atrophy, cortical blindness, congenital stationary night blindness, flecked retina syndrome, and achromatopsia. Although similarly named, LCA should not be confused

358

with Leber optic atrophy. In addition, there are syndromes seen in infancy where visual impairment at birth is a component. A thorough ophthalmologic examination including diagnostic tests measuring retinal function and an accurate documentation of family history can distinguish between these related conditions.

What treatment is available?

Currently, there is no treatment for LCA. However, scientists have isolated four[1] genes that contain mutations that can each cause LCA.[2] Ongoing scientific research is directed toward understanding how these genes function in the retina and toward locating the remaining genes that cause LCA. With this information, scientists can better develop a means of prevention and treatment.

Some individuals with LCA, who have remaining vision, may benefit from the use of low-vision aids, including electronic, computer-based, and optical aids. Orientation and mobility training, adaptive training skills, job placement, and income assistance are available through community resources.

Health Reference Series *Medical Advisor's Notes and Updates*

1. Six genes have now been isolated.

2. Current data suggests that LCA may actually be a group of several diseases, each with different causes, but producing similar symptoms and retinal changes.

Section 43.4

Retinitis Pigmentosa

© 2007 A.D.A.M., Inc. Reprinted with permission.

Definition

Retinitis pigmentosa is an eye disease in which there is damage to the retina. The damage gets worse (progresses) over time. People with this condition have problems with night vision and peripheral vision.

Causes, Incidence, and Risk Factors

Retinitis pigmentosa commonly runs in families. The disorder can be caused by a number of genetic defects.

The cells controlling night vision (rods) are most likely to be affected. However, in some cases, retinal cone cells are damaged the most. The main sign of the disease is the presence of dark pigmented spots in the retina.

As the disease gets worse, peripheral vision is gradually lost. The condition may eventually lead to blindness, but usually not complete blindness. Signs and symptoms often first appear in childhood, but severe visual problems do not usually develop until early adulthood.

The main risk factor is a family history of retinitis pigmentosa. It is an uncommon condition affecting about 1 in 4,000 people in the United States.

Symptoms

- Vision decreased at night or in reduced light
- Loss of peripheral vision
- Loss of central vision (in advanced cases)

Signs and Tests

Tests determine the integrity of the retina:

- Visual acuity
- Refraction test
- Color defectiveness determination
- Pupillary reflex response
- Slit lamp examination
- Intraocular pressure determination
- Retinal examination by ophthalmoscopy
- Ultrasound of the eye
- Retinal photography
- Fluorescein angiography
- Electroretinogram (a record of the action currents of the retina produced by visual stimuli)

Treatment

There is no effective treatment for this condition. The use of sunglasses to protect the retina from ultraviolet light may help preserve vision.

Controversial studies have suggested that treatment with antioxidant agents (such as vitamin A palmitate) may delay the disease from getting worse.

Referral to a low vision specialist is very helpful. Patients should make regular visits to an eye care specialist to screen for the development of cataracts or retinal swelling—both of which can be treated.

Expectations (Prognosis)

The disorder will continue to progress, although slowly. Complete blindness is uncommon.

Complications

Peripheral and central loss of vision will eventually occur. Many other syndromes with features similar to retinitis pigmentosa have been described, including:

- Friedreich ataxia;
- mucopolysaccharidosis;
- muscular dystrophy (myotonic dystrophy);

- Laurence-Moon syndrome (also called Laurence-Moon-Bardet-Biedl syndrome); and

- Usher syndrome.

Calling Your Health Care Provider

Call your health care provider if night vision becomes difficult or if other symptoms of this disorder develop.

Prevention

Genetic counseling may determine the risk of this disease occurring in a person's children.

Section 43.5

Usher Syndrome

Excerpted from "Usher Syndrome Resource Guide" by the
National Eye Institute (NEI, www.nei.nih.gov), part of the National
Institutes of Health, December 2006.

What is Usher syndrome?

Usher syndrome is an inherited condition that causes 1) a serious hearing loss that is usually present at birth or shortly thereafter and 2) progressive vision loss caused by retinitis pigmentosa (RP). RP is a group of inherited diseases that cause night blindness and peripheral (side) vision loss through the progressive degeneration of the retina, the light-sensitive tissue at the back of the eye that is crucial for vision.

Researchers have described three types of Usher syndrome—type I, type II and type III.

- Individuals with Usher syndrome type I are nearly or completely deaf and experience problems with balance from a young age. They usually begin to exhibit signs of RP in early adolescence.

- Individuals with Usher syndrome type II experience moderate to severe hearing impairment, have normal balance, and experience symptoms of RP later in adolescence.

- Individuals with Usher syndrome type III are born with normal hearing but develop RP and then progressive hearing loss.

How is Usher syndrome inherited?

The Usher syndrome types are inherited as an autosomal recessive trait. This means that an affected person receives one abnormal gene from each of his or her parents. A person who inherits a gene from only one parent will be a carrier, but will not develop the disease.

A person with Usher syndrome must pass on one disease gene to each of his or her children. However, unless the person has children with another carrier of Usher genes, the individual's children are not at risk for developing the disease. Currently we cannot reasonably test everyone for carrier status, but this may change in the years ahead.

How is Usher syndrome diagnosed?

Since individuals with Usher syndrome have both hearing and visual symptoms, we perform testing of both systems. This testing includes:

- visual function tests: visual fields and electroretinogram (ERG);

- a retinal examination;

- hearing tests; and

- balance tests for all patients age 10 years and older.

Although some of the genes that cause Usher syndrome have been identified, the diagnosis is still based on ocular and clinical testing.

Is genetic testing for Usher syndrome available?

At this time, genetic testing for Usher syndrome is done only as part of research projects. This is due to many factors. Usher syndrome is not caused by only one gene. So far, 10 Usher genes have been mapped: 7 for type I, 3 for type II, and 1 for type 3. There are still more genes to find. A few of these genes have been sequenced and described. These are MYO7A, harmonin, CDH23, PCDH15, all causing type I. The usherin gene causes type II disease.

Finding the genes is a very important advance in the fight against Usher syndrome. Further study is required to characterize these genes, and determine how the mutated genes cause Usher syndrome. Additional genes that cause Usher syndrome also need to be identified. Several researchers throughout the world are working on Usher syndrome. Findings from this research may one day allow treatments for Usher syndrome to be developed.

Section 43.6

Juvenile Retinoschisis

What is juvenile retinoschisis?

Juvenile retinoschisis is an inherited disease diagnosed in childhood that causes progressive loss of central and peripheral (side) vision due to degeneration of the retina.

What are the symptoms?

Juvenile retinoschisis, also known as X-linked retinoschisis, occurs almost exclusively in males. Although the condition begins at birth, symptoms do not typically become apparent until after the age of 10. About half of all patients diagnosed with juvenile retinoschisis first notice a decline in vision. Other early symptoms of the disease include an inability of both eyes to focus on an object (strabismus) and roving, involuntary eye movements (nystagmus).

Vision loss associated with juvenile retinoschisis is caused by the splitting of the retina into two layers. This retinal splitting most notably affects the macula, the central portion of the retina responsible for fine visual detail and color perception. On examination, the fovea (the center of the macula) has spoke-like streaks. The spaces created by the separated layers are often filled with blisters and ruptured blood vessels that can leak blood into the vitreous body (the transparent, colorless mass of jelly-like material filling the center of the eye). The presence of blood in the vitreous body causes further visual impairment. The vitreous body degenerates and may eventually separate from the retina. The entire retina may also separate from underlying tissue layers causing retinal detachments.

The extent and rate of vision loss vary greatly among patients with juvenile retinoschisis. Central vision is almost always affected. Peripheral (side) vision loss occurs in about half of all cases. Some patients retain useful vision well into adulthood, while others experience a rapid decline during childhood.

Is it an inherited disease?

Juvenile retinoschisis is genetically passed through families by the X-linked pattern of inheritance. In this type of inheritance, the gene for the disease is located on the X chromosome. Females have two X chromosomes and can carry the disease gene on one of their X chromosomes. Because they have a healthy version of the gene on their other X chromosome, carrier females typically are not affected by X-linked diseases such as juvenile retinoschisis. Sometimes, however, when carrier females are examined, the retina shows minor signs of the disease.

Males have only one X chromosome (paired with one Y chromosome) and are therefore genetically susceptible to X-linked diseases. Males cannot be carriers of X-linked diseases. Males affected with an X-linked disease always pass the gene on the X chromosome to their daughters, who then become carriers. Affected males never pass an X-linked disease gene to their sons because fathers pass the Y chromosome to their sons.

Female carriers have a 50 percent chance (or 1 chance in 2) of passing the X-linked disease gene to their daughters, who become carriers, and a 50 percent chance of passing the gene to their sons, who are then affected by the disease.

What treatment is available?

At this time, there is no treatment for juvenile retinoschisis. However, in some cases, surgery can repair retinal detachments.[1] In 1997, researchers identified mutations in a gene on the X chromosome that cause juvenile retinoschisis. Scientists are now studying the gene to determine its function in the retina. This information will greatly enhance efforts to develop treatments for juvenile retinoschisis. [2, 3]

Individuals with juvenile retinoschisis may benefit from the use of low-vision aids, including electronic, computer-based, and optical aids. Orientation and mobility training, adaptive training skills, job placement, and income assistance are available through community resources.

Are there any other related diseases?

Juvenile retinoschisis can resemble other retinal degenerative diseases such as retinitis pigmentosa (RP), Goldman-Favre vitreoretinal dystrophy, Wagner vitreoretinal dystrophy, and Sticklers syndrome. A thorough ophthalmologic examination, including diagnostic tests measuring retinal function and visual field, combined with an accurate documentation of family history, can distinguish between these diseases.

Health Reference Series *Medical Advisor's Notes and Updates*

1. Studies of surgical management of X-linked retinoschisis have generally shown disappointing results.

2. The responsible gene, retinoschisin (RS1), appears to be important in the adherence of retinal cells to one another. Most tested individual with X-linked retinoschisis have a mutation that prevents this protein from functioning normally, and this presumably responsible for the splitting apart of retinal layers in this disease. The identification of the responsible gene has greatly enhanced efforts to develop treatments for juvenile retinoschisis. Mouse models (strains of laboratory mice which develop changes similar to the human disease) have been developed, and are being used to study potential treatments. Gene therapy, which involves delivering normal copies of the gene to retinal cells, has treated the disease successfully in some of these mouse strains. However, this has not been attempted in humans.

3. There have been a few reports of retinoschisis patients improving when treated with a class of medications known as carbonic anhydrate inhibitors. However, no trials of this therapy have been published. Studies in larger numbers of patients will be necessary to determine whether these drugs are actually effective for this condition.

Chapter 44

Retinopathy of Prematurity

Chapter Contents

Section 44.1

What Is Retinopathy of Prematurity?

Excerpted from "Retinopathy of Prematurity (ROP) Resource Guide," by
the National Eye Institute (NEI, www.nei.nih.gov), part of the National
Institutes of Health, December 2006.

What is retinopathy of prematurity?

Retinopathy of prematurity (ROP) is a potentially blinding eye
disorder that primarily affects premature infants weighing about 2
3/4 pounds (1250 grams) or less that are born before 31 weeks of gestation (A full-term pregnancy has a gestation of 38–42 weeks). The
smaller a baby is at birth, the more likely that baby is to develop ROP.
This disorder—which usually develops in both eyes—is one of the most
common causes of visual loss in childhood and can lead to lifelong
vision impairment and blindness. ROP was first diagnosed in 1942.

How many infants have ROP?

Today, with advances in neonatal care, smaller and more premature infants are being saved. These infants are at a much higher risk
for ROP. Not all babies who are premature develop ROP. There are
approximately 3.9 million infants born in the United States each year;
of those, about 28,000 weigh 2 3/4 pounds or less. About 14,000–16,000
of these infants are affected by some degree of ROP. The disease improves and leaves no permanent damage in milder cases of ROP. About
90 percent of all infants with ROP are in the milder category and do
not need treatment. However, infants with more severe disease can
develop impaired vision or even blindness. About 1,100–1,500 infants
annually develop ROP that is severe enough to require medical treatment. About 400–600 infants each year in the United States become
legally blind from ROP.

What causes ROP?

ROP occurs when abnormal blood vessels grow and spread throughout the retina, the tissue that lines the back of the eye. These abnormal

blood vessels are fragile and can leak, scarring the retina and pulling it out of position. This causes a retinal detachment. Retinal detachment is the main cause of visual impairment and blindness in ROP.

Several complex factors may be responsible for the development of ROP. The eye starts to develop at about 16 weeks of pregnancy, when the blood vessels of the retina begin to form at the optic nerve in the back of the eye. The blood vessels grow gradually toward the edges of the developing retina, supplying oxygen and nutrients. During the last 12 weeks of a pregnancy, the eye develops rapidly. When a baby is born full-term, the retinal blood vessel growth is mostly complete (The retina usually finishes growing a few weeks to a month after birth). But if a baby is born prematurely, before these blood vessels have reached the edges of the retina, normal vessel growth may stop. The edges of the retina—the periphery—may not get enough oxygen and nutrients.

Scientists believe that the periphery of the retina then sends out signals to other areas of the retina for nourishment. As a result, new abnormal vessels begin to grow. These new blood vessels are fragile and weak and can bleed, leading to retinal scarring. When these scars shrink, they pull on the retina, causing it to detach from the back of the eye.

How is ROP treated?

The most effective proven treatments for ROP are laser therapy or cryotherapy. Laser therapy "burns away" the periphery of the retina, which has no normal blood vessels. With cryotherapy, physicians use an instrument that generates freezing temperatures to briefly touch spots on the surface of the eye that overlie the periphery of the retina. Both laser treatment and cryotherapy destroy the peripheral areas of the retina, slowing or reversing the abnormal growth of blood vessels. Unfortunately, the treatments also destroy some side vision. This is done to save the most important part of our sight—the sharp, central vision we need for "straight ahead" activities such as reading, sewing, and driving.

Both laser treatments and cryotherapy are performed only on infants with advanced ROP. Both treatments are considered invasive surgeries on the eye, and doctors don't know the long-term side effects of each.

In the later stages of ROP, other treatment options include:

- **Scleral buckle:** This involves placing a silicone band around the eye and tightening it. This keeps the vitreous gel from pulling on the scar tissue and allows the retina to flatten back down onto the wall of the eye. Infants who have had a sclera buckle need to have the band removed months or years later, since the eye continues to grow; otherwise they will become nearsighted. Sclera buckles are usually performed on infants with stage IV or V.

• **Vitrectomy:** Vitrectomy involves removing the vitreous and replacing it with a saline solution. After the vitreous has been removed, the scar tissue on the retina can be peeled back or cut away, allowing the retina to relax and lay back down against the eye wall. Vitrectomy is performed only at stage V.

Can ROP cause other complications?

Yes. Infants with ROP are considered to be at higher risk for developing certain eye problems later in life, such as retinal detachment, myopia (nearsightedness), strabismus (crossed eyes), amblyopia (lazy eye), and glaucoma. In many cases, these eye problems can be treated or controlled.

Section 44.2

Information for Parents with Children with Retinopathy of Prematurity

"Information for Parents," © 2006 Association for Retinopathy of Prematurity and Related Diseases. Reprinted with permission.

Children who are blind or visually impaired need to enjoy the same experiences that all children enjoy. Blind children should not be coddled. All children fall. All children hurt themselves, and many children break bones during their childhood. Blind children walk independently, take care of themselves independently, and should be expected to do household chores. The following common sense ideas are included to get you started if there are no services readily available to you now.

1. Direct indoor lighting or sunlight coming in through the windows may affect any child's ability to use his vision effectively. Always try to place your child in a position where the light is coming from behind him (over his shoulder), but not casting his shadow on his toys.

2. It is much easier to see things that do not have a glare effect. Glare is produced when the light is reflected off of an object. If you have the choice of a bright laminated top or a wood surface to play on, choose the wood; it will not cause glare.

3. When you go to buy things for your child to play with or to decorate her room try to choose objects that are red, blue, green, yellow, or black and white. All young children are attracted to primary colors. Many children see bright red or bright yellow objects most easily. Watch your child to see if there is a color that she responds to more readily, but often red is the color ROP children respond to first.

4. Try to limit the number of toys your child is playing with. Too many toys just cause clutter and make it difficult to focus on a task.

5. Remember that it is easier to see objects if there is an obvious difference between the object and the background on which the object is presented. Try to always provide the most contrast you can as you play. You may have to change the color of the surface you are working on by placing either a light cloth or a dark cloth over it.

6. The more familiar your child is with a toy, the better he will be able to start looking at smaller parts of that toy. Don't expect him to identify parts before he is really familiar with the whole.

Things to Keep in Mind as You Play with Your Child

One of the most important things you can do for your child is to become the "narrator" of the things she cannot see. Talk to your child, even though she may not be old enough to understand what you are saying. This will help you to begin this narrative habit and it will soon become natural for you. This may seem awkward at first, but early conversational skills enhance all learning for all children. As an example, when you are in the supermarket explain to her what you have bought; let her feel the size and weight of the objects. Talk about the difference in temperature as you walk to the freezer aisles. Have fun, talk, and learn from everyday experiences.

Gradually you should start to relate new objects and experiences to familiar ones. Try to use color words to describe things. You can use small models or pictures for things that are too big to touch, but you must always tell your child that the real object is much larger.

It is extremely important to allow your child to spend time playing on the floor. This play time on the floor is very important for all children. This is how children learn to move their own bodies. When she begins to crawl and later to walk, she will learn to create a mental map of her environment. This is the same thing we do, for instance when we give someone directions to our home.

Activities to Do with Infants

- Try to incorporate a multisensory approach to learning. Toys that make noises when they are moved or manipulated are excellent for this. For example, small rubber dog toys have interesting textures and make noise when they are squeezed.

- Explore body parts on yourself and on your child. Take turns touching each other. There are many traditional songs and games which make this a fun activity.

- Go outside in all kinds of weather and explore the textures and smells of nature.

Activities for Toddlers

- Try real-life activities like sorting clothes and silverware.

- Present big and little versions of familiar things like brushes, combs, rocks, and Slinkys.

- Present unfamiliar things like sea shells and other objects with unusual texture to broaden your child's experiences with unfamiliar textures. This will prevent him from being afraid of touching things that are not, like most toys, made of plastic. Having lots of experiences touching a variety of textures will help him learn to want to explore things on his own. Provide objects that are prickly, smooth, bumpy, cold, warm, and sticky and then make comparisons.

While you might assume that people who work with children and adults with visual impairments will know this, it is not always the case. If your child is about to have drops placed in his eyes, or be given a shot, and the medical professional does not appear to be doing this, you should give your child a verbal warning of what is to come. This will help your child, and may also teach that medical professional a new skill! It may also be helpful to lightly, but firmly, touch the area that is to be affected. A very light touch is more difficult to tolerate than a firmer touch. If your young child needs to be hospitalized, you may want to put a sign over her hospital crib or bed which says something like:

Hi!

I am Samantha. I do not see very well. Please talk to me before you do any medical procedure on me. A firm touch of my body at the spot that you are going to do the procedure will help me know what is coming. It's also very nice if you tell me what you are about to do. I also like just hearing people chat with me. Having people talk to me usually makes me happy.

Thanks.

Sometimes it is hard to remember that caregivers with a child who has special needs often need to take care of themselves too. Allow yourselves the right to take breaks from the daily need of caring for your child. There are several links at ropard.org with contacts for respite care.

Section 44.3

Genetics Influence Retinopathy of Prematurity

This information was provided by KidsHealth, one of the largest resources online for medically reviewed health information written for parents, kids, and teens. For more articles like this one, visit www.KidsHealth.org, or www.TeensHealth.org. © 2006 The Nemours Foundation. Reviewed by Steven Dowshen, M.D., December 2006.

Retinopathy of prematurity (ROP), a condition caused by abnormal growth of the blood vessels in an infant's eye, is common in preemies, affecting more than two thirds of babies born under 2.6 pounds. Even with prevention efforts and treatment, ROP accounts for 3% to 11% of blindness in children. Despite the prevalence and seriousness of this visual problem, doctors can't always determine why some preemies develop it and others don't.

To understand more about the factors that contribute to ROP, researchers studied 63 identical and 137 fraternal twins born at or before 32 weeks of gestation. Because identical twins share 100% of the same genetic information and fraternal twins have at least 50% of the same genetic information, researchers could estimate how much genetic material contributes to the development of ROP. In addition, they noted all interventions the twins received at or after birth, including supplemental oxygen, ventilation, and continuous positive airway pressure (CPAP).

Twenty-two percent of the infants were diagnosed with ROP, and the condition was much more prevalent in smaller, lighter infants. The infant's gestational age before birth and the amount of time spent on supplemental oxygen predicted whether the baby would develop ROP. Based on analysis of the twins, researchers determined that there's a strong genetic predisposition for developing ROP.

What This Means to You

The results of this study indicate that genetic factors play a major role in the development of ROP in infants. If you're pregnant, be sure to get early and regular prenatal care for the benefit of your baby's health. If your baby was born with ROP, an ophthalmologist (a doctor who specializes in treating disorders of the eye) can advise you on any treatments or therapies your child may need.

Often, laser treatment is used to reduce the abnormal blood vessels and prevent the retina from pulling away from the wall of the eye. The good news is that according to the American Association for Pediatric Ophthalmology and Strabismus, treatment for ROP is very effective and drastically reduces the risk of visual impairment.

Source: Matthew J. Bizzarro, M.D.; Naveed Hussain, M.D.; Baldvin Jonsson, M.D.; Rui Feng, Ph.D; Laura R. Ment, M.D.; Jeffrey R. Gruen, M.D.; Heping Zhang, Ph.D; Vineet Bhandari, M.D., D.M.; *Pediatrics,* November 2006.

Section 44.4

Early Treatment of Retinopathy of Prematurity Can Prevent Severe Vision Loss

From a news release of the National Eye Institute
(NEI, www.nei.nih.gov), part of the National Institutes of Health,
December 8, 2003.

An important clinical trial, sponsored by the National Eye Institute (NEI), a part of the National Institutes of Health (NIH), has provided doctors with improved prognostic indicators and treatment options for retinopathy of prematurity (ROP), a blinding disease that affects premature, low birthweight infants. ROP spurs the growth of abnormal blood vessels in the back of the eye. These vessels leak fluid and blood and scar the nerve tissue inside the eye, increasing the risk of retinal detachment and severe vision loss in infants.

Because it follows an unpredictable course, ROP presents doctors with difficult treatment decisions. In many infants the disease spontaneously regresses and spares vision. However, in some infants ROP progresses, resulting in serious visual impairment. Although current therapy can stem its progression, many infants are still blinded by the disease. Due to a lack of clinical criteria to predict which patients will ultimately develop severe vision loss from ROP, ophthalmologists were forced previously to defer treatment until it was clearly indicated. Unfortunately, as it turns out, delaying therapy can leave infants who might benefit more from early treatment with poor visual outcomes.

The Early Treatment for Retinopathy of Prematurity (ETROP) study results, published in the December [2003] issue of the *Archives of Ophthalmology*, demonstrated that premature infants, who are at the highest risk for developing vision loss from ROP, will retain better vision when therapy is administered in the early stage of the disease. This treatment approach was found to be better than waiting until ROP has reached the traditional treatment threshold. Just as importantly, the study also established the value of an improved risk assessment model to more accurately identify those infants who are at the highest risk for developing severe vision loss from ROP.

"Premature, low birthweight infants face a host of medical complications with lifelong consequences. The results of this study allow us to improve treatment for ROP and, hopefully, the quality of life for children who most need sight-saving therapy," said Paul A. Sieving, M.D., Ph.D., director of the NEI.

"This is a great step forward in research to treat blinding eye diseases," said National Institutes of Health Director Elias Zerhouni, M.D. "The NIH will continue to look for new ways to treat and even prevent ROP, which is one of the leading causes of severe vision loss in infants and young children."

Each year ROP affects an estimated 14,000 to 16,000 premature, low birthweight infants in the United States and thousands more worldwide, making it a leading cause of vision loss in children. Of these cases, approximately 1,500 infants will develop severe ROP that requires treatment. Despite available treatment, about 400 to 600 infants with ROP still become legally blind each year. Researchers have identified birthweight of 2.75 pounds (1250 grams) or less as a major risk factor for developing ROP.

The previous standard treatment threshold for ROP hinged on the disease having progressed enough that the risk of retinal detachment approached 50 percent. As part of the ETROP study, a new computerized risk model, developed by NEI-supported researchers, was used to identify high-risk infants early in the disease. The risk model assessed birthweight, ethnicity, being a single or multiple birth baby, gestational age, ophthalmic exam findings, and whether the infant had been born in a hospital that participated in the study. "This new risk assessment model proved invaluable in the early detection of infants who have a high risk of blindness and may require treatment. It also allowed us to better identify and monitor those patients who are less likely to require treatment," said Robert J. Hardy, Ph.D., the University of Texas School of Public Health at Houston researcher who led the efforts to develop this improved risk model.

Once identified, the infants were then assigned randomly either to treatment at the standard threshold (50 percent chance of retinal detachment) or to early treatment. Researchers found that early treatment significantly reduced the likelihood of poor vision from 19.5 to 14.5 percent at about one year of age. Early treatment also considerably reduced the likelihood of structural damage to the eye from 15.6 to 9.1 percent.

Current treatments for ROP involve laser therapy or cryotherapy. Laser therapy uses heat from light energy while cryotherapy uses freezing temperatures to retard blood vessel growth. A consequence of these treatments, known clinically as blood vessel ablation, is a partial loss of peripheral or side vision. Nonetheless, treatment is valuable in preserving the most important part of our sight—the sharp, central vision we need to read, see faces, or perform detailed tasks that require hand-eye coordination.

"It is crucial that infants with high-risk ROP be identified early and be given timely treatment," said the chair of the study William Good, M.D., of the Smith-Kettlewell Eye Research Institute in San Francisco. "Early treatment could save infants from a lifetime of visual impairment. The results also clearly indicate that for certain subgroups of eyes, watchful waiting and not immediate treatment is the best approach."

The study will continue to follow these infants until age six to ensure that the benefits of early treatment persist into childhood. "Because visual acuity continues to develop during infancy and early childhood, the long-term effect of early treatment on visual development is not yet fully known. We expect that the significant benefits to vision found in this study will persist into childhood, but we have to be sure," Dr. Good said.

The study was conducted at 26 participating centers in the United States.

Chapter 45

Sjögren Syndrome

What Is Sjögren's Syndrome?

Sjögren's (pronounced SHOW-grins) syndrome is a chronic autoimmune inflammatory disease in which moisture-producing glands are damaged, significantly decreasing the quantity and quality of saliva and tears. The disease was first identified by a Swedish physician, Henrik Sjögren, in 1933.

Although the hallmark symptoms are dry eyes and dry mouth, Sjögren's also may cause dysfunction of other organs, affecting the kidneys, gastrointestinal system, blood vessels, lungs, liver, pancreas, and the nervous system. Patients may experience extreme fatigue and joint pain and have a higher risk of lymphoma. Sjögren's is one of the most prevalent autoimmune disorders, striking as many as 4,000,000 Americans. Nine out of ten patients are women.

About half of the time Sjögren's syndrome occurs alone, and the other half it occurs in the presence of another connective tissue disease such as rheumatoid arthritis, lupus, or scleroderma. When Sjögren's occurs alone, it is referred to as primary Sjögren's. When it occurs with another connective tissue disease, it is referred to as secondary Sjögren's. All instances of Sjögren's syndrome are systemic, affecting the entire body. Symptoms may plateau, worsen, or, uncommonly, go into remission. While some people experience mild discomfort, others suffer debilitating symptoms that greatly impair their functioning. Early diagnosis and proper treatment are important—they may prevent serious complications and greatly improve a patient's quality of life.

What are the symptoms of Sjögren's syndrome?

Symptoms vary from person to person but may include a dry, gritty, or burning sensation in the eyes; dry mouth; difficulty talking, chewing, or swallowing; a sore or cracked tongue; dry or burning throat; dry, peeling lips; a change in taste or smell; increased dental decay; joint pain; vaginal and skin dryness; digestive problems; dry nose; and fatigue.

Who is most likely to develop Sjögren's syndrome?

Nine out of ten Sjögren's patients are women. The average age of diagnosis is the late 40s, although it can occur in all age groups (including in children) and in both sexes.

Is it easy to diagnose Sjögren's syndrome?

Sjögren's syndrome often is undiagnosed or misdiagnosed. The symptoms of Sjögren's syndrome may mimic those of menopause, drug side effects, or medical conditions such as lupus, rheumatoid arthritis, fibromyalgia, chronic fatigue syndrome, and multiple sclerosis. Because all symptoms are not always present at the same time and because Sjögren's can involve several body systems, physicians and dentists sometimes treat each symptom individually and do not recognize that a systemic disease is present. The average time from the onset of symptoms to diagnosis is over six years.

What kind of doctor treats Sjögren's?

Rheumatologists have primary responsibility for managing Sjögren's syndrome. Patients also are seen and treated by specialists such as ophthalmologists, optometrists, dentists, and others.

How is Sjögren's diagnosed?

It can be difficult to diagnose Sjögren's syndrome. No single test will confirm the diagnosis and, since it is a syndrome, Sjögren's syndrome may appear in many different forms in different patients. Physicians may conduct a series of tests and ask about symptoms. An international group of experts has formulated classification criteria for Sjögren's syndrome, which will help your doctor arrive at a diagnosis. These criteria consider dryness symptoms, changes in salivary (mouth) and lacrimal (eye) gland function, and systemic (whole body) findings.

Blood tests you may have include:

- **ANA (anti-nuclear antibody):** Found in 70% of Sjögren's patients and people with other autoimmune diseases.

- **RF (rheumatoid factor):** Antibody found in 60% to 70% of Sjögren's patients and people with rheumatoid arthritis.

- **SS-A (or Ro) and SS-B (or La):** Marker antibodies for Sjögren's. Seventy percent of Sjögren's patients are positive for SS-A and 40% are positive for SS-B. Also found in lupus patients.

- **ESR (erythrocyte sedimentation rate):** Measures inflammation. An elevated ESR can indicate an inflammatory disorder, including Sjögren's syndrome.

- **IGs (immunoglobulins):** Normal blood proteins, usually elevated in Sjögren's.

The eye tests include:

- **Schirmer test:** Measures tear production.

- **Rose bengal and lissamine green:** Use dyes to examine the surface of the eye for dry spots.

The dental tests include:

- **Salivary flow:** Measures the amount of saliva produced over a certain period of time.

- **Salivary scintigraphy:** A nuclear medicine test that measures salivary gland function.

- **Salivary gland biopsy** (usually in the lower lip): Confirms lymphocytic infiltration of the minor salivary glands.

Your physician will consider the results of these tests and his or her examination to arrive at a final diagnosis. Further research is being conducted to refine the diagnostic criteria for Sjögren's syndrome and to help make diagnosis easier and more accurate.

What treatments are available?

Currently, there is no cure for Sjögren's syndrome. However, treatments may improve various symptoms and prevent complications. Prescription medicines for dry eyes and dry mouth are available. A number of over-the-counter products may also be used to alleviate different types of dryness. Immunosuppressive medications are used to treat serious internal organ manifestations.

Will I die from Sjögren's syndrome?

Sjögren's syndrome is serious but generally not fatal if complications are diagnosed and treated early. Sjögren's syndrome patients must be monitored carefully for development of internal organ involvement, related autoimmune diseases, and other serious complications. In particular, patients should be aware that the incidence of lymphomas (cancer of the lymph glands) is significantly higher in people with Sjögren's compared to the general population.

Is there a cure?

Not yet. But with your help, there will be.

Dry Eye and Sjögren's Syndrome

Millions of Americans suffer from dry eye. There are two main causes: decreased secretion of tears by the lacrimal (tear-producing) glands and loss of tears due to excess evaporation. Both can lead to ocular surface discomfort, often described as feelings of dryness, burning, a sandy/gritty sensation, or itchiness. Visual fatigue, sensitivity to light, and blurred vision are also characteristic of dry eye.

Dry eye is a hallmark symptom of Sjögren's syndrome, a chronic systemic autoimmune disorder in which white blood cells mistakenly invade tear- and saliva-producing glands, causing inflammation and reducing secretion. The age of onset for Sjögren's syndrome is typically in the late 40s, and 90% of Sjögren's patients are women. About half of patients with Sjögren's also have other autoimmune disorders such as rheumatoid arthritis, systemic lupus, and systemic sclerosis (scleroderma).

About Tears

Normal healthy tears contain a complex mixture of proteins and other components that are essential for ocular health and comfort. Tears are important because they:

- provide nutrients and support the health of cells in the cornea;

- lubricate the ocular surface; and

- protect the exposed surface of the eye from infections. Clear vision depends on even distribution of tears over the ocular surface.

For Sjögren's syndrome patients, inflammation of tear-secreting glands reduces tear production, resulting in chronic dry eye. In addition, changes in the composition of tears contribute to dry eye. In people with dry eye, thin spots in the tear film may appear and the tears no longer adequately protect and support the health of ocular surface tissues.

Diagnosis of Dry Eye

Treatment options for dry eye depend on its causes and severity, so it is important to be examined by an eye care professional who is trained to diagnose and treat ocular diseases. The doctor may use tests to assess tear production, tear stability, and tear distribution. A slit-lamp examination using dyes that temporarily stain unhealthy tissue will reveal any abnormality or damage to the ocular surface. These tests typically cause little discomfort and are performed in the doctor's office.

Treatments for Dry Eye Disease

Artificial tears are available over the counter. They can provide temporary relief from dry eye symptoms. Artificial tears contain water, salts, and polymers but lack the proteins found in natural tears. Patients who frequently use drops should choose a brand without preservatives or one with special non-irritating preservatives. Artificial tears are used to treat mild forms of dry eye or to supplement other treatments.

Punctal occlusion blocks the small openings in the eyelid that normally drain tears away from the eye. Usually this is done by inserting plugs made of silicone or other materials into the openings. This simple procedure helps to retain the patient's tears on the ocular surface for a longer time. It can improve symptoms and increase comfort for some patients.

Cyclosporine ophthalmic emulsion (Restasis®) treats an underlying cause of chronic dry eye by suppressing the inflammation that disrupts tear secretion. Many patients report a noticeable increase in tear production and comfort with continued use of Restasis®. Topically applied corticosteroids (cortisone) are occasionally prescribed to treat acute episodes of inflammation in dry eye. The use of these medications should be limited in frequency and duration to avoid potential complications of glaucoma and cataract.

Other Treatment Options and Considerations

Cevimeline (Evoxac®) and pilocarpine (Salagen®) are medications taken orally to increase salivation in Sjögren's syndrome patients. Recent studies have shown some improvement in dry eye symptoms; however, tear production was either not increased or not measured in these studies. These medications are approved for treating dry mouth; treatment for dry eye is considered an off-label indication for use.

Because excess evaporation of the tear film can occur when there is irritation of the eyelids (conditions known as blepharitis or meibomian eyelid gland dysfunction), it is often helpful to maintain eyelid hygiene by using warm compresses and eyelid massage. Any infections of the eyelid margin should be treated with appropriate antibiotics as prescribed by the patient's physician. Allergy and certain skin disorders (such as rosacea) also can aggravate dry eye and should be treated appropriately.

There is accumulating evidence to suggest that taking essential fatty acid supplements (omega-3) by mouth may improve dry eye symptoms and signs. Further clinical trials are underway to confirm this potential benefit. Essential fatty acids are also available in flaxseed oil and fish oil supplements and in some over-the-counter products.

Ongoing clinical trials of other dry eye treatments may eventually result in new FDA [Food and Drug Administration]-approved treatments for stimulating the production of specific tear components in dry eye patients.

Coping with Dry Eye

Making changes in your environment, habits, and medications can help minimize dry eye symptoms. Here are some suggestions:

- Avoid environmental stresses that worsen dry eye, such as low humidity, drafts from air conditioners or fans, smoke, dust, or excessive makeup.

- When possible, avoid taking drugs that cause dryness as a side effect, such as certain drugs for blood pressure regulation, anti-depressants, and antihistamines (e.g., Benadryl®). These drugs and others may decrease tear secretion and worsen dry eye. Your eye care professional can help determine whether any drugs you take may be contributing to your condition.

- Try blinking on purpose or taking a short break with your eyes closed when reading or working at a computer. We tend to blink less often during these activities, potentially aggravating dry eye. Wear special glasses or goggles to lessen dry eye. These items decrease tear evaporation by blocking air drafts and increasing humidity around the eyes. Increased humidity has proven to prevent the evaporation of natural and artificial tears.

- Use specially formulated ophthalmic gels or ointments. Although these may blur vision, they can be used overnight to keep eyes moist. Alternatively, use artificial tears before bedtime and in the morning.

- Apply warm compresses on the eyes. Compresses can soothe dry, irritated tissues and improve secretion of oil from meibomian glands in the eyelids. Try applying them after waking in the morning and periodically during the day.

- Keep your eyes lubricated throughout the day, even if you don't have dryness symptoms. Don't wait until your eyes hurt to seek treatment for dry eye because this could lead to damage to the eye. Patients should use one or more of the treatments listed above and ask their eye care professional about any FDA-approved medications.

Chapter 46

Tear System Problems and Their Treatment

Many children are born with an underdeveloped tear-duct system, a problem that can lead to tear-duct blockage, excess tearing, and infection.

Blocked tear ducts are a fairly common problem in infants; as many as one third may be born with this condition. Fortunately, more than 90% of all cases resolve by the time children are 1 year old with little or no treatment. The earlier that blocked tear ducts are discovered, the less likely it is that infection will result or that surgery will be necessary.

What Are Tear Ducts?

Our eyes are continually exposed to dust, bacteria, viruses, and other objects that could cause damage. The eyelids and eyelashes play a key role in preventing these objects from entering our eyes and hurting them. But besides serving as barriers, the lids and lashes also help our eyes stay moist. Without moisture, our corneas, which serve as protective domes for the front of the eyes, would dry out and could become cloudy or injured.

Working with our lids and lashes, the protective system of glands and ducts called the lacrimal system keeps our eyes from drying out.

"Tear-Duct Obstruction and Surgery" was provided by KidsHealth, one of the largest resources online for medically reviewed health information written for kids, teens, and parents. For more articles like this one, visit www.KidsHealth.org, or www.TeensHealth.org. © 2005 The Nemours Foundation. Reviewed by Sharon Lehman, M.D., August 2005.

Small glands at the edge of the eyelid produce an oily film that mixes with the liquid part of our tears and keeps them from evaporating. Lacrimal (or tear-producing) glands secrete the watery part of tears. These glands are located under the brow bone behind the upper eyelid, at the edge of the eye socket, and in the lids.

Eyelids move tears across the eyes. Tears keep the eyes lubricated and clean and contain antibodies that protect the eyes from infection. They drain out of the eyes through two ducts called punctum or lacrimal ducts, one on each of the upper and lower lids. From these ducts, tears enter small tubes called canaliculi, which are located at the inner corner of the eyelids. They pass from the eyes into the lacrimal sac, a small sac that's located next to the inner corner of the eyes (between the eyes and the nose).

From the lacrimal sacs, tears move down through the nasolacrimal duct and drain into the back of the nose. (That's why you usually get a runny nose when you cry—your eyes are producing excess tears, and your nose can't handle the additional flow.) When you blink, the motion forces the lacrimal sacs to compress, squeezing tears out of them, away from the eyes, and into the nasolacrimal duct.

The nasolacrimal duct and the lacrimal ducts are also known as tear ducts. However, it's the nasolacrimal duct that's involved in tear-duct blockage.

What Causes a Blocked Tear Duct?

Many children are born without a fully developed nasolacrimal duct. This is called congenital nasolacrimal duct obstruction or dacryostenosis. Most commonly, an infant is born with a duct that is more narrow than usual and therefore does not drain properly or becomes blocked easily. The majority of children outgrow this condition by the time they are 1 year old.

Less often, a child has a web of tissue over the end of the duct that didn't dissolve during fetal development. This condition is more likely to require surgical probing.

Other causes of blockage in children (especially older children) are rare. Some children have nasal polyps, which are cysts or growths of extra tissue in the nose at the end of the tear duct. A blockage also can be caused by a tumor in the nose, but again, this is unusual in children.

Trauma to the eye area or an eye injury that lacerates (cuts through) the tear ducts could also cause this condition, but reconstructive surgery at the time of the accident or injury may prevent blockage from happening.

Signs of Blocked Tear Ducts

Children with blocked tear ducts usually develop symptoms of the condition between birth and 12 weeks of age, although you may not realize your child has this problem until his or her eyes become infected. The most common signs of blocked tear ducts are excessive tearing, even when a child is not crying (this is called peripheral). You also may notice pus in the corner of your child's eye, or that your child wakes up with a crust over the eyelid or in the eyelashes.

Children with blocked tear ducts can develop an infection in their lacrimal sac called dacryocystitis. Signs of this infection include redness at the inner corner of the eye and a slight tenderness and swelling or bump at the side of the nose.

Another sign that the tear ducts may be blocked can be present at birth or soon after. Some infants are born with a swollen lacrimal sac, causing a blue bump called a dacryocystocele to appear next to the inside corner of the eye. Although this condition should be monitored closely by your child's doctor, it doesn't always lead to infection and can be treated at home with firm massage and topical antibiotics. However, if it becomes infected, the child is usually admitted to the hospital for intravenous antibiotics, followed by surgical probing of the duct.

When to Call Your Child's Doctor

If your child's eyes tear excessively but show no sign of infection, consult with your child's doctor or a pediatric ophthalmologist (eye specialist) to see if your child has a blocked tear duct. Early treatment can prevent the need for surgery. If your child shows signs of infection (such as redness, pus, or swelling), call your child's doctor immediately because the infection can spread to other parts of the face and the blockage can lead to an abscess if not treated.

Treating Blocked Tear Ducts

Children with blocked tear ducts often can be treated at home. Your child's doctor or pediatric ophthalmologist may recommend that you massage the eye several times daily for a couple of months. Before massaging the tear duct, wash your hands. Place your index finger on the side of your child's nose and firmly massage down toward the corner of the nose. You may also want to apply warm compresses to the eye to help promote drainage and ease any discomfort your child may have.

If your child develops an infection as a result of the tear-duct blockage, your child's doctor will prescribe antibiotic eyedrops or ointment to treat the infection. It's important to remember that antibiotics will not get rid of the obstruction. Once the infection has cleared, you can continue massaging the tear duct as your child's doctor recommends.

If your child still has excess tearing after 6 to 8 months, develops a serious infection, or has repeated infections, the doctor may recommend that your child's tear duct be surgically probed. This procedure has an 85% to 95% success rate for children who are 1 year old or younger; the success rate drops as children age.

Surgical probing may be repeated if it's not initially successful. If your child continues to experience blockage, your child's doctor may recommend surgery to widen the tear ducts using tubes that are implanted in your child's tear ducts for 6 months, or a balloon that stretches the tear duct. Both of these surgical procedures have high success rates.

What Happens before and during Surgery?

Surgery should be performed by an ophthalmologist who is familiar with the procedure—your child's doctor should be able to refer you to such a specialist. These surgical procedures are done on an outpatient basis (unless your child is suffering from a severe infection and has already been admitted to the hospital) under general anesthesia.

When a child is referred for a blocked tear duct because of an infection or excessive tearing, a pediatric ophthalmologist will do a complete eye exam to rule out any other eye problems or types of inflammation that might be causing similar symptoms.

A dye disappearance test also may help determine the cause of the problem. This involves placing fluorescein dye in the eye and then examining the tear film (the amount of tear in the eye) to see if it's greater than it should be. Or the doctor will wait to see if dye has drained properly by having the child blow his nose and then checking to see if any of the dye exited through the nose.

A surgical probe takes about 10 minutes. A thin, blunt metal wire is gently passed through the tear duct to open any obstruction. Sterile saline is then irrigated through the duct into the nose to make sure that there is now an open path. Infants experience no pain after the probing. If surgical probing is unsuccessful, your child's doctor may recommend further surgical treatment. The more traditional form of treatment is called silicone tube intubation. In this procedure, silicone tubes are placed in your child's tear ducts to stretch them. The tubes are left in place for 6 months and then removed in another short surgical procedure. A newer form of treatment is balloon catheter dilation (DCP) or LacriCATH. In this procedure, a balloon is inserted through an opening in the corner of the eye and into the tear duct. The balloon is inflated with a sterile solution to expand the tear duct for 90 seconds. It is then deflated and reinflated for 60 seconds before being repositioned slightly higher in the duct and inflated twice again. It's then deflated and removed.

Both of these procedures require that your child be put under anesthesia and are fairly short—your child will be in surgery for less than an hour. Also, both procedures are considered to be generally successful. There is an approximate 80% to 90% success rate in younger children, with the chance of success decreasing if the procedure is done at older ages. It may take up to a week after surgery before your child's symptoms improve. Your child's doctor will give you antibiotic ointment or drops along with specific instructions on how to care for your child.

Chapter 47

Retinal and Lacrimal Gland Changes Often Caused by Aging

Chapter Contents

Section 47.1

Facts about Floaters

From the National Eye Institute (NEI, www.nei.nih.gov), part of the
National Institutes of Health, December 2006.

Floaters are little "cobwebs" or specks that float about in your field
of vision. They are small, dark, shadowy shapes that can look like
spots, thread-like strands, or squiggly lines. They move as your eyes
move and seem to dart away when you try to look at them directly.
They do not follow your eye movements precisely, and usually drift
when your eyes stop moving.

In most cases, floaters are part of the natural aging process and
simply an annoyance. They can be distracting at first, but eventually
tend to "settle" at the bottom of the eye, becoming less bothersome.
They usually settle below the line of sight and do not go away completely. Most people have floaters and learn to ignore them; they are
usually not noticed until they become numerous or more prominent.
Floaters can become apparent when looking at something bright, such
as white paper or a blue sky.

Floaters occur when the vitreous, a gel-like substance that fills about
80 percent of the eye and helps it maintain a round shape, slowly
shrinks. As the vitreous shrinks, it becomes somewhat stringy, and the
strands can cast tiny shadows on the retina. These are floaters.

Floaters are more likely to develop as we age and are more common in people who are very nearsighted, have diabetes, or who have
had a cataract operation. There are other, more serious causes of floaters, including infection, inflammation (uveitis), hemorrhaging, retinal tears, and injury to the eye.

Sometimes a section of the vitreous pulls the fine fibers away from
the retina all at once, rather than gradually, causing many new floaters to appear suddenly. This is called a vitreous detachment, which in
most cases is not sight-threatening and requires no treatment. However, a sudden increase in floaters, possibly accompanied by light flashes
or peripheral (side) vision loss, could indicate a retinal detachment. A
retinal detachment occurs when any part of the retina, the eye's light-
sensitive tissue, is lifted or pulled from its normal position at the back

wall of the eye. A retinal detachment is a serious condition and should always be considered an emergency. If left untreated, it can lead to permanent visual impairment within two or three days or even blindness in the eye. Those who experience a sudden increase in floaters, flashes of light in peripheral vision, or a loss of peripheral vision should have an eye care professional examine their eyes as soon as possible.

For people who have floaters that are simply annoying, no treatment is recommended. On rare occasions, floaters can be so dense and numerous that they significantly affect vision. In these cases, a vitrectomy, a surgical procedure that removes floaters from the vitreous, may be needed. A vitrectomy removes the vitreous gel, along with its floating debris, from the eye. The vitreous is replaced with a salt solution. Because the vitreous is mostly water, you will not notice any change between the salt solution and the original vitreous. This operation carries significant risks to sight because of possible complications, which include retinal detachment, retinal tears, and cataract. Most eye surgeons are reluctant to recommend this surgery unless the floaters seriously interfere with vision.

Section 47.2

Dealing with Dry Eye

This article was written by Michelle Meadows and published in the *FDA Consumer* magazine, a publication of the U.S. Food and Drug Administration (FDA), May-June 2005.

Tears serve as a protective coating for the eyes. They keep the eyes moist, provide essential nutrients, and wash away dust and other particles. When the eyes don't produce enough tears or the right quality of tears, the result is a condition that doctors call keratitis sicca, popularly known as "dry eye."

Just as the name suggests, this condition makes the eyes feel dry, scratchy, and gritty. Other symptoms include burning, stinging, itching, pain, sensitivity to light, redness, blurry vision, and the feeling that there is a speck of dirt in the eye. There may also be a stringy discharge from the eyes. And though it may seem strange, dry eye can cause the eyes to water. "This can happen because the eyes are irritated," says Carolyn Begley, O.D., a professor of optometry at Indiana University in Bloomington. "You may experience excessive tearing the same way you would if something got in your eye."

But these tears won't necessarily make the eyes feel better. Reflex tears—the watery type that are produced in response to injury, irritation, or emotion—don't have the lubricating qualities necessary to prevent dry eye. Tear film is made of water, oil, and mucus, all of which are important for maintaining good eye health. The cornea, which covers the front of the eye, needs these tears continuously to protect it against infection. Most people who have dry eye experience mild irritation with no long-term effects, Begley says. But if the condition is left untreated or becomes severe, eye damage and vision loss can occur. Severe problems with dry eye can cause eye inflammation, corneal infection, and scarring.

"When dry eye symptoms are severe, they can interfere with quality of life," Begley says. "Some people may have trouble keeping their eyes open or they may not be able to work or drive." Fortunately, identifying the cause of the problem and seeking treatment early can make a big difference in easing the discomfort.

Common Causes

Aging is one of the most common causes of dry eye because tear production decreases as we get older. Dry eye affects more women than men because hormonal changes, such as those that occur in pregnancy, menstruation, and menopause, can decrease tear production. Environmental conditions also can play a role. Wind, heat, dust, air conditioning, cigarette smoke, and even hair dryers can make the eyes dry. Some people benefit from avoiding dusty, smoky areas, wearing sunglasses, and using a humidifier to moisten the surrounding air.

Another common culprit is not blinking enough, which happens during activities such as watching TV and computer use. "Each time you blink, it coats the eye with tears," Begley says. "You normally blink about every 12 seconds. But we've done studies of people playing computer games, and found that some people blinked once or twice in three minutes."

Begley says that about half of all people who wear contact lenses complain of dry eye. That's because soft contact lenses, which float on the tear film that covers the cornea, absorb the tears in the eyes. Dry eye also occurs or gets worse after LASIK [laser-assisted in situ keratomileusis] and other refractive surgeries, in which the corneal nerves are cut during creation of a corneal flap. The corneal nerves stimulate tear secretion. Begley says, "If you've had dry eyes from wearing contact lenses or for any other reason and you are thinking about refractive surgery, this is something to consider."

Dry eye also can be caused by certain medications, including antihistamines, some antidepressants, birth control pills, nasal decongestants, and the prescription acne drug Accutane. And some autoimmune diseases, such as lupus, rheumatoid arthritis, and Sjögren syndrome, can attack the tear glands.

Other diseases can also cause dry eye. For example, certain types of thyroid disease can interfere with blinking. Blepharitis, an inflammation of the eyelids, can interfere with the oil glands in the eyes.

Diagnosis and Treatment

Even though many treatments for dry eye are available without a prescription, it's wise to see a health care professional to evaluate the cause of the condition and to help you pick the best treatment.

Eye doctors use a combination of routine clinical exams and other specific tests for dry eye. For example, the Schirmer test uses a tiny strip of paper placed on the edge of the lower eyelids. "This measures how much moisture is in the eye, and it's also useful for determining the severity of the problem," Begley says. Doctors may also use dye, such as fluorescein or rose bengal, which is placed on the eye to stain the surface. This is to see how much the surface of the eye has been affected by dryness. Another test, tear break-up time (TBUT), measures the time it takes for tears to break up in the eye.

The first line of treatment for dry eye is usually over-the-counter demulcent drops, also known as artificial tears. These lubricate the eye and ease symptoms. Commonly found ingredients in these products include hydroxypropyl methylcellulose, the ingredient in Bion Tears and GenTeal, and carboxymethylcellulose, contained in Refresh Plus and Thera Tears. Always read the directions, but these products can generally be used as often as needed throughout the day.

Your health care professional can guide you in choosing the right one for you. "Some people use drops for red eyes, but that can make the eyes even more dry," Begley says. Red eyes could be caused by numerous factors, from allergies to an eye infection, which is why a proper diagnosis is important. If you wear contact lenses, use rewetting drops specifically for contact lenses. Other types of drops may contain ingredients that damage the lens.

Restasis (cyclosporine ophthalmic emulsion) is the only prescription product for chronic dry eyes. Approved by the Food and Drug Administration in 2002, the drug increases tear production, which may be reduced because of inflammation on the eye surface. In a clinical trial involving 1,200 people, Restasis increased tear production in 15 percent of patients, compared with 5 percent of patients in the placebo group, says Wiley Chambers, M.D., deputy director of the FDA's Division of Anti-Inflammatory, Analgesic and Ophthalmologic Drug Products.

Restasis is usually given twice a day, 12 hours apart. It should not be used by people with eye infections or hypersensitivity to the ingredients. It has not been tested in people with herpes viral infections of the eye. The most common side effect is a burning sensation. Other side effects may be eye redness, discharge, watery eyes, eye pain, foreign body sensation, itching, stinging, and blurred vision.

For people who have not found dry eye relief with drugs, punctal plugs may help. "These are reserved for people with moderate or severe dry eye when other medical treatment hasn't been adequate," says Eva Rorer, M.D., a medical officer in the FDA's Division of Ophthalmic and Ear, Nose, and Throat Devices.

In each eye, there are four puncta, little openings that drain tears into the tear ducts. Punctal plugs are inserted into the puncta to block tear drainage. Some doctors try out temporary ones made of collagen first to make sure that permanent ones will not cause excessive tearing. Permanent plugs are usually made of silicone. In recent years, Rorer says, some plugs have been approved that are made of thermally reactive material. "Some of these are inserted into the punctum as a liquid and then they harden and conform to the individual's drainage system." Others start out rigid and become soft and flexible, adapting to the individual's punctal size after they are inserted. Artificial tears are usually still required after punctal plug insertion.

"The risks of punctal plugs are fairly minimal," Rorer says. "There is a risk of eye irritation, excessive tearing, and, in rare cases, infection."

Part Seven

Eye Infections, Muscular Problems, and Malignancies

Chapter 48

Eye Infections

Chapter Contents

Section 48.1

Conjunctivitis (Pinkeye)

"Pinkeye (Conjunctivitis)" was provided by KidsHealth, one of the largest resources online for medically reviewed health information written for kids, teens, and parents. For more articles like this one, visit www .KidsHealth.org, or www.TeensHealth.org. © 2007 The Nemours Foundation. Reviewed by Elana Pearl Ben-Joseph, M.D., January 2007.

Conjunctivitis, commonly known as pinkeye, is an inflammation of the conjunctiva, the clear membrane that covers the white part of the eye and the inner surface of the eyelids.

While pinkeye can sometimes be alarming because it may make the eyes extremely red and can spread rapidly, it's a fairly common condition and usually causes no long-term eye or vision damage. But if your child shows symptoms of pinkeye, it's important to see a doctor. Some kinds of pinkeye go away on their own, but other types require treatment.

Conjunctivitis can be caused by infections (such as bacteria and viruses), allergies, or substances that irritate the eyes.

Causes of Pinkeye

Pinkeye can be caused by many of the bacteria and viruses responsible for colds and other infections—including ear infections, sinus infections, and sore throats—and by the same types of bacteria that cause the sexually transmitted diseases (STDs) chlamydia and gonorrhea.

Pinkeye also can be caused by allergies. These cases tend to happen more frequently among kids who also have other allergic conditions, such as hay fever. Some triggers of allergic conjunctivitis include grass, ragweed pollen, animal dander, and dust mites.

Sometimes a substance in the environment can irritate the eyes and cause pinkeye; for example, chemicals (such as chlorine and soaps) and air pollutants (such as smoke and fumes).

Pinkeye in Newborns

Newborns are particularly susceptible to pinkeye and can be more prone to serious health complications if it goes untreated.

If a baby is born to a mother who has an STD, during delivery the bacteria or virus can pass from the birth canal into the baby's eyes, causing pinkeye. To prevent this, doctors give antibiotic ointment or eye drops to all babies immediately after birth. Occasionally, this preventive treatment causes a mild chemical conjunctivitis, which typically clears up on its own. Doctors also can screen pregnant women for STDs and treat them during pregnancy to prevent transmission of the infection to the baby.

Many babies are born with a narrow or blocked tear duct, a condition which usually clears up on its own. Sometimes, though, it can lead to conjunctivitis.

Symptoms of Pinkeye

The different types of pinkeye can have different symptoms. And symptoms can vary from child to child.

One of the most common symptoms is discomfort in the eye. A child may say that it feels like there's sand in the eye. Many kids have redness of the eye and inner eyelid, which is why conjunctivitis is often called pinkeye. It can also cause discharge from the eyes, which may cause the eyelids to stick together when the child awakens in the morning. Some kids have swollen eyelids or sensitivity to bright light.

In cases of allergic conjunctivitis, itchiness and tearing are common symptoms.

Contagiousness

Cases of pinkeye that are caused by bacteria and viruses are contagious. (Conjunctivitis caused by allergies or environmental irritants are not.)

A child can get pinkeye by touching an infected person or something an infected person has touched, such as a used tissue. In the summertime, pinkeye can spread when kids swim in contaminated water or share contaminated towels. It also can be spread through coughing and sneezing. Doctors usually recommend keeping kids diagnosed with contagious conjunctivitis out of school, day care, or summer camp for a short time.

Someone who has pinkeye in one eye can also inadvertently spread it to the other eye by touching the infected eye, then touching the other one.

Preventing Pinkeye

To prevent pinkeye caused by infections, teach kids to wash their hands often with warm water and soap. They also should not share eye drops, tissues, eye makeup, washcloths, towels, or pillowcases with other people.

Be sure to wash your own hands thoroughly after touching an infected child's eyes, and throw away items like gauze or cotton balls after they've been used. Wash towels and other linens that the child has used in hot water separately from the rest of the family's laundry to avoid contamination.

If you know your child is prone to allergic conjunctivitis, keep windows and doors closed on days when the pollen is heavy, and dust and vacuum frequently to limit allergy triggers in the home. Irritant conjunctivitis can only be prevented by avoiding the irritating causes.

Many cases of pinkeye in newborns can be prevented by screening and treating pregnant women for STDs. A pregnant woman may have bacteria in her birth canal even if she shows no symptoms, which is why prenatal screening is important.

Treating Pinkeye

Pinkeye caused by a virus usually goes away on its own without any treatment. If a doctor suspects that the pinkeye has been caused by a bacterial infection, antibiotic eye drops or ointment will be prescribed.

Sometimes it can be a challenge to get kids to tolerate eye drops several times a day. If you're having trouble, put the drops on the inner corner of your child's closed eye—when the child opens the eye, the medicine will flow into it. If you continue to have trouble with drops, ask the doctor about antibiotic ointment. It can be applied in a thin layer where the eyelids meet, and will melt and enter the eye.

If your child has allergic conjunctivitis, your doctor may prescribe antiallergy medication, which comes in the form of pills, liquid, or eye drops.

Cool or warm compresses and acetaminophen or ibuprofen may make a child with pinkeye feel more comfortable. You can clean the edges of the infected eye carefully with warm water and gauze or cotton balls. This can also remove the crusts of dried discharge that may cause the eyelids to stick together first thing in the morning.

When to Call the Doctor

If you think your child has pinkeye, it's important to contact your doctor to try to determine what's causing it and how to treat it. Other serious eye conditions can mimic conjunctivitis, so a child who complains of severe pain, changes in eyesight, or sensitivity to light should be re-examined. If the pinkeye does not improve after 2 to 3 days of treatment, or after a week when left untreated, call your doctor.

If your child has pinkeye and starts to develop increased swelling, redness, and tenderness in the eyelids and around the eye, along with a fever, call your doctor. Those symptoms may mean the infection has started to spread beyond the conjunctiva and will require additional treatment.

Section 48.2

Herpetic Eye Disease

"Herpetic Eye Disease," © 2006 The Cleveland Clinic Cole Eye Institute, 9500 Euclid Avenue Mail Stop W14, Cleveland, OH 44195, www .clevelandclinic.org/eye. Additional information is available from the Cleveland Clinic Health Information Center, 216-444-3771, toll-free 800-223-2273 extension 43771, or at http://www.clevelandclinic.org/health.

What is herpetic eye disease?

There is a family of viruses that are all called herpesvirus. Two of these viruses can cause infection in the eye, which is called herpetic eye disease. These two viruses are not the same virus that causes genital herpes, and herpetic eye disease is not a sexually transmitted disease.

One of the viruses that cause herpetic eye disease is called the varicella-zoster virus. It is the same virus that causes chickenpox, which is called varicella in medical language, and also the nervous-system disease known as "shingles." When it affects the eye, it is called herpes zoster ophthalmicus.

The other virus that causes herpetic eye disease is called herpes simplex type 1. Herpes simplex type 1 is the same virus that causes cold sores on the lips and mouth. In the eye, it usually causes an infection of the cornea, the clear area in the center of the front surface of the eye. This infection is called herpes simplex keratitis.

It is important to remember that even though both of these problems are called by the name herpes, they are different types of infections that might need different types of treatment.

Why do people get herpetic eye disease?

Like many viruses, the herpes simplex 1 and varicella-zoster viruses are actually present in most adults. The viruses in the herpes family usually live around the nerve fibers in humans without ever causing a problem. Occasionally, the viruses will start to multiply, or they will move from one area of the body to another, and that is when herpetic disease breaks out. This often happens when the immune system of the body is weakened by some other health problem.

How does the doctor know whether someone has herpetic eye disease?

The two different types of herpetic eye disease have different symptoms. One thing they have in common, however, is that they can both be very painful because they affect the nerves directly.

The problem is likely to be herpes zoster ophthalmicus if the doctor finds some or all of these symptoms:

- pain in and around only one eye;
- redness, rash, or sores on the eyelids and around the eyes, especially on the forehead (sometimes the rash breaks out on the tip of the nose);
- redness of the eye; or
- swelling and cloudiness of the cornea.

The problem is likely to be herpes simplex keratitis if the doctor sees these symptoms:

- pain in and around only one eye;
- redness of the eye;
- feeling of dirt or "grit" in the eye;
- overflowing tears;
- pain when looking at bright light; or
- swelling or cloudiness of the cornea.

The doctor might want to use special tests if it looks like herpetic eye disease might be present. The pressure inside the eye will probably be checked, for example. There is also a special dye called fluorescein that the doctor might put into the eye. This dye glows under ultraviolet light and will show the doctor if the virus is causing problems on the surface of the eye.

How is herpes zoster ophthalmicus treated?

Because herpes is a virus, antibiotics such as penicillin are not an effective treatment. The only drugs that will work against herpes infections are antiviral medications.

Depending on how serious the herpes zoster ophthalmicus is and what part of the eye is affected, the doctor will recommend antiviral eye drops, pills, or both. No matter what kind of medication is recommended, it is important to keep using the medicine for as long as your doctor recommends. Even though the eye might start to look or feel better, the infection could come back if you stop taking your medicine too soon.

If the infection is affecting the cornea, another kind of eye drops called corticosteroids might also be recommended. Corticosteroids will help control the disease, but they can also raise the pressure in the eyes of some people. If corticosteroids are being used, it is important for the patient to come back to the doctor's office so the pressure can be checked.

Another type of eye drop might also be prescribed to keep the pupil dilated. This will help the eye's natural fluids flow, which prevents the pressure from increasing.

Unfortunately, herpetic eye disease can be painful even after several days of treatment when the eye is starting to look better. This can be discouraging, but it does not mean that the treatment is a failure. The medications are working, and the pain will go away eventually.

How is herpes simplex keratitis treated?

The same types of eye drops and pills are prescribed to treat herpes simplex keratitis. It is also just as important to use the medications as recommended, and to keep all appointments with your doctor.

Sometimes a herpes virus infection can cause a corneal lesion, which is a small area where the surface of the eye starts to break apart. If this happens, your doctor may recommend a different medication.

Corneal lesions can occasionally become serious enough that an operation to remove part of the cornea might have to be performed. The best way to avoid a serious problem like this is to take all medications as prescribed and to keep all appointments with your doctor.

Section 48.3

Histoplasmosis

Excerpted from "Histoplasmosis," from the National Eye Institute (NEI, www.nei.nih.gov), part of the National Institutes of Health, December 2006.

What is histoplasmosis?

Histoplasmosis is a disease caused when airborne spores of the fungus *Histoplasma capsulatum* are inhaled into the lungs, the primary infection site. This microscopic fungus, which is found throughout the world in river valleys and soil where bird or bat droppings accumulate, is released into the air when soil is disturbed by plowing fields, sweeping chicken coops, or digging holes.

Histoplasmosis is often so mild that it produces no apparent symptoms. Any symptoms that might occur are often similar to those from a common cold. In fact, if you had histoplasmosis symptoms, you might dismiss them as those from a cold or flu, since the body's immune system normally overcomes the infection in a few days without treatment.

However, histoplasmosis, even mild cases, can later cause a serious eye disease called ocular histoplasmosis syndrome (OHS), a leading cause of vision loss in Americans ages 20 to 40.

How does histoplasmosis cause ocular histoplasmosis syndrome?

Scientists believe that *Histoplasma capsulatum* (histo) spores spread from the lungs to the eye, lodging in the choroid, a layer of blood vessels that provides blood and nutrients to the retina. The retina is the light-sensitive layer of tissue that lines the back of the eye. Scientists have not yet been able to detect any trace of the histo fungus in the eyes of patients with ocular histoplasmosis syndrome. Nevertheless, there is good reason to suspect the histo organism as the cause of OHS.

How does OHS develop?

OHS develops when fragile, abnormal blood vessels grow underneath the retina. These abnormal blood vessels form a lesion known as choroidal neovascularization (CNV). If left untreated, the CNV lesion can turn into scar tissue and replace the normal retinal tissue in the macula. The macula is the central part of the retina that provides the sharp, central vision that allows us to read a newspaper or drive a car. When this scar tissue forms, visual messages from the retina to the brain are affected, and vision loss results.

Vision is also impaired when these abnormal blood vessels leak fluid and blood into the macula. If these abnormal blood vessels grow toward the center of the macula, they may affect a tiny depression called the fovea. The fovea is the region of the retina with the highest concentration of special retinal nerve cells, called cones, that produce sharp, daytime vision. Damage to the fovea and the cones can severely impair, and even destroy, this straight-ahead vision. Early treatment of OHS is essential; if the abnormal blood vessels have affected the fovea, controlling the disease will be more difficult. Since OHS rarely affects side, or peripheral vision, the disease does not cause total blindness.

What are the symptoms of OHS?

OHS usually has no symptoms in its early stages; the initial OHS infection usually subsides without the need for treatment. This is true for other histo infections; in fact, often the only evidence that the inflammation ever occurred are tiny scars called "histo spots," which remain at the infection sites. Histo spots do not generally affect vision, but for reasons that are still not well understood, they can result in complications years—sometimes even decades—after the original eye infection. Histo spots have been associated with the growth of the abnormal blood vessels underneath the retina.

In later stages, OHS symptoms may appear if the abnormal blood vessels cause changes in vision. For example, straight lines may appear crooked or wavy, or a blind spot may appear in the field of vision. Because these symptoms indicate that OHS has already progressed enough to affect vision, anyone who has been exposed to histoplasmosis and perceives even slight changes in vision should consult an eye care professional.

Who is at risk for OHS?

Although only a tiny fraction of the people infected with the histo fungus ever develops OHS, any person who has had histoplasmosis should be alert for any changes in vision similar to those described above. Studies have shown the OHS patients usually test positive for previous exposure to histoplasmosis.

In the United States, the highest incidence of histoplasmosis occurs in a region often referred to as the "Histo Belt," where up to 90 percent of the adult population has been infected by histoplasmosis. This region includes all of Arkansas, Kentucky, Missouri, Tennessee, and West Virginia as well as large portions of Alabama, Illinois, Indiana, Iowa, Kansas, Louisiana, Maryland, Mississippi, Nebraska, Ohio, Oklahoma, Texas, and Virginia. Since most cases of histoplasmosis are undiagnosed, anyone who has ever lived in an area known to have a high rate of histoplasmosis should consider having their eyes examined for histo spots.

How is OHS diagnosed?

An eye care professional will usually diagnose OHS if a careful eye examination reveals two conditions: (1) The presence of histo spots, which indicate previous exposure to the histo fungus spores; and (2) Swelling of the retina, which signals the growth of new, abnormal blood vessels. To confirm the diagnosis, a dilated eye examination must be performed. This means that the pupils are enlarged temporarily with special drops, allowing the eye care professional to better examine the retina.

If fluid, blood, or abnormal blood vessels are present, an eye care professional may want to perform a diagnostic procedure called fluorescein angiography. In this procedure, a dye, injected into the patient's arm, travels to the blood vessels of the retina. The dye allows a better view of the CNV lesion, and photographs can document the location and extent to which it has spread. Particular attention is paid to how close the abnormal blood vessels are to the fovea.

How is OHS treated?

The only proven treatment for OHS is a form of laser surgery called photocoagulation. A small, powerful beam of light destroys the fragile, abnormal blood vessels, as well as a small amount of the overlying retinal tissue. Although the destruction of retinal tissue during the procedure can itself cause some loss of vision, this is done in the hope of protecting the fovea and preserving the finely-tuned vision it provides.

What help is available for people who have already lost significant vision from OHS?

Scientists and engineers have developed many useful devices to help people with severe visual impairment in both eyes. These devices, called low vision aids, use special lenses or electronics to create enlarged visual images. An eye care professional can suggest sources that provide information on counseling, training, and special services for people with low vision. Many organizations for people who are blind also serve those with low vision.

Chapter 49

Inflammation of the Eye Structures

Chapter Contents

Section 49.1

Blepharitis: Inflammation of the Eyelids

From "Blepharitis Resource Guide," by the National Eye Institute (NEI, www.nei.nih.gov), part of the National Institutes of Health, December 2006.

What is blepharitis?

Blepharitis (also called granulated eyelids) is a common condition that causes inflammation of the eyelids. The condition can be difficult to manage because it tends to recur.

What causes blepharitis?

Blepharitis occurs in two forms:

- **Anterior blepharitis** affects the outside front of the eyelid, where the eyelashes are attached. The two most common causes of anterior blepharitis are bacteria (Staphylococcus) and scalp dandruff.

- **Posterior blepharitis** affects the inner eyelid (the moist part that makes contact with the eye) and is caused by problems with the oil (meibomian) glands in this part of the eyelid. Two skin disorders can cause this form of blepharitis: acne rosacea, which leads to red and inflamed skin, and scalp dandruff (seborrheic dermatitis).

What are the symptoms of blepharitis?

Symptoms of either form of blepharitis include a foreign body or burning sensation, excessive tearing, itching, sensitivity to light (photophobia), red and swollen eyelids, redness of the eye, blurred vision, frothy tears, dry eye, or crusting of the eyelashes on awakening.

What other conditions are associated with blepharitis?

Complications from blepharitis include:

- **Stye:** A red tender bump on the eyelid that is caused by an acute infection of the oil glands of the eyelid.

- **Chalazion:** This condition can follow the development of a stye. It is a usually painless firm lump caused by inflammation of the oil glands of the eyelid. Chalazion can be painful and red if there is also an infection.

- **Problems with the tear film:** Abnormal or decreased oil secretions that are part of the tear film can result in excess tearing or dry eye. Because tears are necessary to keep the cornea healthy, tear film problems can make people more at risk for corneal infections.

How is blepharitis treated?

Treatment for both forms of blepharitis involves keeping the lids clean and free of crusts. Warm compresses should be applied to the lid to loosen the crusts, followed by a light scrubbing of the eyelid with a cotton swab and a mixture of water and baby shampoo. Because blepharitis rarely goes away completely, most patients must maintain an eyelid hygiene routine for life. If the blepharitis is severe, an eye care professional may also prescribe antibiotics or steroid eyedrops.

When scalp dandruff is present, a dandruff shampoo for the hair is recommended as well. In addition to the warm compresses, patients with posterior blepharitis will need to massage their eyelids to clean the oil accumulated in the glands. Patients who also have acne rosacea should have that condition treated at the same time.

Section 49.2

Uveitis: Inflammation of the Uvea

What Is Uveitis?

Uveitis is inflammation of a part of the eye called the uvea. The uvea (pronounced "you-vay-uh") is a layer of the eye made up of three parts. These are the iris, the ciliary body, and the choroid.

Uveitis can occur in one eye or both eyes. Inflammation of the uvea may involve other parts of the eye, or any part of the eye, including the cornea (the clear, curved front of the eye), the sclera (the white outer part of the eye), the vitreous body, the retina and the optic nerve.

The iris is the colored part of the front of the eye. It controls light that enters the eye by controlling the size of the eye's opening (the pupil).

The ciliary body is a group of muscles and blood vessels that changes the shape of the lens so the eye can focus. It also makes a fluid called aqueous humor. Aqueous humor is a clear, watery fluid that fills and circulates through parts of the front of the eye.

The choroid is a middle layer of the eye. It holds blood vessels that feed other parts of the eye, especially the retina. The retina is the inner layer of the eye. It contains nerve cells that sense color and light and send image information to the brain.

What Causes Uveitis?

Uveitis is inflammation of the eye's uvea. Inflammation is the body's response to injury, or trauma. To treat uveitis, doctors look for the cause of the trauma to the eye. Uveitis can be caused by many different kinds of trauma, including a virus, bacteria infections, or parasites.

Genes can play an important role in uveitis. Also, diseases that damage the body's immune system, such as AIDS [acquired immunodeficiency syndrome], can lower the body's ability to protect itself from infections that can cause uveitis.

In many cases, perhaps as many as a third or half of all uveitis cases, the cause of the inflammation is not known.

Signs of Uveitis

Eye problems other than uveitis may cause signs of uveitis, but if you notice any sign of possible eye problems, you should see an eye doctor for a complete eye exam with dilated pupil.

How Do Doctors Diagnose and Treat Uveitis?

Diagnosis and treatment of uveitis is important for a number of reasons. Uveitis can cause permanent damage to the eyes and vision loss that cannot be reversed. Also, uveitis may be caused by another disease or condition that, if left untreated, can lead to serious illness. For some people, a diagnosis of uveitis is a first step in diagnosing and treating a life-threatening problem.

Eye doctors treat different kinds of uveitis very differently. The cause of uveitis may be very difficult for a doctor to discover, and in many cases the doctor will not be able to find a cause.

In some cases, discovery of the cause of uveitis may take many years as the individual is treated for chronic or recurrent uveitis.

Living with Uveitis

Modern treatments help control uveitis and can often prevent vision loss and blindness if the condition is found and treated early.

You must work with your eye doctor if you have uveitis. Eye doctors know how to treat uveitis, but they have to work with you to find the best way to treat the condition. Stay informed, take your medicines as scheduled, and follow your treatment plan.

You and your doctor must work together to determine the best medicines for you.

What You Do Makes a Difference

- Remember to take notes about how you feel. Write down your questions so you can make the most of your eye doctor visits.

- Explain to your eye doctor how the medicines you are taking affect you.

- Tell all of your other doctors about your eye medicines and all other drugs you're taking.

- Tell the eye doctor about any changes in your physical condition, any changes in your medicine or any side effects.

- Call your eye doctor if you notice any unusual changes in your eyes, your vision or the way you feel in general.

- Schedule regular checkups and follow through with them.

- Take care of yourself—your eyes and the rest of you along with them.

Follow Your Treatment Plan

It's up to you to follow your treatment plan and have follow-up visits as recommended by your eye doctor. Remember to report anything you believe may be a side effect of the medicine you are taking.

Don't Skip Doses

Skipping doses of your medicine may put your vision in danger and mislead your doctor. Be sure to tell your doctor if you've missed any doses.

After evaluating your progress, your doctor may try changing your doses, switching medicines, or changing other parts of your treatment to find the best results for you.

Questions for Your Eye Doctor

You will have many questions as your doctor diagnoses and treats your uveitis. It's helpful to keep a list of these questions, especially if they come to mind in between your doctor appointments.

Write all your questions down and bring the list with you, then discuss them with your doctor. Here are some questions many people have:

- What do the medicines do?

- How much will they cost? Will my insurance help pay for them? (These may be questions for your insurance company, not your doctor).

- What are the possible side effects of my medicines?

- Can I do anything to lower the chance of side effects or reduce the effects?

- When exactly should I take my medicine? Can you please write down a detailed schedule?

- What should I do if I miss a dose?

- Do I need to do anything special to take care of my medicines?

Tips for Taking Your Medicine

- Learn about the medicines you are taking and the best way to use them. Find out whether they need special handling, such as storing them in the refrigerator.

- If you take a combination of drops and ointments, always apply the drops first.

- Schedule your doses around your normal routine, such as when you wake up, when you eat meals, and when you go to bed at night.

- Keep your medicines in plain sight. It's easier to remember to take them.

- Keep medicines in a clean place. For example, if you carry them in your purse, put them in a sealed plastic bag to keep them clean.

- Take your medicines with you when you're away from home. If you're checking luggage at the airport, keep your medicines with you in your carry-on or in your purse.

- If you forget a dose, do not automatically double your next dose. Instead, follow your doctor's instructions on what to do.

- If you can't remember whether you took your medicines, simply use one dose at your next scheduled time.

You Have to Help Save Your Sight

Find support and encouragement from your family, friends, and others. Sometimes it helps to talk to people who have experienced the same thing. It can help you to discuss side effects, share ways to remember your medicines, and celebrate getting your uveitis under control.

Unfortunately, there are a few people who will lose vision despite commitment to working with their eye doctor and following their treatment plan. The future holds great promise for uveitis. New medicines and treatments continue to be developed. In the meantime, take heart in knowing that you're doing everything possible to treat your condition. The doctor/patient team approach, support from others, and promising scientific discoveries will help you look forward toward a bright future.

Chapter 50

Amblyopia and Strabismus

Chapter Contents

Section 50.1

Amblyopia

Excerpted from "Amblyopia Resource Guide," from the National
Eye Institute (NEI, www.nei.nih.gov), part of the National Institutes
of Health, December 2006.

What is amblyopia (lazy eye)?

The brain and the eye work together to produce vision. Light enters the eye and is changed into nerve signals that travel along the optic nerve to the brain. Amblyopia is the medical term used when the vision in one of the eyes is reduced because the eye and the brain are not working together properly. The eye itself looks normal, but it is not being used normally because the brain is favoring the other eye. This condition is also sometimes called lazy eye.

How common is amblyopia?

Amblyopia is the most common cause of visual impairment in childhood. The condition affects approximately 2 to 3 out of every 100 children. Unless it is successfully treated in early childhood, amblyopia usually persists into adulthood, and is the most common cause of monocular (one eye) visual impairment among children and young and middle-aged adults.

What causes amblyopia?

Amblyopia may be caused by any condition that affects normal visual development or use of the eyes. Amblyopia can be caused by strabismus, an imbalance in the positioning of the two eyes. Strabismus can cause the eyes to cross in (esotropia) or turn out (exotropia). Sometimes amblyopia is caused when one eye is more nearsighted, farsighted, or astigmatic than the other eye. Occasionally, amblyopia is caused by other eye conditions such as cataract.

How is amblyopia treated in children?

Treating amblyopia involves making the child use the eye with the reduced vision (weaker eye). Currently, there are two ways used to do this:

- **Atropine:** A drop of a drug called atropine is placed in the stronger eye once a day to temporarily blur the vision so that the child will prefer to use the eye with amblyopia. Treatment with atropine also stimulates vision in the weaker eye and helps the part of the brain that manages vision develop more completely.

- **Patching:** An opaque, adhesive patch is worn over the stronger eye for weeks to months. This therapy forces the child to use the eye with amblyopia. Patching stimulates vision in the weaker eye and helps the part of the brain that manages vision develop more completely.

Previously, eye care professionals often thought that treating amblyopia in older children would be of little benefit. However, surprising results from a nationwide clinical trial show that many children age seven through 17 with amblyopia may benefit from treatments that are more commonly used on younger children. This study shows that age alone should not be used as a factor to decide whether to treat a child for amblyopia.

Can amblyopia be treated in adults?

Studies are very limited at this time and scientists don't know what the success rate might be for treating amblyopia in adults. During the first six to nine years of life, the visual system develops very rapidly. Complicated connections between the eye and the brain are created during that period of growth and development. Scientists are exploring whether treatment for amblyopia in adults can improve vision.

Section 50.2

Strabismus

© 2007 A.D.A.M., Inc. Reprinted with permission.

Alternative Names

Crossed eyes; esotropia; exotropia; squint; walleye

Definition

Strabismus is a disorder that causes one eye to be misaligned with the other when focusing.

Causes, Incidence, and Risk Factors

Strabismus is caused by a lack of coordination between the eyes. As a result, the eyes look in different directions and do not focus at the same time on a single point.

In most cases of strabismus in children, the cause is unknown. In more than half of these cases, the problem is present at or shortly after birth (congenital strabismus).

In children, when the two eyes fail to focus on the same image, the brain may learn to ignore the input from one eye. If this is allowed to continue, the eye that the brain ignores will never see well. This loss of vision is called amblyopia, and it is frequently associated with strabismus.

Some other disorders associated with strabismus in children include:

- retinopathy of prematurity;
- retinoblastoma;
- traumatic brain injury;
- hemangioma near the eye during infancy;
- Apert syndrome;
- Noonan syndrome;

- Prader-Willi syndrome;
- trisomy 18 (a child has 3 copies of chromosome 18, instead of the normal 2 copies);
- congenital rubella;
- incontinentia pigmenti syndrome; and
- cerebral palsy.

Acquired strabismus in adults can be caused by injuries to the orbit of the eye or injuries to the brain, including closed head injuries and strokes. People with diabetes may have loss of circulation, causing a condition known as acquired paralytic strabismus. Loss of vision in one eye from any cause will usually cause the eye to gradually turn outward (exotropia). Because the brains of adults are already developed for vision, the problems associated with amblyopia do not occur with adult strabismus.

Some disorders associated with strabismus in adults include:

- diabetes;
- vision loss from any eye disease or injury;
- stroke;
- traumatic brain injury;
- paralytic shellfish poisoning (PSP);
- Guillain-Barré syndrome; and
- botulism.

A family history of strabismus is a risk factor. Farsightedness may be a contributing factor. In addition, any other disease causing vision loss may produce strabismus as a complication.

Symptoms

- Eyes that appear crossed
- Eyes that do not align in the same direction
- Uncoordinated eye movements (eyes that do not move together)
- Double vision
- Vision in only one eye, with loss of depth perception (depth perception is our ability to see three dimensions, and recognize the order of objects in the space around us)

Signs and Tests

Your child's health care provider will first determine if the child truly has strabismus. If the child has strabismus, a workup will be done to determine the cause.

The physical examination will include a detailed examination of the eyes. The patient may be asked to look through a series of prisms to determine the differences between the eyes. The eye muscles will be tested to determine the strength of the extraocular muscles.

Tests include:

- standard ophthalmic exam;
- visual acuity;
- retinal exam; and
- neurological examination.

Treatment

Initially, strategies to strengthen the weakened muscles and thereby realign the eyes are attempted. Glasses may be prescribed. Eye muscle exercises may be prescribed.

If amblyopia is present, patching of the preferred eye may be done to force the child to use the amblyopic eye. Surgery may be required to realign the eye muscles if strengthening techniques are unsuccessful.

Expectations (Prognosis)

With an early diagnosis, the defect can usually be corrected. With delayed treatment, vision loss in one eye may be permanent.

Complications

- Loss of vision in one eye due to amblyopia
- Embarrassment over facial appearance with eye patch

Calling Your Health Care Provider

Strabismus requires prompt medical evaluation. Call for an appointment with your health care provider or eye doctor if your child exhibits any of the following:

- complains of double vision;

- has difficulty seeing;
- appears to be cross-eyed; or
- the eyes do not appear to fix on the same point.

Also call if there are problems at school, which could possibly be related to the child being unable to see the blackboard or the reading material.

Section 50.3

Older Children Benefit from Patching for Amblyopia

From "Older Children Can Benefit From Treatment For Childhood's Most Common Eye Disorder," a press release by the National Eye Institute (NEI, www.nei.nih.gov), part of the National Institutes of Health, April 11, 2005.

Surprising results from a nationwide clinical trial show that many children age seven through 17 with amblyopia (lazy eye) may benefit from treatments that are more commonly used on younger children.

Treatment improved the vision of many of the 507 older children with amblyopia studied at 49 eye centers. Previously, eye care professionals often thought that treating amblyopia in older children would be of little benefit. The study results, funded by the National Eye Institute (NEI), part of the National Institutes of Health (NIH), appear in the April [2005] issue of *Archives of Ophthalmology*.

"Doctors can now feel confident that traditional treatments for amblyopia will work for many older children," said Paul A. Sieving, M.D., Ph.D., director of the NEI. "This is important because it is estimated that as many as three percent of children in the United States have some degree of vision impairment due to amblyopia. Many of these children do not receive treatment while they are young," he said.

Amblyopia is a leading cause of vision impairment in children and usually begins in infancy or childhood. It is a condition resulting in poor vision in an otherwise healthy eye due to unequal or abnormal visual input while the brain is developing in infancy and childhood. The most common causes of amblyopia are crossed or wandering eye (strabismus) or significant differences between the eyes in refractive error, such as astigmatism, farsightedness, or nearsightedness.

Children in the study were divided randomly into two groups. One group was fitted with new prescription glasses only. The other group was fitted with glasses as well as an eye patch or the eye patch along with special eyedrops to limit use of the unaffected eye. These children were also asked to perform near-vision activities. The patching, near activities, and eyedrops force a child to use the eye with amblyopia. Patching was prescribed for periods of two to six hours daily, while the eyedrops were administered daily for the children seven through 12 years of age.

The study investigators defined successful vision improvement as the ability to read (with the eye with amblyopia) at least two more lines on a standard eye chart. The study investigators found that 53 percent of children age seven through 12 years who received both glasses and treatment with patches and near activity met this standard, while only 25 percent of those children in this age group who received glasses alone met the standard. For children age 13 through 17 years who were treated with both glasses and patches (these children did not get drops), 25 percent met the standard while 23 percent of children of these ages who received only glasses met the standard.

The study also revealed that among children age 13 through 17 years who had not been previously treated for amblyopia, 47 percent of those who were treated with glasses, patching, and near activities improved two lines or more compared with only 20 percent of those treated with glasses alone. Despite the benefits of the treatment, most children, including those who responded to treatment, were left with some visual impairment. They did not obtain "20/20" vision.

"This study shows how important it is to screen children of all ages for amblyopia." said study co-chairman Richard W. Hertle, M.D., Children's Hospital of Pittsburgh.

Commented co-chairman Mitchell M. Scheiman, O.D., Pennsylvania College of Optometry, "This study shows that age alone should not be used as a factor to decide whether or not to treat a child for amblyopia. The opportunity to treat amblyopia does not end with the preschool years."

It is not known, say the authors of the current study, whether vision improvement will be sustained in these children once treatment is discontinued. The NEI is supporting a one-year, follow-up study to determine the percentage of amblyopia that recurs among the children who responded well to treatment, as well as many other clinical studies of amblyopia at eye centers nationwide.

Dr. Sieving also commented that the current study results are "a wonderful example of the adaptability of the human visual system and brain. The NIH is exploring ways to take advantage of this adaptability in order to better understand and treat vision problems and other neurological conditions."

The study described in this release was conducted by the NEI-funded Pediatric Eye Disease Investigator Group. The group focuses on studies of childhood eye disorders that can be implemented by both university-based and community-based practitioners as part of their routine practice. The study was coordinated by the Jaeb Center for Health Research in Tampa, Florida.

Section 50.4

Daily Eye Patching Offers Effective Treatment for Amblyopia

From "Reduced Daily Eye Patching Effectively Treats Childhood's Most Common Eye Disorder," a press release by the National Eye Institute (NEI, www.nei.nih.gov), part of the National Institutes of Health, December 2006.

Patching the unaffected eye of children with moderate amblyopia for two hours daily works as well as patching the eye for six hours. This research finding should lead to better compliance with treatment and improved quality of life for children with amblyopia, or "lazy eye," the most common cause of visual impairment in childhood. These results appear in the May [2003] issue of *Archives of Ophthalmology*.

"These results will change the way doctors treat moderate amblyopia and make an immediate difference in treatment compliance and the quality of life for children with this eye disorder," said Paul A. Sieving, M.D., Ph.D., director of the National Eye Institute, one of the Federal government's National Institutes of Health and the agency that sponsored the study. "This is very important, because it is estimated that as many as three percent of children in the United States have some degree of vision impairment due to amblyopia."

After four months of treatment, children with moderate amblyopia who wore an adhesive patch daily for two hours over their unaffected eye showed the same improvement in vision as those who wore a patch for six hours. Placing an opaque adhesive patch, or eye bandage, over the unaffected eye for six hours daily is considered one of the standard treatments for moderate amblyopia. Both groups of children in the study performed one hour a day of "near" work, such as coloring, tracing, reading, and crafts, while the eye was patched.

Amblyopia, which usually begins in infancy or childhood, is a condition of poor vision in an otherwise healthy eye because the brain has learned to favor the other eye. Although the eye with amblyopia often looks normal, there is interference with normal visual processing that limits the development of a portion of the brain responsible for vision. The most common causes of amblyopia are crossed or wandering eyes or significant differences in refractive error, such as farsightedness or nearsightedness, between the two eyes.

"Prior to these results, many children with amblyopia had to wear an eye patch during school hours," Dr. Sieving said. "For these children, the accompanying social and psychological stigma was very real. Many were stared at and teased by other children, which made them feel different. Now, children can look forward to attending school without the patch. This will make them feel better about themselves."

Dr. Sieving said it is crucial for young children to comply with the recommended treatment because visual impairment can persist into adulthood if amblyopia is not successfully treated in early childhood. Amblyopia is the most common cause of monocular (one eye) visual impairment among children and young and middle-aged adults.

"Because the daily burden to administer treatment for amblyopia falls on the parent, the findings from this study will immediately affect families that have young children with this eye disorder," said study chairman Michael Repka, M.D., professor of ophthalmology and pediatrics at the Wilmer Eye Institute of Johns Hopkins University School of Medicine in Baltimore. "The findings make it much easier for parents to monitor their children and encourage children to successfully comply with treatment. Timely and successful treatment for amblyopia in childhood can prevent lifelong visual impairment."

Patching the unaffected eye has been the mainstay of amblyopia treatment for decades. In March 2002, the same researchers reported the effectiveness of a second treatment, which involved using atropine eye drops that dilated the unaffected eye, temporarily blurring vision. Both treatments force the child to use the eye with amblyopia, stimulating vision improvement in that eye by helping the part of the brain that manages vision to develop more completely. However, with patching, opinions varied widely on the number of daily hours it should be prescribed. No prior study had provided conclusive evidence of the optimal number of patching hours.

In this study, 189 children less than seven years old with moderate amblyopia were randomly assigned to receive either two hours or six hours of daily patching. The average age of the children was 5.2 years. Both groups showed significant improvement in the vision of the eye with amblyopia. "After four months, we found that 79 percent of children in the two-hour group and 76 percent of the patients in the six-hour group could read at least two more lines on the standard eye chart," Dr. Repka said. "The study also found that parents of children who wore the patch for six hours were more concerned about social stigma than the parents of children who wore the patch for two hours."

Dr. Repka said having the child perform one hour of "near," or close-up, work per day while patched was an important part of the prescribed treatment. He said it remains unclear if the same amount of visual improvement would occur with patching alone. "We are planning a clinical trial to address the importance of near work in the treatment of amblyopia," he said.

Dr. Repka noted that these results do not necessarily apply to all children with amblyopia. "Children with more severe amblyopia, or who have amblyopia from causes other than crossed eyes or refractive error, may need a different treatment regimen," he said. "The Pediatric Eye Disease Investigator Group (PEDIG), which conducted this study, is currently conducting a clinical trial on children with severe amblyopia and expects the results will be available in the Fall of 2003."

The study described here was conducted by the PEDIG at 35 clinical sites throughout North America. The PEDIG focuses on studies of childhood eye disorders that can be implemented by both university-based and community-based practitioners as part of their routine practice. The study was funded by the National Eye Institute and coordinated by the Jaeb Center for Health Research in Tampa, Florida.

431

Section 50.5

Botulinum Toxin Injections Used to Treat Adult Strabismus

"Botox (Medical)" is reprinted with permission from www.eyecareamerica.com, © 2007. EyeCare America is a program of the Foundation of the American Academy of Ophthalmology.

What It Is

Botox is a drug that is injected in small amounts to stop muscle spasms. It can help with adult strabismus, or lazy eye.

What You Can Expect

The treatment takes a few minutes. Botox starts working within a few hours or days. The effects last up to three months.

Who Is a Good Candidate?

You could be a good candidate if you are physically healthy and you are not pregnant or nursing.

What It's For

Strabismus (pronounced struh-BIZ-mus) is a condition in which the eyeballs point in different directions. This means the eyes are misaligned.

Adults with strabismus may experience any or all of these symptoms: eye fatigue, double vision, overlapped or blurred images, a pulling sensation around the eyes, reading difficulty, or loss of depth perception.

If an overactive eye muscle is the cause of the strabismus, Botox injections can help. In small amounts, Botox temporarily paralyzes muscles. It can last several months and may even cause a permanent change in eye alignment.

How It Works

Botox is the brand name for botulinum toxin, which is extracted from the bacteria *Clostridia botulinum*. For years Botox has been used as a nonsurgical treatment for uncontrollable facial spasms and disorders of the eye. It was approved as a therapy for strabismus in adults in 1989.

Using a very fine needle, your ophthalmologist (Eye M.D.) will inject the Botox directly into the targeted eye muscles. A topical anesthetic cream may be applied to your skin to decrease the sensation of the injection. Botox is thought to work on strabismus by lengthening the injected muscle while shortening the opposing muscle.

Botox treatments take only a few minutes during a typical office visit. You should be able to return to your normal activities immediately. The effects usually last about three months. As long as you don't have an allergic reaction, Botox treatment can be repeated as necessary.

Risks

Botox is a toxin and can be potent in high concentrations. Only small, diluted amounts of Botox are used in treatments. The most common side effects from Botox are headache and temporary redness or bruising of the skin at the injection site.

More serious complications are rare but possible. There is a chance that nearby muscles could be affected and weakened. If Botox seeps below the eyebrow and into the muscle that controls eyelid function, the eyelid might droop. This is called ptosis. Though the effect is not permanent and will eventually go away as the Botox wears off, drooping eyelids may temporarily obstruct your ability to see.

Having an Eye M.D. perform your Botox treatment helps to ensure the safety of your eyes and your vision.

You should inform your doctor of your medical history and all medications, vitamins, and/or herbal supplements you are currently taking before having Botox treatments.

Chapter 51

Involuntary Eye and Eyelid Movements

Chapter Contents

Section 51.1

Understanding Nystagmus

"Understanding Nystagmus," by Richard L. Windsor, O.D., F.A.A.O., and Laura K. Windsor, O.D., F.A.A.O., The Low Vision Centers of Indiana, © 2000. Reviewed 2007. Reprinted with permission.

Nystagmus is an involuntary rhythmic shaking or wobbling of the eyes. The term nystagmus is derived from the Greek word, "nystagmus," which was used to describe the wobbly head movements of a sleepy or inebriated individual. Nystagmus has also been described as "dancing eyes" or "jerking eyes." Doctors and researchers classify nystagmus by the characteristics of the eye movements like: do they move back and forth like a pendulum or do they move slowly in one direction and then rapidly in another? Do the eyes move laterally or vertically and by how much? How fast do the eyes move?

There are various methods of classifying nystagmus. Traditionally nystagmus has been divided into two groups. Sensory nystagmus is related to vision loss and motor nystagmus is related to the control of muscle function. There are over 45 types of nystagmus. To simplify our explanation of nystagmus, we will divide nystagmus into two basic types. The first is nystagmus that begins very early in life and is associated with vision loss. The second is called acquired nystagmus and is associated with neurological disorders occurring later in life.

Nystagmus from Early in Life

Early onset nystagmus often accompanies vision loss acquired at birth or soon after and may be one of the first signs that a child has a loss of vision. Studies suggest 1 in every 1,000 children have nystagmus. In 80–90% of cases, it is a side effect of vision loss from eye diseases such as albinism, aniridia, optic nerve hypoplasia, achromatopsia congenital cataracts, coloboma, or retinopathy of prematurity. This type of nystagmus is usually observed around the sixth to eighth week of life and is rarely seen before then. In about 10–20% of cases, it presents with mild vision loss not associated with other diagnosed ocular diseases. The discovery of nystagmus in a child is reason for an immediate examination.

The typical nystagmus related to vision loss during childhood is a pendular nystagmus. The eyes rotate back and forth evenly, much like a pendulum. Patients with early onset nystagmus do not notice the movement of their vision when their eyes shake. Although nystagmus is associated with early vision loss, it may vary from stress, emotional status, and direction of view. It is uncommon to permanently worsen over time. In fact, nystagmus often improves mildly from childhood to adulthood.

Most cases of early onset nystagmus are associated with ocular disease, many of which are inherited conditions. Genetic counseling can help the patient and family understand the odds of passing the condition to their children. Not all cases of early onset nystagmus are hereditary.

Nystagmus Arising Later in Life

While vision loss before birth will result in nystagmus, loss of vision occurring later in life does not usually cause nystagmus. Thus, a patient with age-related macular degeneration would not show nystagmus while a child with achromatopsia would develop this condition.

Nystagmus can be acquired later in life due to neurological dysfunction such as a head injury, multiple sclerosis, or brain tumors. Unlike nystagmus acquired from early in life, patients with late onset nystagmus usually notice movement in their vision related to the movement of their eyes. This is called oscillopsia. Oscillopsia causes a person to have vertigo or dizziness related to the new movement they experience in their vision.

Late onset nystagmus is more likely to be directional. The eye will move slowly in one direction, then quickly move back. The nystagmus may change as the patient looks in different directions. The unexplained onset of nystagmus in an adult may indicate a serious neurological disorder and an immediate examination is indicated.

Medications and Nystagmus

Some medications may cause nystagmus. For example, Dilantin and Phenobarbital, medications given to prevent seizures, may cause nystagmus. This acquired condition may cause the patient to experience oscillopsia, a sensation of movement in their vision that causes a vertigo effect. When it occurs vertically, the patient may describe a rolling of the vision in front of them.

Fluctuations in Vision

Nystagmus patients often experience fluctuations in their vision. A change in the speed of the nystagmus leading to a decrease in vision can be related to stress, the patient's emotional state, fatigue, the direction of view or when one eye is covered. Understanding these issues allows the patient and teachers to create a better environment.

The Null Position: Unusual Head and Eye Positions

Patients with nystagmus often find a unique position of their head and eyes that slows the nystagmus allowing them to have better vision. This is called a null position and varies with each person. Teachers, friends, and family must understand and support the patient's unusual head or eye position.

Balance and Binocular Vision

Patients with nystagmus may report problems with balance. Impairment to binocular vision is common with early onset nystagmus and depth perception is indirectly impaired in many patients. Nystagmus acquired later in life may cause vertigo or dizziness like effects from the sensation of motion in the vision. Nystagmus may decrease when the eyes converge to read. Low vision specialists can add prism to induce convergence artificially and thus reduce the nystagmus in some patients.

Examining the Nystagmus Patient

Patients with nystagmus have many unique problems that should be evaluated by a low vision specialist or eye doctor skilled in treating nystagmus. Simple tests like visual acuity can be misleading as the vision may decrease if the patient is under stress or has latent nystagmus, which causes an increase in nystagmus in both eyes when one eye is covered. The visual acuity testing requires special steps to ensure an accurate measurement.

Low vision specialists also use special testing techniques during the refraction to measure the eyeglass prescription and prevent inaccurate results from latent nystagmus. Reducing stress during testing is another method used by low vision specialists to obtain the best results.

Nystagmus and Eyeglasses

Patients with nystagmus frequently have other vision problems such as astigmatism that require prescription eyeglasses. This is particularly true of patients with albinism and retinopathy of prematurity. Eyeglasses, however, do not cure nystagmus. Prisms may be added to the eyewear to improve the patient's cosmetic appearance by changing the null position to a slightly more normal position. Prisms may also be used to induce more convergence, turning in of the eyes, which may reduce nystagmus slightly. When bifocals are prescribed, the null position must be considered. Placing a small bifocal in the normal position may not be usable in a patient who must turn his or her eyes far to the left to have the best vision.

Nystagmus and Contact Lenses

Contact lenses have been shown to aid some nystagmus patients. One theory is that the tactile feedback of feeling the contact lenses on the eyes may lead to better control of the movement and allow the patient better vision. Another benefit of contact lenses is that they move with the eyes and thus provide better image quality.

Medical and Surgical Treatments

Several surgical procedures have been developed to reduce null positions and thus improve a patient's cosmetic appearance. Botox, botulinum toxin, has been used to paralyze ocular muscles and thus reduce nystagmus. It has not become a practical treatment since the effect of this drug lasts only three to four months and requires injection into the ocular muscles under general anesthesia. Baclofen has also been used to lessen certain forms of nystagmus. Additionally, biofeedback has also been used to treat nystagmus.

Social Issues

Not only do nystagmus patients have vision loss, but they also are faced with cosmetic problems from the constant eye movements and often an unusual head/eye position. Patients may be teased about their appearance or chastised and told to hold their head correctly.

School Issues

The teacher of a child with nystagmus needs to understand how to aid a child with nystagmus and associated vision loss. Timed tests may create emotional stress that can cause the nystagmus to increase and the child's vision to temporarily decrease. The teacher must understand the need for the child to turn his eyes or head in a specific manner. Allowing the child to sit at the front of the classroom is also needed. Depending on the level of vision, low vision adaptation may be required including large print books, closed circuit television, optical low vision aids, etc. Low vision children should always have their own books and worksheets. Sharing materials is difficult for low vision patients. Materials should be enlarged and of high contrast. A simple clear yellow acetate sheet with a black line across it may be helpful in keeping one's place especially when looking away to the chalkboard or to a computer screen.

Summary

Nystagmus, an involuntary shaking or jerking of the eyes is a very complex ocular condition. It can occur early in life secondary to various ocular diseases or can be acquired later in life in patients who have neurological disorders. Patients with nystagmus often have an abnormal head position called a null position in which their vision is improved. Low vision specialists or other nystagmus specialists may be able to provide special care, eyewear, and contact lenses to help patients with nystagmus.

Internet Resources on Nystagmus

American Nystagmus Network: www.nystagmus.org

Low Vision Gateway to the Internet: www.lowvision.org

Section 51.2

Blepharospasm

Excerpted from "Blepharospasm Resource Guide," from the
National Eye Institute (NEI, www.nei.nih.gov), part of the National
Institutes of Health, December 2006.

What are other names for blepharospasm?

Benign essential blepharospasm, hemifacial spasm

What is blepharospasm?

Blepharospasm is an abnormal, involuntary blinking or spasm of
the eyelids.

What causes blepharospasm?

Blepharospasm is associated with an abnormal function of the
basal ganglion from an unknown cause. The basal ganglion is the part
of the brain responsible for controlling the muscles. In rare cases,
heredity may play a role in the development of blepharospasm.

What are the symptoms of blepharospasm?

Most people develop blepharospasm without any warning symptoms. It may begin with a gradual increase in blinking or eye irritation. Some people may also experience fatigue, emotional tension, or
sensitivity to bright light. As the condition progresses, the symptoms
become more frequent, and facial spasms may develop. Blepharospasm
may decrease or cease while a person is sleeping or concentrating on
a specific task.

How is blepharospasm treated?

To date, there is no successful cure for blepharospasm, although
several treatment options can reduce its severity.

In the United States and Canada, the injection of Oculinum (botulinum toxin, or Botox) into the muscles of the eyelids is an approved

treatment for blepharospasm. Botulinum toxin, produced by the bacterium *Clostridium botulinum*, paralyzes the muscles of the eyelids.

Medications taken by mouth for blepharospasm are available but usually produce unpredictable results. Any symptom relief is usually short term and tends to be helpful in only 15 percent of the cases.

Myectomy, a surgical procedure to remove some of the muscles and nerves of the eyelids, is also a possible treatment option. This surgery has improved symptoms in 75 to 85 percent of people with blepharospasm.

Alternative treatments may include biofeedback, acupuncture, hypnosis, chiropractic, and nutritional therapy. The benefits of these alternative therapies have not been proven.

Chapter 52

Surgery for Eyelid Drooping or Excess Skin

Complete eye health includes having healthy eyes and healthy eyelids. Common eyelid problems include excess eyelid skin, droopy eyelids, or eyelids that turn inward or outward. These problems can cause eye discomfort, limit vision, and affect appearance. Fortunately, they can be corrected with surgery.

Ptosis: Upper Eyelid Drooping

Ptosis (pronounced: toe-sis) can either be apparent at birth (congenital) or develop with age (involutional).

A child with congenital ptosis may tilt his or her head backward in order to see, so the condition does not always lead to poor vision. However, children with ptosis should be examined by an ophthalmologist (Eye M.D.) because they may have other associated eye problems.

Surgery to correct ptosis is commonly recommended in the preschool years to improve appearance and make it easier for the child to see. The type of surgery varies, depending upon how much the eyelids droop.

Involutional ptosis develops with aging. It may worsen after other types of eye surgery or eyelid swelling. Ptosis may limit your side or even your central vision. If ptosis occurs in one eye, it may create an

"Eyelid Surgery," © 2005 American Academy of Ophthalmology. Reprinted with permission.

uneven appearance. Surgical shortening of the muscle that opens the eyelid will often lead to better vision and improved appearance.

Excess Eyelid Skin

Over time, many people develop excess eyelid skin. Eyelid skin is the thinnest skin of the body, so it tends to stretch.

In the upper eyelid, this stretched skin may limit your side vision. The same problem causes "bags" to form in the lower eyelids.

The excess skin in the upper eyelids can be removed surgically by a procedure called blepharoplasty. It improves side vision and other symptoms. Removal of the excess skin in either the upper or lower eyelids also may improve appearance. If excess fatty tissue is present, it may be removed at the same time.

Ectropion: Outward Turning of the Lower Eyelid

Stretching of the lower eyelid from age may cause the eyelid to droop downward and turn outward. This condition is called ectropion. Eyelid burns or skin disease also can cause this problem. Ectropion can cause dryness of the eyes, excessive tearing, redness, and sensitivity to light and wind.

Surgery usually restores the normal position of the eyelid, improving these symptoms.

Entropion: Inward Turning of the Lower Eyelid

Entropion also occurs most commonly as a result of aging. Infection and scarring inside the eyelid are other causes of entropion. When the eyelid turns inward, the eyelashes and skin rub against the eye, making it red, irritated, watery, and sensitive to light and wind.

If entropion is not treated, an infection may develop on the clear surface of the eye called the cornea.

With surgery, the eyelid can be turned outward to its normal position, protecting the eye and improving these symptoms.

Eyelid Plastic Surgery

Eyelid plastic surgery is almost always performed on an outpatient basis using local anesthesia.

Before surgery, your ophthalmologist will perform an eye examination and make recommendations.

Photographs and side-vision testing are often required by insurance companies before blepharoplasty and ptosis surgery.

If you are planning to have surgery, be sure to tell your ophthalmologist if you are taking aspirin or aspirin-containing drugs or blood thinners or if you have a bleeding problem.

This surgery is generally safe; however, as with any surgery, there are some risks.

- The ophthalmic surgeon will attempt to make both eyes look similar, but differences in healing between the eyes may cause some unevenness in appearance following surgery.

- A black eye is common but will resolve quickly.

- The eye may feel dry after surgery because it may be more difficult to close your eyes completely. This irritation can be treated and generally disappears as the eyelids heal.

- Serious complications are rare. The risk of losing vision is estimated to be less than one in 5,000 surgeries. Infections and excessive scarring occur infrequently.

Eyelid plastic surgery procedures can be done safely in an outpatient setting by your ophthalmologist. The improvement in vision, comfort, and appearance can be very gratifying.

Chapter 53

Malignancies of the Eye

Chapter Contents

Section 53.1

Cancer of the Eye and Orbit

Excerpted from a fact sheet from Surveillance Epidemiology and End Results (SEER), part of the National Cancer Institute (NCI, www.cancer .gov), 2006. For tables and references, visit seer.cancer.gov.

It is estimated that 2,340 men and women (1,310 men and 1,030 women) will be diagnosed with and 220 men and women will die of cancer of the eye and orbit in 2007.

Incidence and Mortality

From 2000 to 2004, the median age at diagnosis for cancer of the eye and orbit was 60 years of age. Approximately 14.1% were diagnosed under age 20; 3.4% between 20 and 34; 7.6% between 35 and 44; 14.6% between 45 and 54; 18.2% between 55 and 64; 19.2% between 65 and 74; 17.3% between 75 and 84; and 5.7% 85+ years of age.

The age-adjusted incidence rate was 0.8 per 100,000 men and women per year. These rates are based on cases diagnosed in 2000 to 2004 from 17 Surveillance Epidemiology and End Results [SEER] geographic areas.

U.S. Mortality

From 2000 to 2004, the median age at death for cancer of the eye and orbit was 69 years of age. Approximately 5.3% died under age 20; 1.5% between 20 and 34; 4.3% between 35 and 44; 11.6% between 45 and 54; 18.8% between 55 and 64; 21.0% between 65 and 74; 24.5% between 75 and 84; and 13.1% 85+ years of age.

The age-adjusted death rate was 0.1 per 100,000 men and women per year. These rates are based on cases diagnosed in 2000 to 2004 from 17 SEER geographic areas.

Survival and Stage

Survival rates can be calculated by different methods for different purposes. The survival rates presented are based on the relative survival rate, which measures the survival of the cancer patients in comparison to the general population to estimate the effect of cancer. The overall 5-year relative survival rate for 1996 to 2003 from 17 SEER geographic areas was 83.7%. Five-year relative survival rates by race and sex were: 83.5% for white men; 82.9% for white women; 75.6% for black men; and 91.2% for black women.

The stage distribution based on historic stage shows that 77% of eye and orbit cancer cases are diagnosed while the cancer is still confined to the primary site (localized stage); 7% are diagnosed after the cancer has spread to regional lymph nodes or directly beyond the primary site; 4% are diagnosed after the cancer has already metastasized (distant stage) and for the remaining 12% the staging information was unknown. The corresponding 5-year relative survival rates were: 86.5% for localized; 69.3% for regional; 69.7% for distant; and 77.7% for unstaged.

Section 53.2

Intraocular Melanoma

Excerpted from "General Information About Intraocular (Eye) Melanoma," from the National Cancer Institute (NCI, www.cancer.gov), January 9, 2007.

Intraocular melanoma is a disease in which malignant (cancer) cells form in the tissues of the eye.

Intraocular melanoma begins in the middle of three layers of the wall of the eye. The outer layer includes the white sclera (the white of the eye) and the clear cornea at the front of the eye. The inner layer has a lining of nerve tissue, called the retina, which senses light and sends images along the optic nerve to the brain.

The middle layer, where intraocular melanoma forms, is called the uvea or uveal tract, and has three main parts:

- **Iris:** The iris is the colored area at the front of the eye (the eye color). It can be seen through the clear cornea. The pupil is in the center of the iris and it changes size to let more or less light into the eye.

- **Ciliary body:** The ciliary body is a ring of tissue with muscle fibers that change the size of the pupil and the shape of the lens. It is found behind the iris. Changes in the shape of the lens help the eye focus. The ciliary body also makes the clear fluid that fills the space between the cornea and the iris.

- **Choroid:** The choroid is the layer of blood vessels that bring oxygen and nutrients to the eye. Most intraocular melanomas begin in the choroid.

Intraocular melanoma is a rare cancer, but it is the most common eye cancer in adults.

Age and sun exposure may increase the risk of developing intraocular melanoma.

Anything that increases your risk of getting a disease is called a risk factor. Risk factors for intraocular melanoma include the following:

- older age;
- having a fair complexion (blond or red hair, fair skin, green or blue eyes); or
- being exposed to a lot of sunlight or to certain chemicals.

Possible signs of intraocular melanoma include a dark spot on the iris or blurred vision.

Intraocular melanoma may not cause any early symptoms. It is sometimes found during a routine eye exam when the doctor dilates the pupil and looks into the eye. The following symptoms may be caused by intraocular melanoma or by other conditions. A doctor should be consulted if any of these problems occur:

- a dark spot on the iris;
- blurred vision;
- a change in the shape of the pupil; or
- a change in vision.

Glaucoma may develop if the tumor causes the retina to separate from the eye. If this happens, there may be no symptoms, or symptoms may include the following:

- eye pain;

- blurred vision;

- eye redness; or

- nausea.

Tests that examine the eye are used to help detect (find) and diagnose intraocular melanoma.

The following tests and procedures may be used:

- **Eye exam with dilated pupil:** An examination of the eye in which the pupil is dilated (enlarged) with medicated eye drops to allow the doctor to look through the lens and pupil to the retina. The inside of the eye, including the retina and the optic nerve, is examined using an instrument that produces a narrow beam of light. This is sometimes called a slit-lamp exam. The doctor may take pictures over time to keep track of changes in the size of the tumor and how fast it is growing.

- **Indirect ophthalmoscopy:** An examination of the inside of the back of the eye using a small magnifying lens and a light.

- **Ultrasound exam of the eye:** A procedure in which high-energy sound waves (ultrasound) are bounced off the internal tissues of the eye to make echoes. Eye drops are used to numb the eye and a small probe that sends and receives sound waves is placed gently on the surface of the eye. The echoes make a picture of the inside of the eye. The picture, called a sonogram, shows on the screen of the ultrasound monitor.

- **Transillumination of the globe and iris:** An examination of the iris, cornea, lens, and ciliary body with a light placed on either the upper or lower lid.

- **Fluorescein angiography:** A procedure to look at blood vessels and the flow of blood inside the eye. An orange fluorescent dye (fluorescein) is injected into a blood vessel in the arm. As the dye travels through blood vessels of the eye, a special camera takes pictures of the retina and choroid to detect any blockage or leakage.

Certain factors affect prognosis (chance of recovery) and treatment options.

The prognosis (chance of recovery) and treatment options depend on the following:

- the type of melanoma cells (how they look under a microscope);
- the size of the tumor;
- which part of the eye the tumor is in (the iris, ciliary body, or choroid);
- whether the tumor has spread within the eye or to other places in the body;
- the patient's age and general health; and
- whether the tumor has recurred (come back) after treatment.

In patients with small tumors that have not spread, intraocular melanoma can be cured and vision can usually be saved.

There are different types of treatments for patients with intraocular melanoma.

Five types of standard treatment are used:

- surgery;
- watchful waiting;
- radiation therapy;
- photocoagulation; and
- thermotherapy.

New types of treatment are being tested in clinical trials.

Section 53.3

Retinoblastoma

Excerpted from "General Information About Retinoblastoma," by the
National Cancer Institute (NCI, www.cancer.gov), December 21, 2005.

Retinoblastoma is a disease in which malignant (cancer) cells form in the tissues of the retina.

The retina is the nerve tissue that lines the inside of the back of
the eye. The retina senses light and sends images to the brain by way
of the optic nerve.

Although retinoblastoma may occur at any age, it usually occurs
in children younger than 5 years of age. The tumor may be in one eye
or in both eyes. Retinoblastoma rarely spreads from the eye to nearby
tissue or other parts of the body. Retinoblastoma is usually found in
only one eye and can usually be cured.

Retinoblastoma is sometimes caused by a gene mutation passed from the parent to the child.

Retinoblastoma is sometimes inherited (passed from the parent to
the child). Retinoblastoma that is caused by an inherited gene mutation
is called hereditary retinoblastoma. It usually occurs at a younger age
than retinoblastoma that is not inherited. Retinoblastoma that occurs
in only one eye is usually not inherited. Retinoblastoma that occurs in
both eyes is always inherited. When hereditary retinoblastoma first occurs in only one eye, there is a chance it will develop later in the other
eye. After diagnosis of retinoblastoma in one eye, regular follow-up exams of the healthy eye should be done every 2 to 4 months for at least
28 months. After treatment for retinoblastoma is finished, it is important that follow-up exams continue until the child is 7 years of age.

Treatment for both types of retinoblastoma should include genetic
counseling (a discussion with a trained professional about inherited
diseases). Brothers and sisters of a child who has retinoblastoma should
also have regular checkups and genetic counseling about the risk of
developing the cancer.

A child who has hereditary retinoblastoma is at risk for developing trilateral retinoblastoma and other cancers.

A child who has hereditary retinoblastoma is at risk for developing pineal tumors in the brain. This is called trilateral retinoblastoma. Regular follow-up exams to check for this rare condition are important during treatment and for at least 4 years after the child is diagnosed with retinoblastoma. Hereditary retinoblastoma also increases the child's risk of developing other types of cancer in later years. Regular follow-up exams are important.

Possible signs of retinoblastoma include "white pupil" and eye pain or redness.

These and other symptoms may be caused by retinoblastoma. Other conditions may cause the same symptoms. A doctor should be consulted if any of the following problems occur:

- pupil of the eye appears white instead of red when light shines into it. This may be seen in flash photographs of the child;
- eyes appear to be looking in different directions; or
- pain or redness in the eye.

Tests that examine the retina are used to detect (find) and diagnose retinoblastoma.

The following tests and procedures may be used:

- **Physical exam and history:** An exam of the body to check general signs of health, including checking for signs of disease, such as lumps or anything else that seems unusual. A history of the patient's health habits and past illnesses and treatments will also be taken. The doctor will ask if there is a family history of retinoblastoma.

- **Eye exam with dilated pupil:** An exam of the eye in which the pupil is dilated (opened wider) with medicated eye drops to allow the doctor to look through the lens and pupil to the retina. The inside of the eye, including the retina and the optic nerve, is examined with a light. Depending on the age of the child, this exam may be done under anesthesia.

- **Ultrasound exam:** A procedure in which high-energy sound waves (ultrasound) are bounced off internal tissues or organs and make echoes. The echoes form a picture of body tissues called a sonogram.

- **CT scan (CAT scan):** A procedure that makes a series of detailed pictures of areas inside the body, such as the eye, taken from different angles. The pictures are made by a computer linked to an x-ray machine. A dye may be injected into a vein or swallowed to help the organs or tissues show up more clearly. This procedure is also called computed tomography, computerized tomography, or computerized axial tomography.

- **MRI (magnetic resonance imaging):** A procedure that uses a magnet, radio waves, and a computer to make a series of detailed pictures of areas inside the body, such as the eye. This procedure is also called nuclear magnetic resonance imaging (NMRI).

Retinoblastoma is usually diagnosed without a biopsy (removal of cells or tissues so they can be viewed under a microscope to check for signs of cancer).

Certain factors affect prognosis (chance of recovery) and treatment options.

The prognosis (chance of recovery) and treatment options depend on the following:

- the stage of the cancer;
- how likely it is that vision can be saved in one or both eyes;
- the size and number of tumors; and
- whether trilateral retinoblastoma occurs.

There are different types of treatment for patients with retinoblastoma.

Children with retinoblastoma should have their treatment planned by a team of doctors with expertise in treating cancer in children.

Some cancer treatments cause side effects months or years after treatment has ended. Six types of standard treatment are used:

- enucleation;
- radiation therapy;
- cryotherapy;

455

- photocoagulation;
- thermotherapy; and
- chemotherapy.

New types of treatment are being tested in clinical trials. These include the following:

- subtenon chemotherapy; and
- high-dose chemotherapy with stem cell transplant.

Section 53.4

Similar Survival Rates Found for Eye Cancer Therapies

"Similar Survival Rates Found for Eye Cancer Therapies" is a press release from the National Cancer Institute (NCI), May 28, 2006.

Researchers with the Collaborative Ocular Melanoma Study (COMS) have found that the survival rates for two alternative treatments for primary eye cancer—radiation therapy and removal of the eye—are about the same.

Also as a consequence of this research, the capability of doctors nationwide to provide more accurate diagnoses and state-of-the-art treatments for eye cancer has been greatly expanded. Mortality data from this, the second of two COMS clinical trials, are compared in the July 2001 issue of the *Archives of Ophthalmology*.

"These findings are reassuring to patients with medium-sized eye tumors who have to choose between the option of radiation therapy versus removal of the eye," said Paul A. Sieving, M.D., Ph.D., director of the National Eye Institute (NEI). "Patients now know that their choice will not impact their survival."

COMS was supported by the NEI and the National Cancer Institute (NCI), components of the federal government's National Institutes of Health. "The COMS findings are a striking example of the role that clinical trials play in improving patient care," said Richard Klausner, M.D., director of the NCI.

With the data showing similar survival rates for radiation therapy versus removal of the eye, quality of life issues become important factors when deciding between the two treatment options.

"Most patients who received the radiation therapy had some vision loss, and some eyes receiving radiation therapy were later removed because of tumor regrowth or other complications," said Stuart Fine, M.D., chairman of the Department of Ophthalmology at the University of Pennsylvania in Philadelphia and chair of the COMS clinical trial. "However, many people diagnosed with primary eye cancer may consider these problems worth risking in comparison to immediate loss of the eye."

For more than a century, removal of the eye has been the standard treatment for primary eye cancer, also known as ocular melanoma. During the past 25 years, interest in radiation therapy has increased because of the potential for saving the eye—and with it, some vision. However, many in the medical community questioned whether patients treated with eye-conserving radiation therapy experienced higher death rates than those whose eyes were removed.

In 1998, researchers from the first of two separate but related randomized COMS trials released results concerning whether a type of preoperative radiation therapy, called external beam radiation, prolonged life for patients whose ocular melanoma tumors were so large that removal of the eye was a medical necessity. Researchers reported that patients had similar survival rates regardless of whether their eyes were treated with external beam radiation prior to removal of the eye, or had their eyes removed without prior radiation therapy.

In the second randomized COMS trial, patients with medium-sized tumors were studied to determine which of two treatments—radiation therapy or removal of the eye—was more likely to prolong survival.

The affected eyes of one group received a form of radiation therapy called I-125 brachytherapy in which a small plaque containing radioactive iodine pellets is placed over the tumor. The other group had the eye removed. Approximately one third of the patients have been followed for 10 years; over 80 percent were followed for five years. Researchers found that the survival rates were essentially the same in the two groups.

COMS researchers also found that the five-year survival rate of patients who were treated with either radiation therapy or eye removal was 82 percent, considerably better than the 70 percent five-year survival rate that had been projected when the study was designed in

1985. Moreover, there is no evidence that either treatment causes harm to the other eye. All patients in the study will continue to be followed for up to 15 years.

COMS researchers have launched a parallel study to assess the quality of life for patients enrolled in the COMS clinical trial. The findings of the quality-of-life study—when released in a few years—"should provide more information on which to base a treatment decision," said Fine.

The type of eye cancer studied by COMS researchers is choroidal melanoma, a tumor of the eye that arises from pigmented cells of the choroid, a layer of tissue in the back of the eye. Although it is rare, choroidal melanoma is the most common primary eye cancer in adults. These tumors enlarge over time and may lead to vision loss.

More importantly, these tumors can spread, or metastasize, to other parts of the body; once metastasis is clinically detected, death typically occurs within months. Because there is no cure for metastatic melanoma, treatment is aimed at keeping the cancer confined to the eye. Researchers estimate that between 1,600 and 2,400 new cases of ocular melanoma are diagnosed annually in the United States and Canada, a rate of about six-to-eight new cases per million people each year. Choroidal melanoma is much more common in whites of northern European descent.

The COMS trials were conducted at 43 institutions, including medical schools, hospitals, and doctors' offices, throughout the United States and Canada.

Part Eight

Disorders with Eye-Related Complications

Chapter 54

Eye Allergies

Similar to processes that occur with other types of allergic responses, the eye may overreact to a substance perceived as harmful even though it may not be. For example, dust that is harmless to most people can cause excessive production of tears and mucus in eyes of overly sensitive, allergic individuals. Eye allergies are often hereditary.

Allergies can trigger other problems, such as conjunctivitis (pinkeye) and asthma. Most of the more than 22 million Americans who suffer from allergies also have allergic conjunctivitis, according to the American Academy of Ophthalmology.

Allergy Symptoms and Signs

Common signs of allergies include: red, swollen, tearing or itchy eyes; runny nose; sneezing; coughing; difficulty breathing; itchy nose, mouth or throat; and headache from sinus congestion.

What Causes Eye Allergies?

Many allergens are in the air, where they come in contact with your eyes and nose. Airborne allergens include pollen, mold, dust, and pet dander. Other causes of allergies, such as certain foods or bee stings,

"Eye Allergies," by Gina White, reviewed by Dr. Vance Thompson, is reprinted with permission from www.allaboutvision.com. © 2007 Access Media Group, LLC.

do not typically affect the eyes the way airborne allergens do. Adverse reactions to certain cosmetics or drugs such as antibiotic eyedrops also may cause eye allergies.

What Causes Watery Eyes?

Two common causes of excessively watery eyes are allergies and dry eye syndrome—two very different problems. With allergies, your body's release of histamine causes your eyes to water, just as it may cause your nose to run. It may not seem to make sense that watery eyes would result from dry eye syndrome, but this is sometimes true, because the excessive dryness works to overstimulate production of the watery component of your eye's tears.

Eye Allergies Self-Test

Take this quiz to see if you might have eye allergies. Always consult your doctor if you suspect you have an eye condition needing care.

- Do allergies run in your family?
- Do your eyes often itch, particularly during spring pollen season?
- Have you ever been diagnosed with pinkeye (conjunctivitis)?
- Are you allergic to certain animals such as cats?
- Do you often need antihistamines and/or decongestants to control sneezing, coughing, and congestion?
- When pollen is in the air, are your eyes less red and itchy when you stay indoors under an air conditioner?
- Do your eyes begin tearing when you wear certain cosmetics or lotions, or when you're around certain strong perfumes?

If you answered "yes" to most of these questions, then you may have eye allergies. Make an appointment with an optometrist or ophthalmologist to determine the best course of action.

Eye Allergy Treatment

Avoidance: The most common "treatment" is to avoid what's causing your eye allergy. Itchy eyes? Keep your home free of pet dander and dust, and stay inside with the air conditioner on when a lot of pollen is in the air. Air conditioners filter out allergens, though you must clean the filters from time to time.

Medications: If you're not sure what's causing your eye allergies, or you're not having any luck avoiding them, your next step will probably be medication to alleviate the symptoms.

Over-the-counter and prescription medications each have their advantages; for example, over-the-counter products are often less expensive, while prescription ones are often stronger.

Eyedrops are available as simple eye washes, or they may have one or more active ingredients such as antihistamines, decongestants or mast cell stabilizers. *Antihistamines* relieve many symptoms caused by airborne allergens, such as itchy, watery eyes, runny nose, and sneezing.

Decongestants clear up redness. They contain vasoconstrictors, which simply make the blood vessels in your eyes smaller, lessening the apparent redness. They treat the symptom, not the cause.

In fact, with extended use, the blood vessels can become dependent on the vasoconstrictor to stay small. When you discontinue the eyedrops, the vessels actually get bigger than they were to begin with. This process is called rebound hyperemia, and the result is that your red eyes get worse over time.

Some products have ingredients that act as mast cell stabilizers, which alleviate redness and swelling. *Mast cell stabilizers* are similar to antihistamines, but while antihistamines are known for their immediate relief, mast cell stabilizers are known for their long-lasting relief.

Antihistamines, decongestants and mast cell stabilizers are available in pill form, but pills don't work as quickly as eyedrops or gels to bring eye relief.

Nonsteroidal anti-inflammatory drug (NSAID) eyedrops may be prescribed to decrease swelling, inflammation, and other symptoms associated with seasonal allergic conjunctivitis, otherwise known as hay fever. Prescription corticosteroid eyedrops also may provide similar, quick relief. However, steroids have been associated with side effects such as increased inner eye pressure (intraocular pressure) leading to glaucoma, which can damage the optic nerve. Steroids also have been known to cause the eye's natural lens to become cloudy, producing cataracts.

Check the product label or insert for a list of side effects of over-the-counter medications. For prescription medication, ask your doctor. In some cases, combinations of medications may be used.

Immunotherapy: You may benefit from immunotherapy, in which an allergy specialist injects you with small amounts of the allergen to help you gradually build up immunity.

Eye Allergies and Contact Lenses

Even if you are generally a successful contact lens wearer, allergy season can make your contacts uncomfortable. Airborne allergens can get on your lenses, causing discomfort. Allergens can also stimulate the excessive production of natural substances in your eyes, which bind to your contacts and also become uncomfortable.

Ask your eye doctor about eyedrops that can help relieve your symptoms and keep your contact lenses clean: certain drops can discolor or damage certain lenses, so it makes sense to ask first before trying out a new brand. Another alternative is daily disposable contact lenses, which are discarded nightly. Because you replace them so frequently, these types of lenses are unlikely to develop irritating deposits that can build up over time and cause or heighten allergy-related discomfort.

Chapter 55

Diabetic Retinopathy

Diabetic Eye Disease: How Much Do You Know?

Do you know that diabetic eye disease is a leading cause of blindness? If you have diabetes, do you know how to reduce your risk of visual loss? To determine what your Eye-Q is, answer the following questions.

People with diabetes are more likely than people without diabetes to develop certain eye diseases.

True. Diabetic eye disease includes diabetic retinopathy—a leading cause of blindness in adults—cataract, and glaucoma. The longer someone has diabetes, the more likely he or she will develop diabetic eye disease.

Diabetic eye disease usually has early warning signs.

False. Often there are none in the early stages of the disease. Vision may not change until the disease becomes severe.

The information under the heading "Diabetic Eye Disease: How much do you know? Quiz," is from the National Eye Institute (NEI, www.nei.nih.gov), part of the National Institutes of Health, November 2006. The information under the heading "Diabetic Retinopathy Defined" is excerpted from "Diabetic Retinopathy," from the NEI, April 2006. The information under "Prevent Diabetes Problems: Keep Your Eyes Healthy," is excerpted from the National Institute on Diabetes and Digestive and Kidney Diseases (NIDDK, www.niddk.nih.gov), January 2007.

People with diabetes should have yearly eye examinations.

True. Everyone with diabetes should get an eye examination through dilated pupils at least once a year. Because diabetic eye disease usually has no symptoms, regular eye exams are important for early detection and timely treatment.

Diabetic retinopathy is caused by changes in the blood vessels in the eye.

True. In some people, blood vessels in the retina may swell and leak fluid. In other people, abnormal new blood vessels grow on the surface of the retina.

People with diabetes are at low risk for developing glaucoma.

False. Glaucoma is almost twice as likely to occur in people with diabetes than in those without the disease. Glaucoma can usually be treated with medications or laser or other surgery.

Laser surgery can be used to halt the progression of diabetic retinopathy.

True. In laser surgery, a special beam of light is used to shrink the abnormal blood vessels or seal leaking blood vessels. Laser surgery has been proved to reduce the five-year risk of vision loss from advanced diabetic retinopathy by more than 90 percent.

People with diabetes should have regular eye examinations through dilated pupils.

True. An eye examination through dilated pupils is the best way to detect diabetic eye disease, in which drops are used to enlarge the pupils. This allows the eye care professional to see more of the inside of the eye to check for signs of the disease.

Cataracts are common among people with diabetes.

True. People with diabetes are twice as likely to develop cataracts and to develop them at an earlier age than are those without diabetes. Cataracts can usually be treated with surgery.

People who have good control of their diabetes are not at high risk for diabetic eye disease.

False. Even with good control of blood glucose, there is still a risk of developing diabetic eye disease. However, studies show that careful management of blood sugar levels slows the onset and progression of diabetic retinopathy.

The risk of blindness from diabetic eye disease can be reduced.

True. With early detection and timely treatment, the risk of blindness from diabetic eye disease can be reduced.

If you got 9 or 10 answers right, congratulations! You know a lot about diabetic eye disease. If you missed some, review the answers so you can share your knowledge with your family and friends who have diabetes.

Diabetic Retinopathy Defined

What is diabetic eye disease?

Diabetic eye disease refers to a group of eye problems that people with diabetes may face as a complication of diabetes. All can cause severe vision loss or even blindness.

Diabetic eye disease may include:

- **diabetic retinopathy:** Damage to the blood vessels in the retina;

- **cataract:** Clouding of the eye's lens. Cataracts develop at an earlier age in people with diabetes; and

- **glaucoma:** Increase in fluid pressure inside the eye that leads to optic nerve damage and loss of vision. A person with diabetes is nearly twice as likely to get glaucoma as other adults.

What is diabetic retinopathy?

Diabetic retinopathy is the most common diabetic eye disease and a leading cause of blindness in American adults. It is caused by changes in the blood vessels of the retina.

In some people with diabetic retinopathy, blood vessels may swell and leak fluid. In other people, abnormal new blood vessels grow on the surface of the retina. The retina is the light-sensitive tissue at the back of the eye. A healthy retina is necessary for good vision.

If you have diabetic retinopathy, at first you may not notice changes to your vision. But over time, diabetic retinopathy can get worse and cause vision loss. Diabetic retinopathy usually affects both eyes.

What are the stages of diabetic retinopathy?

Diabetic retinopathy has four stages:

1. **Mild nonproliferative retinopathy:** At this earliest stage, microaneurysms occur. They are small areas of balloon-like swelling in the retina's tiny blood vessels.

2. **Moderate nonproliferative retinopathy:** As the disease progresses, some blood vessels that nourish the retina are blocked.

3. **Severe nonproliferative retinopathy:** Many more blood vessels are blocked, depriving several areas of the retina with their blood supply. These areas of the retina send signals to the body to grow new blood vessels for nourishment.

4. **Proliferative retinopathy.** At this advanced stage, the signals sent by the retina for nourishment trigger the growth of new blood vessels. This condition is called proliferative retinopathy. These new blood vessels are abnormal and fragile. They grow along the retina and along the surface of the clear, vitreous gel that fills the inside of the eye. By themselves, these blood vessels do not cause symptoms or vision loss. However, they have thin, fragile walls. If they leak blood, severe vision loss and even blindness can result.

How does diabetic retinopathy cause vision loss?

Blood vessels damaged from diabetic retinopathy can cause vision loss in two ways:

1. Fragile, abnormal blood vessels can develop and leak blood into the center of the eye, blurring vision. This is proliferative retinopathy and is the fourth and most advanced stage of the disease.

2. Fluid can leak into the center of the macula, the part of the eye where sharp, straight-ahead vision occurs. The fluid makes

the macula swell, blurring vision. This condition is called macular edema. It can occur at any stage of diabetic retinopathy, although it is more likely to occur as the disease progresses. About half of the people with proliferative retinopathy also have macular edema.

Who is at risk for diabetic retinopathy?

All people with diabetes—both type 1 and type 2—are at risk. That's why everyone with diabetes should get a comprehensive dilated eye exam at least once a year. The longer someone has diabetes, the more likely he or she will get diabetic retinopathy. Between 40 to 45 percent of Americans diagnosed with diabetes have some stage of diabetic retinopathy. If you have diabetic retinopathy, your doctor can recommend treatment to help prevent its progression.

During pregnancy, diabetic retinopathy may be a problem for women with diabetes. To protect vision, every pregnant woman with diabetes should have a comprehensive dilated eye exam as soon as possible. Your doctor may recommend additional exams during your pregnancy.

What can I do to protect my vision?

If you have diabetes get a comprehensive dilated eye exam at least once a year and remember:

- Proliferative retinopathy can develop without symptoms. At this advanced stage, you are at high risk for vision loss.

- Macular edema can develop without symptoms at any of the four stages of diabetic retinopathy.

- You can develop both proliferative retinopathy and macular edema and still see fine. However, you are at high risk for vision loss.

- Your eye care professional can tell if you have macular edema or any stage of diabetic retinopathy. Whether or not you have symptoms, early detection and timely treatment can prevent vision loss.

If you have diabetic retinopathy, you may need an eye exam more often. People with proliferative retinopathy can reduce their risk of blindness by 95 percent with timely treatment and appropriate follow-up care.

The Diabetes Control and Complications Trial (DCCT) showed that better control of blood sugar levels slows the onset and progression of retinopathy. The people with diabetes who kept their blood sugar levels as close to normal as possible also had much less kidney and nerve disease. Better control also reduces the need for sight-saving laser surgery.

This level of blood sugar control may not be best for everyone, including some elderly patients, children under age 13, or people with heart disease. Be sure to ask your doctor if such a control program is right for you.

Other studies have shown that controlling elevated blood pressure and cholesterol can reduce the risk of vision loss. Controlling these will help your overall health as well as help protect your vision.

Does diabetic retinopathy have any symptoms?

Often there are no symptoms in the early stages of the disease, nor is there any pain. Don't wait for symptoms. Be sure to have a comprehensive dilated eye exam at least once a year.

Blurred vision may occur when the macula—the part of the retina that provides sharp central vision—swells from leaking fluid. This condition is called macular edema.

If new blood vessels grow on the surface of the retina, they can bleed into the eye and block vision.

What are the symptoms of proliferative retinopathy if bleeding occurs?

At first, you will see a few specks of blood, or spots, "floating" in your vision. If spots occur, see your eye care professional as soon as possible. You may need treatment before more serious bleeding occurs. Hemorrhages tend to happen more than once, often during sleep.

Sometimes, without treatment, the spots clear, and you will see better. However, bleeding can reoccur and cause severely blurred vision. You need to be examined by your eye care professional at the first sign of blurred vision, before more bleeding occurs.

If left untreated, proliferative retinopathy can cause severe vision loss and even blindness. Also, the earlier you receive treatment, the more likely treatment will be effective.

How are diabetic retinopathy and macular edema detected?

Diabetic retinopathy and macular edema are detected during a comprehensive eye exam that includes:

- **Visual acuity test:** This eye chart test measures how well you see at various distances.

- **Dilated eye exam:** Drops are placed in your eyes to widen, or dilate, the pupils. This allows the eye care professional to see more of the inside of your eyes to check for signs of the disease. Your eye care professional uses a special magnifying lens to examine your retina and optic nerve for signs of damage and other eye problems. After the exam, your close-up vision may remain blurred for several hours.

- **Tonometry:** An instrument measures the pressure inside the eye. Numbing drops may be applied to your eye for this test.

Your eye care professional checks your retina for early signs of the disease, including:

- leaking blood vessels;

- retinal swelling (macular edema);

- pale, fatty deposits on the retina—signs of leaking blood vessels;

- damaged nerve tissue; and

- any changes to the blood vessels.

If your eye care professional believes you need treatment for macular edema, he or she may suggest a fluorescein angiogram. In this test, a special dye is injected into your arm. Pictures are taken as the dye passes through the blood vessels in your retina. The test allows your eye care professional to identify any leaking blood vessels and recommend treatment.

How is diabetic retinopathy treated?

During the first three stages of diabetic retinopathy, no treatment is needed, unless you have macular edema. To prevent progression of diabetic retinopathy, people with diabetes should control their levels of blood sugar, blood pressure, and blood cholesterol.

Proliferative retinopathy is treated with laser surgery. This procedure is called scatter laser treatment. Scatter laser treatment helps to shrink the abnormal blood vessels. Your doctor places 1,000 to 2,000 laser burns in the areas of the retina away from the macula, causing the abnormal blood vessels to shrink. Because a high number of laser burns are necessary, two or more sessions usually are required to complete treatment. Although you may notice some loss of your side vision, scatter laser treatment can save the rest of your sight. Scatter laser treatment may slightly reduce your color vision and night vision.

Scatter laser treatment works better before the fragile, new blood vessels have started to bleed. That is why it is important to have regular, comprehensive dilated eye exams. Even if bleeding has started, scatter laser treatment may still be possible, depending on the amount of bleeding.

If the bleeding is severe, you may need a surgical procedure called a vitrectomy. During a vitrectomy, blood is removed from the center of your eye.

How is a macular edema treated?

Macular edema is treated with laser surgery. This procedure is called focal laser treatment. Your doctor places up to several hundred small laser burns in the areas of retinal leakage surrounding the macula. These burns slow the leakage of fluid and reduce the amount of fluid in the retina. The surgery is usually completed in one session. Further treatment may be needed.

A patient may need focal laser surgery more than once to control the leaking fluid. If you have macular edema in both eyes and require laser surgery, generally only one eye will be treated at a time, usually several weeks apart.

Focal laser treatment stabilizes vision. In fact, focal laser treatment reduces the risk of vision loss by 50 percent. In a small number of cases, if vision is lost, it can be improved. Contact your eye care professional if you have vision loss.

What happens during laser treatment?

Both focal and scatter laser treatment are performed in your doctor's office or eye clinic. Before the surgery, your doctor will dilate your pupil and apply drops to numb the eye. The area behind your eye also may be numbed to prevent discomfort.

The lights in the office will be dim. As you sit facing the laser machine, your doctor will hold a special lens to your eye. During the procedure, you may see flashes of light. These flashes eventually may create a stinging sensation that can be uncomfortable. You will need someone to drive you home after surgery. Because your pupil will remain dilated for a few hours, you should bring a pair of sunglasses.

For the rest of the day, your vision will probably be a little blurry. If your eye hurts, your doctor can suggest treatment.

Laser surgery and appropriate follow-up care can reduce the risk of blindness by 90 percent. However, laser surgery often cannot restore vision that has already been lost. That is why finding diabetic retinopathy early is the best way to prevent vision loss.

What is a vitrectomy?

If you have a lot of blood in the center of the eye (vitreous gel), you may need a vitrectomy to restore your sight. If you need vitrectomies in both eyes, they are usually done several weeks apart.

A vitrectomy is performed under either local or general anesthesia. Your doctor makes a tiny incision in your eye. Next, a small instrument is used to remove the vitreous gel that is clouded with blood. The vitreous gel is replaced with a salt solution. Because the vitreous gel is mostly water, you will notice no change between the salt solution and the original vitreous gel.

You will probably be able to return home after the vitrectomy. Some people stay in the hospital overnight. Your eye will be red and sensitive. You will need to wear an eye patch for a few days or weeks to protect your eye. You also will need to use medicated eyedrops to protect against infection.

Are scatter laser treatment and vitrectomy effective in treating proliferative retinopathy?

Yes. Both treatments are very effective in reducing vision loss. People with proliferative retinopathy have less than a five percent chance of becoming blind within five years when they get timely and appropriate treatment. Although both treatments have high success rates, they do not cure diabetic retinopathy.

Once you have proliferative retinopathy, you always will be at risk for new bleeding. You may need treatment more than once to protect your sight.

What can I do if I already have lost some vision from diabetic retinopathy?

If you have lost some sight from diabetic retinopathy, ask your eye care professional about low vision services and devices that may help you make the most of your remaining vision. Ask for a referral to a specialist in low vision. Many community organizations and agencies offer information about low vision counseling, training, and other special services for people with visual impairments. A nearby school of medicine or optometry may provide low vision services.

The National Eye Institute (NEI) is conducting and supporting research that seeks better ways to detect, treat, and prevent vision loss in people with diabetes. This research is conducted through studies in the laboratory and with patients.

For example, researchers are studying drugs that may stop the retina from sending signals to the body to grow new blood vessels. Someday, these drugs may help people control their diabetic retinopathy and reduce the need for laser surgery.

Prevent Diabetes Problems: Keep Your Eyes Healthy

What should I do each day to stay healthy with diabetes?

- Follow the healthy eating plan that you and your doctor or dietitian have worked out.

- Be active a total of 30 minutes most days. Ask your doctor what activities are best for you.

- Take your medicines as directed.

- Check your blood glucose every day. Each time you check your blood glucose, write the number in your record book.

- Check your feet every day for cuts, blisters, sores, swelling, redness, or sore toenails.

- Brush and floss your teeth every day.

- Control your blood pressure and cholesterol.

- Don't smoke.

What can I do to prevent diabetes eye problems?

- Keep your blood glucose and blood pressure as close to normal as you can.

- Have an eye care professional examine your eyes once a year. Have this exam even if your vision is OK. The eye care professional will use drops to make the black part of your eyes—pupils—bigger. This process is called dilating your pupil, which allows the eye care professional to see the back of your eye. Finding eye problems early and getting treatment right away will help prevent more serious problems later on.

- Ask your eye care professional to check for signs of cataracts and glaucoma.

- If you are pregnant and have diabetes, see an eye care professional during your first 3 months.

- If you are planning to get pregnant, ask your doctor if you should have an eye exam.

- Don't smoke.

Chapter 56

Vision Problems Associated with Stroke and Traumatic Brain Injury

According to the National Center for Health Statistics, there are over 8 million head injuries each year with over 1.5 million of them classified as major injuries. The vast majority of people are saved by advances in modern medicine while only about 100,000 suffer fatal injuries. Another 500,000 people suffer from strokes each year, and it is estimated that there are over 3 million stroke survivors in the United States alone.

Millions of stroke and traumatic brain injury survivors suffer from visual problems. These visual problems range from dry eyes to visual field loss to double vision. Each case is different and the difficulty each patient has depends on the severity and location of the injury. Unfortunately, many patients with visual problems after a stroke or head injury fail to receive adequate vision rehabilitation.

Brain injury may affect vision in many ways. Here are some of the most common visual problems associated with stroke and traumatic brain injury.

Loss of Visual Field

A common visual effect of brain injury is the loss of one's visual field or our ability to see to the side. There are many types of visual field losses that can occur, but the most common form is a homonymous

"Common Vision Problems from Stroke or Traumatic Brain Injury," by Richard L. Windsor, O.D., F.A.A.O., and Laura K. Windsor, O.D., F.A.A.O., The Low Vision Centers of Indiana, © 2001. Reviewed 2007. Reprinted with permission.

hemianopsia or loss of half of the field of vision in each eye. If the posterior portion of the brain is damaged on one side of the brain, a loss of visual field occurs to the opposite side in both eyes. Patients often mistakenly believe the loss is just in one eye.

Patients frequently bump into objects and easily trip or fall over objects in their field loss. Going into crowded stores may become quite difficult, because people and objects suddenly appear in front of them from the blind side. Patients become afraid of leaving their homes and may even experience panic attacks. Additionally, the loss of visual field may also cause patients to miss words and have difficulty reading.

Patients with hemianoptic field loss may benefit from the Visual Field Awareness System developed by Dr. Daniel Gottlieb or the Peli Lens developed by Dr. Eli Peli, senior researcher at Harvard. Both of these systems increase the patient's ability to detect objects on the side of their vision loss. Training the patient in scanning techniques is also an important part of the treatment.

Visual Spatial Disorders and Visual Neglect

Patients may experience a variety of visual spatial disorders. When certain portions of the brain are damaged, the patient may fail to appreciate space to one side, which is usually to the left. Unlike visual field loss, this problem is not a physical loss of sensation, but rather a loss of attention to the area. A man with neglect may no longer shave one side of his face. Patients with visual neglect have more difficulties than those with only visual field loss. Unfortunately, both neglect and field loss may occur together. Other visual-spatial disorders may occur as well. Patients may experience difficulty navigating themselves even in familiar areas. Patients also misjudge the straight-ahead position and can confuse right versus left.

Vertigo, Dizziness, and Impaired Eye Movements

Smooth and accurate eye movements are essential in reading, tracking objects, and compensating for body movements. Following injury to the brain, movements may become more jerky in nature. As we move or tilt our head, our inner ears sense the angle at which we are tilting and cause compensatory eye movements. After head injury, these compensatory movements may become impaired. Nystagmus, a jerky motion of the eyes, may also occur. When acquired later in life, nystagmus results in a vertigo-like sensation or a feeling that the world is moving. Damage to the brain stem often results in dizziness.

Double Vision

Our eyes must point precisely at the same point in space to prevent diplopia or double vision. Each eye has six external muscles that move the eyes together as a team. If control is impaired to one or more muscles, the eyes cannot maintain alignment in all positions of gaze. This may occur due to damage to the control centers for the III, IV, and VI cranial nerves. Double vision may be constant or intermittent. The patient may experience normal single vision in the straight-ahead position, but suddenly have double vision on looking to one side.

Eyestrain and Difficulty in Reading

As we bring reading material close to our eyes, both eyes must turn in together as a team. It is called ocular convergence. This ability is frequently impaired in brain injury resulting in fatigue or discomfort while reading. Orthoptic therapy and prism lenses may aid this problem.

After injury, younger patients may experience more problems focusing at near. This may present simply as difficulty in reading. This is usually due to damage to the oculomotor nerve (CN III). This nerve is responsible for controlling the eye's ability to focus by changing the shape of the crystalline lens. Patients benefit from the use of bifocals to help compensate.

Eye movements called saccades are used to jump from word to word as we read. Impairments in saccades may result in difficulty reading smoothly along a line of print. Visual field loss may also impair reading. When the loss of field borders on the central area of the retina used in reading, patients may lose their place or have difficulty in reading long words. Impairments in cognitive skills and memory may also limit reading. Some patients may acquire an alexia, a loss of reading ability. Therapists may be able to rebuild reading skills in some patients. For those still unable to read, electronic scanner/reading machines like the Kurweil Omni system can read to the patient.

Light Sensitivity

Light sensitivity is quite variable. Some patients experience no problems while others have severe light sensitivity. Much like the volume control on a radio being broken, patients seem to have difficulty adjusting to the various lighting levels. Tinted eyewear, especially amber filters, may aid the patient and light sensitivity may improve with treatment of other vision problems.

Dry Eyes

Dry, burning, or gritty eyes may occur after brain injury. It may result from a decrease in the blink rate or poor closure of the lids. Artificial tears or tear duct plugs will usually control the problem.

Visual Hallucinations

Visual hallucinations may be formed objects such as a person or figure or may be unformed such as flashes of lights, stars, or flickering distortions.

Impaired Visual Memory

Memory is often impaired after stroke or head injury. In rare cases very specific types of memory processing is impaired. A patient may no longer be able to recognize faces, objects, or letters.

Summary

The visual problems of acquired brain injury may affect nearly all aspects of vision and can hinder normal recovery. Early vision evaluation is crucial. A clinician skilled in both low vision and brain injury is often needed to understand the interaction of all of these visual problems in order to make the appropriate low vision rehabilitation plan for each patient with acquired brain injury. The long road back from brain injury requires the teamwork of many doctors and therapists and most of all time and patience throughout the rehabilitative process.

About the Authors

Drs. Richard and Laura Windsor are a father and daughter team of low vision specialists at the Low Vision Centers of Indiana. Dr. Laura Windsor was recently honored with the 2001 National Essilor Award. Her father is past recipient of the American Optometric Association's National Optometrist of the Year 1999. They are currently completing a book chapter on low vision care for the acquired brain injury patient. They have also prepared a videotape on rehabilitation of hemianoptic visual field loss which is common in brain injury patients. Their work has recently been featured on *Breakthroughs in Science* television segment broadcast around the United States. You may reach them Dr. Richard L. Windsor at richw@eyeassociates.com and Dr. Laura K. Windsor at drlaura@eyeassociates.com.

Chapter 57

Hereditary Disorders That Affect Vision

Chapter Contents

Section 57.1

Albinism and Its Effect on Vision

"Albinism: Low Vision Considerations," by Richard L. Windsor, O.D.,
F.A.A.O., and Laura K. Windsor, O.D., F.A.A.O., The Low Vision Centers
of Indiana, © 2001. Reviewed 2007. Reprinted with permission.

Albinism is a set of inherited disorders that result from the inability of the body to produce melanin pigment. Melanin is dark pigment that protects our tissues from ultraviolet radiation. The process of forming melanin in the body takes many steps and may be affected by genes on six different chromosomes. Due to the many genetic variations causing this condition many different forms of albinism may occur. The most severe form of albinism presents with little or no pigmentation of the skin, hair, and eyes. These individuals present with white/platinum hair, pink skin, and often a pinkish eye color. Other forms of albinism may affect only the eyes. These individuals will present with many of the eye and vision problems related to albinism, but have normal skin and hair pigmentation.

Effects of Albinism

- **Reduced vision and macular/foveal hypoplasia:** Patients with albinism have reduced visual acuity primarily from an underdevelopment of the center of the retina. The macula is where the best vision is located and it contains a very sensitive area called the foveal pit. The pit fails to develop in albinism and causes mild to moderate reduction of central vision.

- **Photophobia:** The melanin pigment absorbs stray light and protects our eyes and skin from ultraviolet light. This pigment coats most of the internal layer of the eye allowing light to enter only through the pupil, and the pigment in the retina normally absorbs stray light. Failure of the eye to develop pigmentation in albinism results in extreme light sensitivity. Thus the patient may not only have too much light entering the eye, but also have no way to handle the excess stray light once in the eye.

- **Sunburn:** Patients with albinism are at risk for severe sunburn. Children must be taught to protect their skin. Sunscreens and adequate clothing are essential. Sun may pass through clothing, especially wet clothing, and burn the skin. Increased risk of sunburn occurs at higher altitudes, and may occur at lower latitudes around reflective surroundings such as sand and water.

- **Nystagmus:** In congenital forms of vision loss it is common for patients to have nystagmus. Nystagmus is an involuntary rhythmic oscillation of the eyes. It is often the first sign that parents recognize an infant has a vision loss. Nystagmus can occur in many forms and can lead to a decrease in vision just from the rhythmic movement.

- **The null position—unusual head and/or eye position:** Patients may also show a tilt or turning of their head or eyes to where they achieve their best vision. This is called the null position. It is crucial that family and teachers allow a child with albinism to tilt or turn their head or eyes to the position that lets them see the best. When bifocals are prescribed, the low vision specialist must select the type and position that works with the patient's null position.

- **Fluctuating vision:** A patient's nystagmus often fluctuates when under stress or when tired or fatigued. As the nystagmus increases, the vision may blur further. Children with nystagmus may not do well with timed tests that may place the child under stress. Even covering one eye may cause a change in the vision of the viewing eye due to an increase in nystagmus.

- **Strabismus (Crossing or turning out):** The loss of binocular vision is common in albinism, and this results in reduced depth perception.

- **Stable condition:** Albinism is a stable condition. In fact, some patients show slight improvement in visual acuity by the time they are young adults. This may be related to increased pigmentation or a better control of the nystagmus.

- **Systemic issues:** Albinism has been linked in rare cases with systemic diseases. The most common is Hermansky-Pudlak syndrome (HPS). HPS occurs throughout the world, but is most commonly associated with patients of Puerto Rican descent. Abnormalities of the granules in the blood platelets cause a bleeding disorder and an accumulation of a chemical called ceroid. Lung and gastrointestinal problems may develop including the inability to full expand the lungs and colitis. To diagnose HPS, the electron microscope must be used to examine the blood platelets. The Hermansky-Pudlak Syndrome Network, Inc. may be reached on the internet at www.hpsnetwork.org. Albinism has also been associated with Chediak-Higashi syndrome (CHS), Prader-Willi syndrome, and Angelman syndrome.

- **Emotional aspects:** Patients with albinism must deal with the emotional aspect of appearing different. Pink skin and eyes, white or platinum hair, unusual head or eye null positions, thick eyewear, and the need to hold reading material very close unfortunately cause these patients to stand out more. Adding to the problem, Hollywood has frequently exploited albinism in movies picturing "albinos" as evil or sinister characters. The Albinism in Popular Culture website at www.lunaeterna.net/popcult discusses how albinism has been viewed by society.

Low Vision Care

- **Low vision care for albinism:** Patients with albinism are excellent candidates for low vision care. Albinism is a mild to moderate, stable central vision loss. These patients have excellent residual side vision. Simple magnification, correction of refractive errors, light and glare control, and use of adaptive aids may all benefit albinism patients.

- **Filters and sun protection:** Tints, selective filters, and hats may aid the albinism patient. The low vision specialist must consider the need for adequate filters both inside and out. Sunlight may be 100 times brighter than inside light. Filters for general wear are usually not adequate for outside wear. Some patients may benefit from Transitions Xtra lenses that darken in the sun. Additionally, adequate education on the use of sunscreens, hats, and clothing is necessary in all albinism patients.

- **Refractive error:** Albinism usually results in significant amounts of farsightedness or nearsightedness combined with astigmatism. Most albinism patients require prescription eyewear. Refracting the nystagmus patient requires special techniques to reduce stress and avoid increasing the nystagmus. Every child with albinism should be carefully refracted by the low vision specialist at an early age.

- **Close reading distance:** With a mild to moderate loss of visual acuity, an albinism patient may require holding materials closer. Parents and teachers often worry about the close distance, but the patient should be allowed to read at the distance where they see the best. Most albinism patients benefit from bifocals to reduce the strain of focusing at such a close distance. Bifocals should be considered in all school-age children with albinism.

- **Reading vision:** At an early age bifocals may help patients with albinism by reducing fatigue and eye strained caused by the very close working distance. Magnifiers, strong reading glasses, and closed circuit television system may be helpful.

- **Contact lenses:** Contact lenses can be used to correct the refractive error (myopia, farsightedness, and astigmatism) of an albinism patient and in some cases an improvement in visual acuity is obtained. Contact lenses have been shown to aid some patients with nystagmus. One theory is that the tactile feedback of feeling the contact lenses on the eyes may lead to better control of the movement and allow the patient better vision. Another benefit of contact lenses is that they move with the eyes and provide better image quality.

- **Bioptic driving:** The vision loss from albinism is moderate and is usually a stable condition. Albinism patients are usually excellent candidates for bioptic driving. Bioptic driving requires the use of a bioptic telescopic system for spotting signs and lights. Extensive training is required to make sure the patient is using the bioptic correctly and that his/her skills behind the wheel are adequate. NOAH, National Organization of Albinism and Hypopigmentation, offers an internet discussion group on bioptic driving. Their website is at www.albinism.org.

Support and Information about Albinism

NOAH, the National Organization of Albinism and Hypopigmentation (NOAH), is a wonderful resource for information on albinism. They have handouts on all aspects of albinism and offer periodic national meetings that serve both as educational experiences and also an opportunity for individuals with albinism and their families to meet.

The International Albinism Center is a located at the University of Minnesota. You may access their website at http://albinism.med.umn .edu. It contains a wealth of information and a scientific database on albinism. You may access online the article "Facts on Albinism" written by Drs. Richard A. King, C. Gail Summers, James W. Haefemeyer, and Bonnie LeRoy.

Section 57.2

Alström Syndrome: A Genetic Condition That Causes Progressive Loss of Vision

Excerpted from "Alström Syndrome," Genetics Home Reference
(ghr.nlm.nih.gov), a service of the U.S. National Library of Medicine,
October 2006.

What is Alström syndrome?

Alström syndrome is a rare condition that affects many body systems. Signs and symptoms of this condition begin in infancy or early childhood. Alström syndrome is characterized by a progressive loss of vision and hearing, enlargement of the heart and weakening of the heart muscle (cardiomyopathy), obesity, type 2 diabetes mellitus (the most common form of diabetes), and short stature. This disorder can also affect the liver, kidneys, bladder, and lungs. Some individuals with Alström syndrome have a skin condition called acanthosis nigricans, which causes the skin in body folds and creases to become thick, dark, and velvety. The signs and symptoms of Alström syndrome vary in severity, and affected individuals may not have all of the characteristic features of the disorder.

How common is Alström syndrome?

This condition is rare; only about 425 people worldwide are known to be affected.

What genes are related to Alström syndrome?

Mutations in the ALMS1 gene cause Alström syndrome. The ALMS1 gene provides instructions for making a protein whose function is unknown. Mutations in this gene probably lead to the production of an abnormally short, nonfunctional version of the ALMS1 protein. This protein is normally present at low levels in most tissues, so a loss of the protein's normal function may help explain why the signs and symptoms of Alström syndrome affect a variety of body systems.

How do people inherit Alström syndrome?

This condition is inherited in an autosomal recessive pattern, which means two copies of the gene in each cell are altered. The parents of an individual with Alström syndrome are carriers of one copy of the altered gene, but do not show signs and symptoms of the disorder.

What other names do people use for Alström syndrome?

- Alstrom-Hallgren syndrome
- Alstrom syndrome

Section 57.3

Anophthalmia and Microphthalmia

Excerpted from the "Anophthalmia and Microphthalmia Resource Guide," by the National Eye Institute (NEI, www.nei.nih.gov), part of the National Institutes of Health, December 2006.

What are anophthalmia and microphthalmia?

Anophthalmia and microphthalmia are often used interchangeably. Microphthalmia is a disorder in which one or both eyes are abnormally small, while anophthalmia is the absence of one or both eyes. These rare disorders develop during pregnancy and can be associated with other birth defects.

What causes anophthalmia and microphthalmia?

Causes of these conditions may include genetic mutations and abnormal chromosomes. Researchers also believe that environmental factors, such as exposure to X-rays, chemicals, drugs, pesticides, toxins, radiation, or viruses, increase the risk of anophthalmia and microphthalmia, but research is not conclusive. Sometimes the cause in an individual patient cannot be determined.

Can anophthalmia and microphthalmia be treated?

There is no treatment for severe anophthalmia or microphthalmia that will create a new eye or restore vision. However, some less severe forms of microphthalmia may benefit from medical or surgical treatments. In almost all cases improvements to a child's appearance are possible. Children can be fitted for a prosthetic (artificial) eye for cosmetic purposes and to promote socket growth. A newborn with anophthalmia or microphthalmia will need to visit several eye care professionals, including those who specialize in pediatrics, vitreoretinal disease, orbital and oculoplastic surgery, ophthalmic genetics, and prosthetic devices for the eye. Each specialist can provide information and possible treatments resulting in the best care for the child and family. The specialist in prosthetic diseases for the eye will make conformers, plastic structures that help support the face and encourage the eye socket to grow. As the face develops, new conformers will need to be made. A child with anophthalmia may also need to use expanders in addition to conformers to further enlarge the eye socket. Once the face is fully developed, prosthetic eyes can be made and placed. Prosthetic eyes will not restore vision.

How do conformers and prosthetic eyes look?

A painted prosthesis that looks like a normal eye is usually fitted between ages one and two. Until then, clear conformers are used. When the conformers are in place the eye socket will look black. These conformers are not painted to look like a normal eye because they are changed too frequently. Every few weeks a child will progress to a larger size conformer until about two years of age. If a child needs to wear conformers after age two, the conformers will be painted like a regular prosthesis, giving the appearance of a normal but smaller eye. The average child will need three to four new painted prostheses before the age of 10.

How is microphthalmia managed if there is residual vision in the eye?

Children with microphthalmia may have some residual vision (limited sight). In these cases, the good eye can be patched to strengthen vision in the microphthalmic eye. A prosthesis can be made to cap the microphthalmic eye to help with cosmetic appearance, while preserving the remaining sight.

Section 57.4

Bietti Crystalline Dystrophy

Excerpted from "Bietti's Crystalline Dystrophy Resource Guide," by the National Eye Institute (NEI, www.nei.nih.gov), part of the National Institutes of Health, December 2006.

What is Bietti crystalline dystrophy?

Bietti crystalline dystrophy (BCD) is an inherited eye disease named for Dr. G. B. Bietti, an Italian ophthalmologist, who described three patients with similar symptoms in 1937. The symptoms of BCD include: crystals in the cornea (the clear covering of the eye); yellow, shiny deposits on the retina; and progressive atrophy of the retina, choriocapillaries, and choroid (the back layers of the eye). This tends to lead to progressive night blindness and visual field constriction. BCD is a rare disease and appears to be more common in people with Asian ancestry.

People with BCD have crystals in some of their white blood cells (lymphocytes) that can be seen by using an electron microscope. Researchers have been unable to determine exactly what substance makes up these crystalline deposits. Their presence does not appear to harm the patient in any other way except to affect vision.

What causes Bietti crystalline dystrophy?

From family studies, we know that BCD is inherited primarily in an autosomal recessive fashion. This means that an affected person receives one nonworking gene from each of his or her parents. A person who inherits a nonworking gene from only one parent will be a carrier, but will not develop the disease. A person with BCD syndrome will pass on one gene to each of his or her children. However, unless the person has children with another carrier of BCD genes, the individual's children are not at risk for developing the disease.

In September 2000, NEI researchers reported that the BCD gene had been localized to chromosome #4. In this region of chromosome #4 there are hundreds of genes. Researchers are now looking for which of the genes in this region of chromosome #4 causes BCD. Finding the gene may shed light on the composition of the crystals found in the corneas of patients with BCD and on what causes the condition.

Can Bietti crystalline dystrophy be treated?

At this time, there is no treatment for BCD. Scientists hope that findings from gene research will be helpful in finding treatments for patients with BCD.

Section 57.5

Color Blindness

Definition

Color blindness is the inability to see certain colors in the usual way.

Causes, Incidence, and Risk Factors

Color blindness occurs when there is a problem with the color-sensing materials (pigments) in certain nerve cells of the eye. These cells are called cones. They are found in the retina, the light-sensitive layer of tissue at the back of the inner eye.

If you are missing just one pigment, you might have trouble telling the difference between red and green. This is the most common type of color blindness. Other times, people have trouble seeing blue-yellow colors. People with blue-yellow color blindness almost always have problems identifying reds and greens, too.

The most severe form of color blindness is achromatopsia. A person with this rare condition cannot see any color. Achromatopsia is often associated with lazy eye, nystagmus (small, jerky eye movements), severe light sensitivity, and extremely poor vision.

Most color blindness is due to a genetic problem. About 1 in 10 men have some form of color blindness. Very few women are color blind.

The drug hydroxychloroquine (Plaquenil) can also cause color blindness. It is used to treat rheumatoid arthritis, among other conditions.

Symptoms

Symptoms vary from person to person, but may include:

- Trouble seeing colors and the brightness of colors in the usual way

- Inability to tell the difference between shades of the same or similar colors

Often, the symptoms may be so mild that some persons do not know they are color blind. A parent may notice signs of color blindness when a child is learning his or her colors.

Rapid, side-to-side eye movements and other symptoms may occur in severe cases.

Signs and Tests

Your doctor or eye specialist can check your color vision in several ways. Testing for color blindness is commonly done during an eye exam.

Treatment

There is no known treatment.

Expectations (Prognosis)

Color blindness is a life-long condition. Most persons are able to adjust without difficulty or disability.

Complications

Those who are colorblind may not be able to get a job that requires color vision. For example, a pilot needs to be able to see colors.

Calling Your Health Care Provider

Make an appointment with your health care provider or ophthalmologist if you think you (or your child) have color blindness.

Section 57.6

Duane Syndrome: Congenital Eye Movement Disorder

"Learning about Duane Syndrome," is from the National Human
Genome Research Institute, part of the National Institutes of Health,
March 2007.

What is Duane syndrome?

Duane syndrome (DS) is a rare, congenital (present from birth) eye movement disorder. Most patients are diagnosed by the age of 10 years and DS is more common in girls (60 percent of the cases) than boys (40 percent of the cases).

DS is a miswiring of the eye muscles, causing some eye muscles to contract when they shouldn't and other eye muscles not to contract when they should. People with DS have a limited (and sometimes absent) ability to move the eye outward toward the ear (abduction) and, in most cases, a limited ability to move the eye inward toward the nose (adduction).

Often, when the eye moves toward the nose, the eyeball also pulls into the socket (retraction), the eye opening narrows and, in some cases, the eye will move upward or downward. Many patients with DS develop a face turn to maintain binocular vision and compensate for improper turning of the eyes.

In about 80 percent of cases of DS, only one eye is affected, most often the left. However, in some cases, both eyes are affected, with one eye usually more affected than the other.

Other names for this condition include: Duane retraction syndrome (or DR syndrome), eye retraction syndrome, retraction syndrome, congenital retraction syndrome, and Stilling-Turk-Duane syndrome.

In 70 percent of DS cases, this is the only disorder the individual has. However, other conditions and syndromes have been found in association with DS. These include malformation of the skeleton, ears, eyes, kidneys and nervous system, as well as:

- Okihiro syndrome, an association of DS with forearm malformation and hearing loss;

- Wildervanck syndrome, fusion of neck vertebrae and hearing loss;

- Holt-Oram syndrome, abnormalities of the upper limbs and heart;

- Morning Glory syndrome, abnormalities of the optic disc or "blind spot"; and

- Goldenhar syndrome, malformation of the jaw, cheek, and ear, usually on one side of the face.

What are the symptoms of Duane syndrome?

Clinically, Duane syndrome is often subdivided into three types, each with associated symptoms.

- **Type 1:** The affected eye, or eyes, has limited ability to move outward toward the ear, but the ability to move inward toward the nose is normal or nearly so. The eye opening narrows and the eyeball pulls in when looking inward toward the nose, however the reverse occurs when looking outward toward the ear. About 78 percent of all DS cases are Type 1.

- **Type 2:** The affected eye, or eyes, has limited ability to move inward toward the nose, but the ability to move outward toward the ear is normal or nearly so. The eye opening narrows and the eyeball pulls in when looking inward toward the nose. About 7 percent of all DS cases are Type 2.

- **Type 3:** The affected eye, or eyes, has limited ability to move both inward toward the nose and outward toward the ears. The eye opening narrows and the eyeball pulls in when looking inward toward the nose. About 15 percent of all DS cases are Type 3.

Each of these three types can be further classified into three subgroups, depending on where the eyes are when the individual looks straight (the primary gaze):

- Subgroup A: The affected eye is turned inward toward the nose (esotropia).

- Subgroup B: The affected eye is turned outward toward the ear (exotropia).

- Subgroup C: The eyes are in a straight, primary position.

What causes Duane syndrome?

Common thought is that Duane syndrome (DS) is a miswiring of the medial and the lateral rectus muscles, the muscles that move the eyes. Also, patients with DS lack the abducens nerve, the sixth cranial nerve, which is involved in eye movement. However, the etiology or origin of these malfunctions is, at present, a mystery.

Many researchers believe that DS results from a disturbance—either by genetic or environmental factors—during embryonic development. Since the cranial nerves and ocular muscles are developing between the third and eighth week of pregnancy, this is most likely when the disturbance happens.

Presently, it appears that several factors may be involved in causing DS. Therefore it is doubtful that a single mechanism is responsible for this condition.

What do we know about heredity and Duane syndrome?

Most likely, both genetic and environmental factors play a role in the development of Duane syndrome (DS). For those cases that show evidence of having a genetic cause, both dominant and recessive forms of DS have been found. (When a gene is dominant, only one gene from one parent is needed for the individual to express it physically. However, when a gene is recessive, a copy of the gene from both parents is needed for expression.)

The chromosomal location of the proposed gene for this syndrome is currently unknown. Some research shows that more than one gene may be involved. There is evidence that a gene involved in the development of DS is located on chromosome 2. Also, deletions of chromosomal material from chromosomes 4 and 8, as well as the presence of an extra marker chromosome thought to be derived from chromosome 22, have been linked to DS.

Section 57.7

Norrie Disease: An Inherited Eye Disorder That Leads to Blindness

Excerpted from "Norrie Disease," Genetics Home Reference
(ghr.nlm.nih.gov), a service of the U.S. National Library of Medicine,
April 2007.

What is Norrie disease?

Norrie disease is an inherited eye disorder that leads to blindness in male infants at birth or soon after birth. It causes abnormal development of the retina, the layer of sensory cells that detect light and color, with masses of immature retinal cells accumulating at the back of the eye. As a result, the pupils appear white when light is shone on them, a sign called leukocoria. The irises (colored portions of the eyes) or the entire eyeballs may shrink and deteriorate during the first months of life, and cataracts (cloudiness in the lens of the eye) may eventually develop.

About one third of individuals with Norrie disease develop progressive hearing loss, and more than half experience developmental delays in motor skills such as sitting up and walking. Other problems may include mild to moderate mental retardation, often with psychosis, and abnormalities that can affect circulation, breathing, digestion, excretion, or reproduction.

How common is Norrie disease?

Norrie disease is a rare disorder; its exact incidence is unknown. It is not associated with any specific racial or ethnic group.

What genes are related to Norrie disease?

Mutations in the NDP gene cause Norrie disease.

The NDP gene provides instructions for making a protein called norrin. Norrin participates in the Wnt cascade, a sequence of steps that affect the way cells and tissues develop. In particular, norrin seems to

495

play a critical role in the specialization of retinal cells for their unique sensory capabilities. It is also involved in the establishment of a blood supply to tissues of the retina and the inner ear, and the development of other body systems.

In order to initiate the Wnt cascade, norrin must bind (attach) to another protein called frizzled-4. Mutations in the norrin protein interfere with its ability to bind to frizzled-4, resulting in the signs and symptoms of Norrie disease.

How do people inherit Norrie disease?

This condition is inherited in an X-linked recessive pattern. A condition is considered X-linked if the mutated gene that causes the disorder is located on the X chromosome, one of the two sex chromosomes. In males (who have only one X chromosome), one altered copy of the gene in each cell is sufficient to cause the condition. In females (who have two X chromosomes), a mutation must be present in both copies of the gene to cause the disorder. Males are affected by X-linked recessive disorders much more frequently than females. A striking characteristic of X-linked inheritance is that fathers cannot pass X-linked traits to their sons.

In X-linked recessive inheritance, a female with one altered copy of the gene in each cell is called a carrier. She can pass on the gene, but generally does not experience signs and symptoms of the disorder. In rare cases, however, carrier females have shown some retinal abnormalities or mild hearing loss associated with Norrie disease.

What other names do people use for Norrie disease?

- Anderson-Warburg syndrome
- Atrophia bulborum hereditaria
- congenital progressive oculo-acoustico-cerebral degeneration
- Episkopi blindness
- Fetal iritis syndrome
- Norrie's disease
- Norrie syndrome
- Norrie-Warburg syndrome
- Oligophrenia microphthalmos
- pseudoglioma congenita
- Whitnall-Norman syndrome

Chapter 58

Other Disorders with Eye-Related Complications

Chapter Contents

Section 58.1

Behçet Disease of the Eye

Excerpted from "Behçet's Disease of the Eye Resource Guide,"
by the National Eye Institute (NEI, www.nei.nih.gov), part of the
National Institutes of Health, December 2006.

What is Behçet disease?

Behçet disease is an autoimmune disease that results from damage to blood vessels throughout the body, particularly veins. In an autoimmune disease, the immune system attacks and harms the body's own tissues.

What causes Behçet disease?

The exact cause is unknown. It is believed that an autoimmune reaction may cause blood vessels to become inflamed, but it is not clear what triggers this reaction.

What are the symptoms of Behçet disease?

Behçet disease affects each person differently. The four most common symptoms are mouth sores, genital sores, inflammation inside of the eye, and skin problems. Inflammation inside of the eye (uveitis, retinitis, and iritis) occurs in more that half of those with Behçet disease and can cause blurred vision, pain, and redness.

Other symptoms may include arthritis, blood clots, and inflammation in the central nervous system and digestive organs.

How is Behçet disease treated?

There is no cure for Behçet disease. Treatment typically focuses on reducing discomfort and preventing serious complications. Corticosteroids and other medications that suppress the immune system may be prescribed to treat inflammation.

What is the prognosis for someone with Behçet disease?

Behçet is a chronic disease that recurs. However, patients may have periods of time when symptoms go away temporarily (remission). How severe the disease is varies from patient to patient. Some patients may live normal lives, but others may become blind or severely disabled.

Section 58.2

Graves Disease: Thyroid Eye Disease

Also known as Graves disease, thyroid eye disease is the most common orbital disorder in adults.

What Is Thyroid Eye Disease?

Thyroid eye disease is an autoimmune condition that is associated with hyperthyroidism or Graves disease. It is the most common orbital disorder in adults. Thyroid eye disease is also known as thyroid-associated ophthalmopathy.

The most important risk factor is the presence of hyperthyroidism. Other risk factors can include advanced age, gender (more prevalent in women), smoking, and radioactive treatment of a hyperthyroid state. Some patients can present with thyroid eye disease before any systemic thyroid disease is identified.

Symptoms of Thyroid Eye Disease

The most common symptoms of thyroid eye disease are:

- eyes may initially feel dry, gritty, and irritated;
- eyelid swelling and retraction;
- bulging of the eyes;
- development of double vision when glancing upward or downward;
- appearance of staring;

499

- face has unbalanced appearance; and
- vision loss.

Treatment for Thyroid Eye Disease

Treatment for thyroid eye disease is complex and often involves several physicians including a neuro-ophthalmologist, an orbital specialist, and an endocrinologist.

There are two phases of thyroid eye disease. The first phase can last as long as 36 months during which time symptoms occur gradually and may even wax and wane. After this time, eye symptoms usually stabilize. During this initial phase, treatment concerns managing and treating the underlying hyperthyroidism as well as reducing discomfort, avoiding double vision, and preserving sight.

Treatments can include:

- using artificial tears at night;
- corticosteroids to reduce swelling;
- radiation treatment to the orbit;
- patching one eye or using prism glasses (to manage double vision); or
- orbital decompression surgery for vision loss from optic nerve compression.

During the second phase of thyroid eye disease the eye symptoms stabilize and treatment concerns correcting any unacceptable permanent changes such as protrusion of the eyes and the appearance of staring, which can be corrected surgically. If double vision continues after the initial stage, this can also be corrected through eye muscle surgery.

Most patients do well and 75% of patients require only supportive therapy. Most patients do not develop sight-threatening complications. The disease runs a self-limited course of 18 to 36 months and up to two thirds of patients with thyroid eye disease will improve spontaneously. However, it is very important that an ophthalmologist monitors one's vision to avoid vision loss from optic neuropathy, a rare but serious potential complication of thyroid eye disease.

Section 58.3

Holmes-Adie Syndrome

"Holmes-Adie Syndrome Information Page," is from the National Institute of Neurological Disorders and Stroke (NINDS, www.ninds.nih.gov), part of the National Institutes of Health, February 13, 2007.

What is Holmes-Adie syndrome?

Holmes-Adie syndrome (HAS) is a neurological disorder affecting the pupil of the eye and the autonomic nervous system. It is characterized by one eye with a pupil that is larger than normal and constricts slowly in bright light (tonic pupil), along with the absence of deep tendon reflexes, usually in the Achilles tendon. HAS is thought to be the result of a viral or bacterial infection that causes inflammation and damage to neurons in the ciliary ganglion, an area of the brain that controls eye movements, and the spinal ganglion, an area of the brain involved in the response of the autonomic nervous system. HAS begins gradually in one eye, and often progresses to involve the other eye. At first, it may only cause the loss of deep tendon reflexes on one side of the body, but then progress to the other side. The eye and reflex symptoms may not appear at the same time. People with HAS may also sweat excessively, sometimes only on one side of the body. The combination of these three symptoms—abnormal pupil size, loss of deep tendon reflexes, and excessive sweating—is usually called Ross syndrome, although some doctors will still diagnosis the condition as a variant of HAS. Some individuals will also have cardiovascular abnormalities. The HAS symptoms can appear on their own, or in association with other diseases of the nervous system, such as Sjögren syndrome or migraine. It is most often seen in young women. It is rarely an inherited condition.

Is there any treatment?

Doctors may prescribe reading glasses to compensate for impaired vision in the affected eye, and pilocarpine drops to be applied three times daily to constrict the dilated pupil. Thoracic sympathectomy, which severs the involved sympathetic nerve, is the definitive treatment for excessive sweating.

What is the prognosis?

Holmes-Adie syndrome is not life-threatening or disabling. The loss of deep tendon reflexes is permanent. Some symptoms of the disorder may progress. For most individuals, pilocarpine drops and glasses will improve vision.

What research is being done?

The National Institute of Neurological Disorders and Stroke (NINDS), and other institutes of the National Institutes of Health (NIH), conduct research related to HAS in laboratories at the NIH, and also support additional research through grants to major medical institutions across the country. Much of this research focuses on finding better ways to prevent, treat, and ultimately cure disorders, such as HAS.

Section 58.4

Ocular Rosacea

While red, teary or scratchy eyes might sometimes be shrugged off as simple irritation from harsh winter weather, these may actually be warning signs of ocular rosacea, a potentially serious condition that many people do not associate with a skin disorder.

"The effects of rosacea on the eyes may easily be overlooked because they often develop after, and sometimes before, the disorder affects the skin," said Dr. Bryan Sires, associate professor and acting chair of ophthalmology at the University of Washington. "In most cases, ocular rosacea is a mild, irritating condition, but it can develop into a permanently debilitating one—including loss of vision—without proper care."

Although as many as 58 percent of rosacea patients have been found to have ocular symptoms in clinical studies, he noted that the condition may be easily controlled if diagnosed and treated before it becomes severe.

An eye affected by rosacea often appears to be watery or bloodshot. Patients may feel a gritty or foreign body sensation in the eye, or have a dry, burning, or stinging sensation.

Dr. Sires added that in the majority of ocular rosacea patients, beyond mild irritation there is a feeling of fullness in the eyelid. This is often the result of thickened secretions of the meibomian or Zeis glands along the eyelid margin. The fatty secretions help to avoid evaporation of the watery layer of the tears. The plugging of these glands may lead to dry eye or styes, both common manifestations of ocular rosacea.

"Severe symptoms result when the cornea becomes infected," he said. "These patients have a deep boring pain. At this point, an aggressive treatment approach is necessary to avoid the need for a more invasive procedure like corneal transplantation."

Left untreated, patients with severe ocular rosacea could endure scarring within the eyelid, vision loss from corneal ulcers, and potential loss of the eye if an ulcer progresses beyond the cornea.

Ocular rosacea is diagnosed by an overall examination of both the facial skin and eyes. Ophthalmologists also frequently use a biomicroscope, which allows the detection of tiny visible blood vessels along the eyelid margin and any plugging of the meibomian glands—both signs of ocular rosacea.

Treatment for ocular rosacea is typically a combination of local and systemic therapy as well as cleansing and tearing agents, all of which may be adjusted over time.

For mild cases, patients are often instructed to use warm compresses several times a day on the eyelids. Lid hygiene may include gentle cleansing with a Q-Tip and baby shampoo. For moderate cases, topical medications may be prescribed, along with eyedrops for lubrication.

"For more severe cases, patients are placed on oral antibiotics such as doxycycline," Dr. Sires said. "This is at regular doses for a two-week period and then at a maintenance dose for several months thereafter."

As with facial rosacea, ocular rosacea patients are also encouraged to identify and avoid any lifestyle or environmental factors that may trigger or aggravate their individual condition. Common trigger factors include emotional stress, hot or cold weather, wind, spicy food, alcohol, heated beverages, and many others.

Part Nine

Protecting Vision by Avoiding Injury

Chapter 59

Eye Emergencies

Chapter Contents

Section 59.1

Types of Eye Emergencies

Definition

Eye emergencies include cuts, scratches, objects in the eye, burns, chemical exposure, and blunt injuries to the eye or eyelid. Since the eye is easily damaged, any of these conditions can lead to vision loss if left untreated.

Considerations

It is important to get medical attention for all significant eye or eyelid injuries and problems. An injury to the eyelid may be a sign of severe injury to the eye itself. Many eye problems (such as a painful red eye) that are not due to injury still need urgent medical attention.

A chemical injury to the eye can be caused by a work-related accident or by common household products, such as cleaning solutions, garden chemicals, solvents, or many other types of chemicals. Fumes and aerosols can also cause chemical burns.

With acid burns, the haze on the cornea often clears with a good chance of recovery. However, alkaline substances—such as lime, lye, commercial drain cleaners, and sodium hydroxide found in refrigeration equipment—may cause permanent damage to the cornea. Ongoing damage may occur in spite of prompt treatment. It is important to flush the eye with clean water or saline while seeking urgent medical care.

Dust, sand, and other debris can easily enter the eye. Persistent pain and redness indicate that professional treatment is needed. A foreign body may threaten your vision if the object enters the eye itself or damages the cornea or lens. Foreign bodies propelled at high speed by machining, grinding, or hammering metal on metal present the highest risk.

A black eye is usually caused by direct trauma to the eye or face. Certain types of skull fractures can result in bruising around the eyes, even without direct trauma to the eye. The bruise is caused by bleeding under the skin. The tissue surrounding the eye turns black and blue, gradually becoming purple, green, and yellow over several days. The abnormal coloring disappears within 2 weeks. Usually, swelling of the eyelid and tissue around the eye also occurs.

Occasionally, serious damage to the eye itself occurs from the pressure of the swollen tissue. Bleeding inside the eye can reduce vision, cause glaucoma, or damage the cornea.

Causes

- Head injury
- Foreign object in the eye
- Chemical injury
- Blow to the eye
- Eyelid and eye cuts
- Conjunctivitis
- Glaucoma
- Orbital cellulitis
- Iritis
- Corneal abrasion

Symptoms

- Eye pain
- Loss of vision
- Decreased vision
- Double vision
- Redness—bloodshot appearance
- Sensitivity to light
- Bleeding
- Bruising
- Cuts or wounds
- Headache
- Itchy eyes
- Pupils of unequal size
- Stinging and burning
- Sensation of something in the eye

First Aid

Take prompt action and follow the steps below if you or someone else has an eye-related injury.

Small Object on the Eye or Eyelid

The eye will often clear itself of tiny objects, like eyelashes and sand, through blinking and tearing. If not, take these steps:

1. Tell the person not to rub the eye. Wash your hands before examining it.

2. Examine the eye in a well-lighted area. To find the object, have the person look up and down, then side to side.

3. If you can't find the object, grasp the lower eyelid and gently pull down on it to look under the lower eyelid. To look under the upper lid, you can place a cotton-tipped swab on the outside of the upper lid and gently flip the lid over the cotton swab.

4. If the object is on an eyelid, try to gently flush it out with water. If that does not work, try touching a second cotton-tipped swab to the object to remove it.

5. If the object is on the eye, try gently rinsing the eye with water. It may help to use an eye dropper positioned above the outer corner of the eye. **Do not** touch the eye itself with the cotton swab.

A scratchy feeling or other minor discomfort may continue after removing eyelashes and other tiny objects. This will go away within a day or two. If the person continues to have discomfort or blurred vision, get medical help.

Object Stuck or Embedded in Eye

1. Leave the object in place. **Do not** try to remove the object. **Do not** touch it or apply any pressure to it.

2. Calm and reassure the person.

3. Wash your hands.

4. Bandage both eyes. If the object is large, place a paper cup or cone over the injured eye and tape it in place. Cover the uninjured eye with gauze or a clean cloth. If the object is small,

cover both eyes with a clean cloth or sterile dressing. Even if only one eye is affected, covering both eyes will help prevent eye movement.

5.   Get medical help immediately.

Chemicals in the Eye

1.   Flush with cool tap water immediately. Turn the person's head so the injured eye is down and to the side. Holding the eyelid open, allow running water from the faucet to flush the eye for 15 minutes.

2.   If both eyes are affected, or if the chemicals are also on other parts of the body, have the victim take a shower.

3.   If the person is wearing contact lenses and the lenses did not flush out from the running water, have the person try to remove the contacts **after** the flushing procedure.

4.   Continue to flush the eye with clean water or saline while seeking urgent medical attention.

5.   After following the above instructions, seek medical help immediately.

Eye Cuts, Scratches, or Blows

1.   If the eyeball has been injured, get medical help immediately.

2.   Gently apply cold compresses to reduce swelling and help stop any bleeding. **Do not** apply pressure to control bleeding.

3.   If blood is pooling in the eye, cover both of the person's eyes with a clean cloth or sterile dressing, and get medical help.

Eyelid Cuts

1.   Carefully wash the eye. Apply a thick layer of bacitracin or mupirocin ointment on the eyelid. Place a patch over the eye. Seek medical help immediately.

2.   If the cut is bleeding, apply gentle pressure with a clean, dry cloth until the bleeding subsides.

3.   Rinse with water, cover with a clean dressing, and place a cold compress on the dressing to reduce pain and swelling.

Do Not

- Do not press or rub an injured eye.

- Do not remove contact lenses unless rapid swelling is occurring, there is a chemical injury and the contacts did not come out with the water flush, or you cannot get prompt medical help.

- Do not attempt to remove a foreign body that appears to be embedded in any part of the eye. Get medical help immediately.

- Do not use cotton swabs, tweezers, or anything else on the eye itself. Cotton swabs should only be used on the eyelid.

- Do not attempt to remove an embedded object.

Call Immediately for Emergency Medical Assistance If

Seek emergency medical care if:

- there appears to be any visible scratch, cut, or penetration of your eyeball;

- any chemical gets into your eye;

- the eye is painful and red;

- nausea accompanies the eye pain; or

- you have any trouble seeing (such as blurry vision).

Prevention

- Supervise children carefully. Teach them how to be safe.

- Always wear protective eye wear when using power tools, hammers, or other striking tools.

- Always wear protective eye wear when working with toxic chemicals.

Section 59.2

Corneal Abrasion and Erosion

What is the cornea?

The cornea is the clear front window of the eye. It covers the iris
(colored portion of the eye) and the round pupil, much like a watch
crystal covers the face of a watch. The cornea is composed of five layers. The outermost layer is called the epithelium.

What is a corneal abrasion?

A corneal abrasion is an injury (a scratch, scrape or cut) to the
epithelium. Abrasions are commonly caused by fingernail scratches,
paper cuts, makeup brushes, scrapes from tree or bush limbs, and
rubbing of the eye. Some eye conditions, such as dry eye, increase the
chance of an abrasion. You may experience the following symptoms
with corneal abrasion:

- feeling of having something in your eye;
- pain and soreness of the eye;
- redness of the eye;
- sensitivity to light;
- tearing; and
- blurred vision.

To detect an abrasion on the cornea, your ophthalmologist (Eye
M.D.) will use a special dye called fluorescein to illuminate the injury.

How is a corneal abrasion treated?

Treatment may include the following:

- patching the injured eye to prevent eyelid blinking from irritating the injury;

- applying lubricating eye drops or ointment to the eye to form a soothing layer between the eyelid and the abrasion;

- using antibiotics to prevent infection;

- dilating (widening) the pupil to relieve pain; or

- wearing a special contact lens to help healing.

Minor abrasions usually heal within a day or two; larger abrasions usually take about a week. It is important not to rub the eye while it is healing. Do not wear contact lenses while the eye is healing; ask your ophthalmologist when you may start wearing your lenses again.

What is corneal erosion?

Corneal erosion is a wearing away of the epithelium layer of the cornea, often at the site of an earlier abrasion. It may occur spontaneously, often after awakening in the morning. Erosion also may occur in dry eyes. Symptoms are similar to those of a corneal abrasion: the feeling of something in your eye, pain and soreness of the eye, redness of the eye, sensitivity to light, tearing, and blurred vision.

How is corneal erosion treated?

Treatment is the same as for corneal abrasion, with the addition of salt solution eye drops or ointment.

If the corneal erosion keeps occurring, further treatment may be needed, including:

- use of a special contact lens to reduce pain and encourage healing;

- gentle removal of the damaged epithelium;

- removal of a small layer of corneal cells using a laser; or

- performing a procedure called anterior stromal puncture, which involves making tiny holes on the surface of the cornea to promote stronger attachments between the top layer of corneal cells and the layer of the cornea underneath.

How can corneal abrasion and erosion be prevented?

For maximum protection:

- Use proper eyewear when using power tools, mowing the lawn and performing other yard work, playing sports, and while working around wood and steel.

- Regularly clip your infant's or young child's fingernails.

- Follow your ophthalmologist's instructions on how to care for and wear your contact lenses.

Section 59.3

Sports Eye Injuries

"Sports Eye Injuries," © 2005 University of Illinois Eye Center, Department of Ophthalmology and Visual Sciences (www.uic.edu/com/eye). Reprinted with permission.

Sports and recreational activities cause more than 40,000 eye injuries each year, according to the American Academy of Ophthalmology—and most of these accidents are preventable. Indeed, Prevent Blindness America reports that 90% of sports-related eye injuries can be prevented.

Basketball and baseball cause the most eye injuries, followed by water sports and racquet sports.

The majority of all eye injuries occur in persons under thirty years of age. Children are especially vulnerable as they often have underdeveloped depth perception and may have difficulty judging the position of a flying ball. It's not uncommon for a child to misjudge a ball in flight, miss it, and take a blow to the face instead. Safety goggles are advised for children who play softball and baseball.

The severity of sports-induced eye injuries varies from mild scrapes of the cornea to severe trauma that can cause visual impairment or even blindness.

Types of Injury

Three types of eye trauma can result from sports injuries: corneal abrasion, blunt injuries, and penetrating injuries.

Corneal abrasion, a scrape of the outer surface of the eye, usually is painful but not severe. The most common cause, in sports and recreation, is a scratch from a fingernail. Many professional basketball players wear goggles when they play to protect themselves from such an injury.

Blunt injuries occur when impact from an object (tennis ball, racquet, fist, elbow, etc.) causes sudden compression of the eye.

Mild blunt injuries sometimes only result in bleeding of the eyelids, or a black eye. Also, a subconjunctival hemorrhage may develop. This involves bleeding from the delicate blood vessels of the conjunctive, which lie on top of the white outer coat of the eye. Neither of these types of bleeding poses a threat to the eye itself. However, these injuries may be seen in more severe cases in which the eye is damaged. As symptoms of severe injury are not always obvious, it is crucial that all cases of eye trauma get a thorough eye examination from an ophthalmologist.

One of the common results of more severe blunt trauma is bleeding in the front of the eye between the clear cornea and colored iris. This condition is known as a hyphema. In addition, blunt injury may cause a cut or tear of the eyelids, which may need special suturing. Also, the bony walls surrounding the eye may be fractured by severe blunt trauma. Severe blunt trauma also may damage important structures inside the eye, such as the retina or optic nerve, resulting in potentially permanent visual loss. Therefore, if you suffer a blunt injury to the eye, see an ophthalmologist as soon as possible.

Penetrating injuries occur when a foreign object pierces the eye. A common cause of these injuries in children is BB pellets. Also, a piece of glass from spectacles shattered during sports play sometimes can penetrate the eye. Penetrating injuries often cause severe, sight-threatening damage; they are true emergencies and must be evaluated promptly by an ophthalmologist.

Symptoms and Evaluation

The warning signs of potentially serious eye injury include:

- visual loss;
- bleeding on the surface or inside the eye;
- tears in the outer ocular walls; and
- a foreign body inside the eye.

The evaluation of sports-related eye injuries is the same as for other types of eye trauma. More emergent injuries, such as head trauma with loss of consciousness, are always treated first.

Treatment

Prompt first aid after eye injury may greatly improve the chance of preserving vision. The recommended first aid involves placing a protective cover over the eye to prevent further damage. (If no shield is available, tape the bottom of a paper cup over the eye.) Seek emergency care as soon as possible.

The type of treatment given depends on the injury. Surgery may be required to repair blunt or penetrating injuries.

Prevention

The best treatment is prevention, as the old adage goes. The best prevention of eye injury while involved in sports and recreation is to wear specially designed protective eyewear. Such eye guards, while they cannot eliminate risk, greatly reduce the chance of ocular injury. Regular eyeglasses and contact lenses do not offer adequate protection from sports injuries. As already mentioned, glass lenses may even shatter and cut the eye.

Racquet sports: Stricter standards for eyewear for racquet sports have helped reduce the number of eye injuries from these activities. Research done at the UIC [University of Illinois at Chicago] Eye Center and elsewhere has led to the improvement of these eye protection devices.

Today, the standard eye guard designed for use in sports such as racquetball, baseball and basketball is made of polycarbonate (plastic) and has closed lenses and sports frames. Avoid open lenses, as a small ball traveling at high speed can be compressed through the opening and cause severe eye damage.

Collision sports: Total head and face protection is essential for any collision sport, for example, a helmet in football and a face mask in hockey. In hockey the risk of eye injury is not so much from collision as from a flying puck. The standardization and use of face masks in organized amateur ice hockey in Canada led to a 66 percent reduction in eye injuries.

The identification of patterns in sports eye trauma is important in helping prevent many of these injuries. The National Eye Trauma System (NETS) is collecting data on the frequency and types of eye injuries, including those due to sports. The UIC Eye Center is one of 50 regional eye trauma centers that are sending the data to NETS.

Chapter 60

Eye Injuries: What to Do

You can treat many minor eye irritations by flushing the eye, but more serious injuries require medical attention. Injuries to the eye are the most common preventable cause of blindness, so when in doubt, err on the side of caution and call your child's doctor for help.

What to Do: Routine Irritations (Sand, Dirt, and Other Foreign Bodies on the Eye Surface)

- Wash your hands thoroughly before touching the eyelids to examine or flush the eye.

- Do not touch, press, or rub the eye itself, and do whatever you can to keep the child from touching it (a baby can be swaddled as a preventive measure).

- Do not try to remove any foreign body except by flushing, because of the risk of scratching the surface of the eye, especially the cornea.

- Tilt the child's head over a basin with the affected eye down and gently pull down the lower lid, encouraging the child to open his

"Eye Injuries" was provided by KidsHealth, one of the largest resources online for medically reviewed health information written for kids, teens, and parents. For more articles like this one, visit www.KidsHealth.org, or www.TeensHealth.org. © 2004 The Nemours Foundation. Reviewed by Sharon Lehman, M.D., May 2004.

or her eyes as wide as possible. For an infant or small child, it's helpful to have a second person hold the child's eyes open while you flush.

- Gently pour a steady stream of lukewarm water (do not heat the water) from a pitcher across the eye. Sterile saline solution can also be used.

- Flush for up to 15 minutes, checking the eye every 5 minutes to see if the foreign body has been flushed out.

- Because a particle can scratch the cornea and cause an infection, the eye should be examined by a doctor if there continues to be any irritation afterward.

- If a foreign body is not dislodged by flushing, it will probably be necessary for a trained medical professional to flush the eye.

Embedded Foreign Body (An Object Penetrates the Globe of the Eye)

- Call for emergency medical help.

- Cover the affected eye. If the object is small, use an eye patch or sterile dressing. If the object is large, cover the injured eye with a small cup taped in place. The point is to keep all pressure off the globe of the eye.

- Keep your child (and yourself) as calm and comfortable as possible until help arrives.

Chemical Exposure

- Many chemicals, even those found around the house, can damage an eye. If your child gets a chemical in the eye and you know what it is, look on the product's container for an emergency number to call for instructions.

- Flush the eye (see above) with lukewarm water for 15 to 30 minutes. If both eyes are affected, flush them in the shower.

- Call for emergency medical help.

- Call your local poison control center for specific instructions. Be prepared to give the exact name of the chemical, if you have it. However, do not delay flushing the eye first.

Black Eye, Blunt Injury, or Contusion

A black eye is often a minor injury, but it can also appear when there is significant eye injury or head trauma. A visit to your child's doctor or an eye specialist may be required to rule out serious injury, particularly if you're not certain of the cause of the black eye.

For a black eye:

- Apply cold compresses intermittently: 5 to 10 minutes on, 10 to 15 minutes off. If you use ice, make sure it's covered with a towel or sock to protect the delicate skin on the eyelid. If you aren't at home when the injury occurs and there's no ice available, a cold soda will do to start.

- Use cold compresses for 24 to 48 hours, then switch to applying warm compresses intermittently. This will help the body reabsorb the leakage of blood and may help reduce discoloration.

- If the child is in pain, give acetaminophen—not aspirin or ibuprofen, which can increase bleeding.

- Prop the child's head with an extra pillow at night, and encourage him or her to sleep on the uninjured side of his or her face (pressure can increase swelling).

- Call your child's doctor, who may recommend an in-depth evaluation to rule out damage to the eye. Call immediately if any of the following symptoms are noted:
  - increased redness;
  - drainage from the eye;
  - persistent eye pain;
  - any changes in vision;
  - any visible abnormality of the eyeball; or
  - visible bleeding on the white part (sclera) of the eye, especially near the cornea.

If the injury occurred during one of your child's routine activities such as a sport, follow up by investing in an ounce of prevention—protective goggles or unbreakable glasses are vitally important.

Chapter 61

Preventing Eye Injuries at Work and Play

Chapter Contents

Section 61.1

Ten Ways to Prevent Occupational Eye Injuries

Nearly one million Americans have lost some degree of their sight due to an eye injury. More than 700,000 Americans injure their eyes at work each year. Luckily, 90% of all workplace eye injuries can be avoided by using proper safety eyewear.

Here are 10 ways that you can help prevent an eye injury in your workplace.

Assess

Look carefully at plant operations. Inspect all work areas, access routes, and equipment for hazards to eyes. Study eye accident and injury reports. Identify operations and areas the present eye hazards.

Test

Uncorrected vision problems can cause accidents. Provide vision testing during routine employee physical exams.

Protect

Select protective eyewear that is designed for the specific duty or hazard. Protective eyewear must meet the current standards from the Occupational Safety and Health Act of 1970 and later revisions.

Participate

Create a 100% mandatory program for eye protection in all operation areas of your plant. A broad program prevents more injuries and is easier to enforce than one that limits eye protection to certain departments, areas, or jobs.

Fit

Workers need protective eyewear that fits well and is comfortable. Have eyewear fitted by an eye care professional or someone trained to do this. Provide repairs for eyewear and require each worker to be in charge of his or her own gear.

Plan for an Emergency

Set up first-aid procedures for eye injuries. Have eyewash stations that are easy to get to, especially where chemicals are used. Train workers in basic first aid and identify those with more advanced training.

Educate

Conduct ongoing educational programs to create, keep up, and highlight the need for protective eyewear. Add eye safety to your regular employee training programs and to new employee orientation.

Support

Management support is key to having a successful eye safety program. Management can show their support for the program by wearing protective eyewear whenever and wherever needed.

Review

Regularly review and update your accident prevention policies. Your goal should be **no** eye injuries or accidents!

Put It in Writing

Once your safety program is created, put it in writing. Display a copy of the policy in work and employee gathering areas. Include a review of the policy in new employee orientation.

Section 61.2

Avoiding Computer-Related Eye Discomfort

"Computer Eyestrain" was provided courtesy of, and is copyrighted, by Lighthouse International, www.Lighthouse.org, a leading non-profit organization that helps people of all ages overcome the challenge of vision loss. © 2007.

Computers have become an indispensable part of everyday life both at work and for personal use. Yet, for many people this also means experiencing eyestrain, a sign that your eyes are fatigued from overuse. Fortunately, the symptoms are usually temporary and not indicative of eye damage. Even better, there are things you can do to reduce or prevent eye discomfort.

Common Symptoms

- Tired or itching eyes
- Red, watery, or dry eyes
- Blurry vision
- Headache
- Discomfort when shifting focus between the monitor and your paper documents
- Color fringes or afterimages when you look away from the monitor
- Increased sensitivity to light

What You Can Do

- Take frequent breaks to give your eyes a rest. A five-minute break every hour is a good rule of thumb. Move around or just close your eyes for a few moments.
- Try blinking more frequently to lubricate your eyes or use artificial tears. People tend to blink less frequently when working at a computer, which can lead to dry eyes.

- Make sure your eyeglass or contact lenses prescription is right for computer work. You may benefit from a prescription that is geared specifically for your work situation.

- Position your monitor so that the top of the screen is at the same level as your eyes or slightly below, and at a distance of approximately 25 inches. Many people find that putting the screen at arm's length is a good rule of thumb.

- Place your keyboard directly in front of your monitor. If it's at an angle or to the side, your eyes have to focus at different distances from the screen, which can cause visual discomfort.

- Use a document holder beside your monitor and at the same level, angle and distance from your eyes as the monitor. This way your eyes will not have to constantly readjust.

- Adjust lighting. Bright light can make it difficult to see the screen and also strain your eyes. To minimize exterior light, close windows, blinds and shades. Consider reducing or eliminating indoor overhead lights and use an adjustable desk lamp. Position the lamp so that the light does not shine on the computer screen or in your eyes.

- Reduce glare. You can check for glare by looking at the monitor when it is off so that you can see reflected light and images. The worst glare is generally from sources above or behind you such as fluorescent lights and sunlight. Position your monitor so that the brightest light sources are off to the side, at a right angle to your monitor. And avoid placing your monitor directly in front of a window or white wall.

- Adjust the contrast and brightness levels of your computer screen so that it's comfortable for you. A glare-reducing screen on the monitor can also help.

- Keep your computer screen free from dust by wiping it down regularly. Dust can reduce contrast and may contribute to glare and reflection problems.

By making a few simple adjustments, you can keep your eyes rested and ready. However, if eye problems persist, see your eye doctor as this could be a sign of a more serious problem.

Sources: Mayo Foundation for Medical Education and Research and American Academy of Ophthalmology

Section 61.3

Impact Protection and Polycarbonate Lenses

Prevent Blindness America believes that all eyewear should protect eyes from impact hazards. Recognizing that the use of polycarbonate materials can help to greatly reduce the frequency and severity of impact injuries to eyes, Prevent Blindness America recommends: When safety is a major issue, lenses in plano and prescription glasses, sunglasses, fashion and occupational eyewear, and the lenses and frames for sports eyewear should be made from polycarbonate materials to provide additional protection for wearers.

The Need for Safety

Today's active lifestyles have placed more Americans at risk of injury, particularly eye injury. Work, sports, recreational activities and hobbies—even routine tasks—expose eyes to a variety of hazards. The lenses in all glasses (prescription, sunglasses, and fashion eyewear) must meet FDA [Food and Drug Administration] minimal impact standards established in 1971. While they do provide some protection for the wearer, they do not provide adequate protection for many common impact hazards. These include hazards at work, as well as during sports or recreational activities. Hazardous situations require the use of eyewear, both lenses and frames, that meet higher level safety standards. Currently, lenses made from polycarbonate materials provide the highest level of impact protection.

Facts about Eye Injuries

Nearly one million Americans have lost some degree of sight (a chronic or permanent disability) due to an eye injury.

- About 7% have a severe impairment and about 9% are blind in one eye. Eye injuries account for 40,000 to 50,000 new cases of impaired vision each year. In 90% of these cases, the injury could have been prevented, or at least could have been less severe, if the victim had been wearing protective eyewear.[1]

- The U.S. Occupational Safety and Health Act (OSHA) of 1970 (Public Law 91-596) requires that "workers' vision be protected." The standard that applies to protective eyewear used in the industrial environment is titled *The American National Standard Practice for Occupational and Educational Eye and Face Protection* (ANSI Z-87.1).[2] Protective eyewear designed to conform to ANSI Z-87 must meet strict safety and performance criteria. Yet despite this requirement, as many as 2,000 eye injuries occur each day in the workplace.[3]

- Information from a 1988 study conducted by the National Institutes for Occupational Safety and Health (NIOSH) indicates that between 600,000-700,000 occupational eye injuries occur per year, with 16% in the construction industry.[4]

- According to the Optical Manufacturers Association, an estimated 60% of Americans wear prescription lenses. Since 1970, the U.S. Food and Drug Administration has required that lenses in prescription glasses, sunglasses, and fashion eyewear meet minimal impact standards. Prior to 1970, there were an estimated 120,000 lens-related injuries each year.[5]

- According to 2002 statistics, there were an estimated 262,000 product-related eye injuries treated in U.S. hospital emergency rooms. The categories contributing to the highest injuries were related to household (124,998), workplace (96,938), and sports (35,633).[6]

- Several types of materials are currently used to make lenses. The most common are treated glass, alloy resin plastic (CR-39, registered trademark of PPG Industries), and polycarbonate. Each of these materials can be used in a manner to satisfy the various regulations (i.e., FDA and OSHA) and standards (i.e., ASTM [American Society for Testing and Materials] and ANSI [American National Standards Institute]).[7]

Recommendations

- Plano and prescription polycarbonate lenses offer the best impact protection and should be used whenever possible.

- Certain lens coatings may reduce the impact effectiveness of polycarbonate and some lens tints may be difficult or impossible to apply. In these and other such situations, alternative lens materials should be used.

- For everyday prescription eyewear, polycarbonate lenses should meet or exceed the requirements of American National Standards Institute (ANSI), *Recommendations for Prescription Ophthalmic Lenses* (ANSI Z-80.1, latest edition).

- For sunglasses and fashion eyewear, polycarbonate lenses should meet or exceed the requirements of ANSI, *Requirements for Non-prescription Sunglasses and Fashion Eyewear* (ANSI Z-80.3, latest edition).

- For occupational use, polycarbonate lenses and frames must meet or exceed the requirements of ANSI, *American National Standard Practice for Occupational and Educational Eye and Face Protection* (ANSI Z-87.1, latest edition).

- For sports use, polycarbonate lenses must be used with protectors that meet or exceed the requirements of American Society for Testing and Materials (ASTM), *Standard Specification for Eye Protectors for Use by Players of Racquet Sports* (ASTM F803, latest edition); *Standard Specification for Eye Protective Devices—Alpine Skiing* (ASTM F659, latest edition); *Standard Safety Specification for Eye and Face Protective Equipment for Hockey Players* (ASTM F513, latest edition); *Standard Specification for Face Guards for Youth Baseball* (ASTM F910, latest edition); or other applicable standard specifications for eye and face protection in sports.

References

1. National Society to Prevent Blindness, *Vision Problems in the U.S.*, New York, NY, 1980.

2. Occupational Safety and Health Administration (OSHA), *Occupational Safety and Health Act* (Public Law 91-596) Washington, DC, 1970.

3. Prevent Blindness America, *Guide to Controlling Eye Injuries in Industry*, Schaumburg, IL, 1991.

4. National Institutes for Occupational Safety and Health (NIOSH), *National Health Interview Survey Occupation Health Supplement*, Washington, DC, 1988.

5. Waller, Julian A. M.D., M.P.H., *Injury Control—A Guide to the Causes and Prevention of Trauma,* Lexington Books, Lexington, MA, 1985.

6. U.S. Consumer Product Safety Commission, Directorate for Epidemiology; National Injury Information Clearinghouse; National Electronic Injury Surveillance System (NEISS), *Product Summary Report—Eye Injuries Only*, 2002, Washington, DC, 2003.

7. Davis, John K., Perspectives on Impact Resistance and Polycarbonate Lenses, *International Ophthalmology Clinics*, Vol. 28, No. 3, Little, Brown and Company, Boston, MA, 1988.

Section 61.4

Recommended Sports Eye Protectors

Each year, more than 40,000 people are treated for eye injuries related to sports activities. Using the right kind of eye protection while playing sports can help prevent serious eye injuries and even blindness.

For sports use, polycarbonate lenses must be used with protectors that meet or exceed the requirements of the American Society for Testing and Materials (ASTM). Each sport has a specific ASTM code, so look for the ASTM label on the product before making a purchase.

Baseball

Type of eye protection:

- Face guard (attached to helmet) made of polycarbonate material
- Sports eye guards

Eye injuries prevented:

- Scratches on the cornea
- Inflamed iris
- Blood spilling into the eye's anterior chamber
- Traumatic cataract
- Swollen retina

Basketball

Type of eye protection:

- Sports eye guards

Eye injuries prevented:

- Fracture of the eye socket
- Scratches on the cornea
- Inflamed iris
- Blood spilling into the eye's anterior chamber
- Swollen retina

Soccer

Type of eye protection:

- Sports eye guards

Eye injuries prevented:

- Inflamed iris
- Blood spilling into the eye's anterior chamber
- Swollen retina

Football

Type of eye protection:

- Polycarbonate shield attached to face guard
- Sports eye guards

Eye injuries prevented:

- Scratches on the cornea
- Inflamed iris
- Blood spilling into the eye's anterior chamber
- Swollen retina

Hockey

Type of eye protection:

- Wire or polycarbonate mask
- Sports eye guards

Eye injuries prevented:

- Scratches on the cornea
- Inflamed iris
- Blood spilling into the eye's anterior chamber
- Traumatic cataract
- Swollen retina

Section 61.5

Most Dangerous Toys to Children's Eyes

In 2003, thousands of children age 14 and younger suffered serious eye injuries, even blindness, from toys. Many of these injuries were caused by guns—both toy and recreational and playground equipment. This is what Prevent Blindness America recommends: Protect your children's eyes by not buying them guns or toys not meant for their age. You can also keep your children safe by showing them how to use toys, and if necessary, by watching them when they play. Below are toys linked with the most eye injuries in children age 14 and younger.

Table 61.1. Toys Linked to the Most Eye Injuries in Children 14 and Younger

Toy Weapons	Number of Eye Injuries
Guns: Air, BB, and Spring	1,293
Toy Weapons (combined types)	325
Slingshots and Sling-Propelled toys	110
Total Toy Weapons	**1,728**
Other Toy Products	
Toys (other and unclassified)	4,371
Fireworks (classified as toys)	802
Playground Equipment	733
Bicycles	558
Art Supplies and Crayons/Chalk	386
Trampolines	240
Scooters, Skateboards, Powered Riding Toys	171
Go-Karts	170
Toy Sports Equipment	155
All other categories combined	736
Total	**10,050**

Source: Prevent Blindness America. Based on statistics provided by the U.S. Consumer Product Safety Commission, Directorate for Epidemiology; National Injury Information Clearinghouse; National Electronic Injury Surveillance System (NEISS). Product Summary Report—Eye Injuries Only—Calendar Year 2003. NEISS data and estimates are based on injuries treated in hospital emergency rooms that patients say are related to products. Therefore, it is incorrect when using NEISS data to say the injuries were caused by the product.

Chapter 62

Preventing Eye Injuries throughout the Year

Chapter Contents

Section 62.1

Winter Eye Safety

As you gaze outside your window this winter, don't lose sight of what brings every wonderland to light—your eyes. By taking precautions this season, you can preserve your vision and guarantee that you will enjoy the sights of the holiday seasons to come. To do so, you need to understand how winter weather creates hazards for the eyes.

"Winter enthusiasts look forward to this time of year," explains Carlo J. DiMarco, D.O., an osteopathic ophthalmologist practicing in Erie, Pennsylvania. "They spend their days happily racing down the slopes, but they do not realize the amount of time they are exposed to intense reflected sunlight."

Overexposure to the winter sun's powerful ultraviolet (UV) rays without proper eye protection can temporarily harm the eyes or even cause photokeratitis. This condition is like sunburning sensitive tissues of the eyeball. Although photokeratitis may heal with time, the best way to safeguard vision is to avoid excessive UV ray exposure.

"It's not just the skiers that need to worry about photokeratitis," warns Dr. DiMarco, a member of the American Osteopathic Association Board of Trustees. "Appropriate eye protection should be worn when shoveling snow; putting up or taking down holiday decorations; or just going for a walk."

Dr. DiMarco further explains that while many people associate winter with gray skies, the sun often comes out unexpectedly. Since sunglasses are left behind, many people are subjected to exposure without the proper protection.

"UV light has been proven to cause certain types of cataracts and has been implicated in age-related macular degeneration," he explains. "These are two of the most common eye health problems experienced in older adults."

In terms of protection, Dr. DiMarco recommends lenses that block 99 percent to 100 percent of both UV-A and UV-B radiation. Ski goggles, which cover the eyes as well as the surrounding skin, are another option. Goggles are the preferred protection for snowmobilers as well as downhill and cross-country skiers, since they block harmful sunlight while preventing debris and snow from blowing into the eyes.

The sun is not winter's only eye hazard. Cool winds and dry air can irritate eyes, even in warmer climates. Harsh weather can make eyes constantly dry and irritated, especially for those who wear contact lenses. Dry eyes can be trouble inside as well, since indoor heat tends to eliminate moisture from the air.

"Although most cases of indoor irritation are mild, it frequently provokes excessive rubbing and further scratching of the eye," explains Dr. DiMarco.

To add moisture to eyes, he recommends eyedrops, like artificial tears, a few times a day. In addition, he suggests installing humidifiers throughout the house to increase indoor levels of humidity.

"Simple preventive measures for your eyes this winter will allow you to enjoy a beautiful spring," stresses Dr. DiMarco.

Section 62.2

Protect Your Eyes from the Sun: What to Look for in a Pair of Sunglasses

"What to Look For in a Pair of Sunglasses," by Michelle Meadows, was published in *FDA Consumer* magazine (www.fda.gov/fdac), by the U.S. Food and Drug Administration, July-August 2002. Reviewed by David A. Cooke, M.D., July 2007.

As you slather on sunscreen to protect your skin this summer, don't forget sunglasses to protect your eyes. The same harmful rays that damage skin can also increase your risk of developing eye problems, such as cataracts—a clouding of the eye's lens that develops over years.

In the short-term, people who spend long hours on the beach or in the snow without adequate eye protection can develop photokeratitis, reversible sunburn of the cornea. This painful condition can result in temporary loss of vision. When sunlight reflects off of snow, sand, and water, it further increases exposure to ultraviolet (UV) radiation. These invisible high-energy rays lie just beyond the violet end of the visible light spectrum.

Everyone is at risk for eye damage from the sun year-round. The risk is greatest from about 10 a.m. to 4 p.m. Fishermen, farmers, beach-goers, and others who spend time in the sun for extended periods are at highest risk.

UV radiation in sunlight is commonly divided into UVA and UVB, and your sunglasses should block both forms. Don't assume that you get more UV protection with pricier sunglasses or glasses with a darker tint. Look for a label that specifically states that the glasses offer 99 percent to 100 percent UV protection. You could also ask an eye-care professional to test your sunglasses if you're not sure of their level of UV protection.

Sunglasses should be dark enough to reduce glare, but not dark enough to distort colors and affect the recognition of traffic signals. Tint is mainly a matter of personal preference. For best color perception, Prevent Blindness America, a volunteer eye health and safety organization dedicated to fighting blindness and saving sight, recommends lenses that are neutral gray, amber, brown, or green. People who wear contact lenses that offer UV protection should still wear sunglasses.

Children also should wear sunglasses. They shouldn't be toy sunglasses, but real sunglasses that indicate the UV-protection level just as with adults. Polycarbonate lenses are generally recommended for children because they are the most shatter-resistant.

Sheryl Berman, M.D., a medical officer in the FDA's Division of Ophthalmic and Ear, Nose, and Throat Devices, says that wearing sunglasses reduces the risk of eye damage due to sun exposure, but doesn't completely eliminate it.

"Even when we talk about 100 percent UV protection, light still enters from the sides of sunglasses and can be reflected into the eye," she says. Some people choose sunglasses that wrap all the way around the temples. A hat with a three-inch brim can help block sunlight that comes in from overhead.

The FDA's Center for Devices and Radiological Health regulates nonprescription sunglasses as over-the-counter medical devices. Sunglasses are normally exempt from the FDA's premarket notification procedures. But sunglasses manufacturers who claim their products are of substantial importance in preventing health problems would be required to submit proof to the FDA. The only medical claim manufacturers are allowed to make on sunglasses is that they may reduce eye strain or eye fatigue due to glare.

Even though sunglasses are exempt from premarket notification, they remain subject to several regulations. Sunglasses regulated by the FDA must comply with impact-resistant requirements, for example. This doesn't mean that the glasses are shatterproof, but that they can withstand moderate impact. Sunglasses are not intended to function as protective eyewear in high-impact sports.

Manufacturers of sunglasses also must follow the FDA's labeling regulations. The FDA has issued warning letters to manufacturers about unsubstantiated performance claims, such as those relating to UV-absorbing sunglasses.

For Your Information: UVA and UVB

- **UVA:** UVA is ultraviolet radiation with wavelengths from 320 to 400 nanometers. It passes through the Earth's ozone layer and can cause early aging of the skin.

- **UVB:** UVB is ultraviolet radiation with wavelengths of 280 to 320 nanometers. The ozone layer absorbs most of the sun's UVB, but even a small amount can do substantial damage. UVB causes skin cancer and may contribute to cataracts.

Source: Centers for Disease Control and Prevention

Section 62.3

Fireworks Eye Safety

There is no safe way for nonprofessionals to use fireworks. It is only safe to enjoy the splendor and excitement of fireworks at a professional display.

According to the U.S. Consumer Product Safety Commission, fireworks were involved in an estimated 10,800 injuries treated in U.S. hospital emergency rooms in 2005.

An estimated 6,500 injuries were treated in hospital emergency rooms during the one month period surrounding the Fourth of July.

The following data is from the 6,500 estimate:

- Eyes were the second most commonly injured part of the body, with an estimated 1,600 fireworks-related eye injuries treated in the same one-month period of 2005.

- Firecrackers accounted for 26% of all injuries followed by rockets (17%), and sparklers (17%).

- Sparklers caused the greatest number of injuries in children 14 and younger, followed by firecrackers and rockets.

- Of the 1,100 estimated sparkler injuries, 500 were to children age 5 and younger.

- 2,900 of the injuries were to children under age 15.

Fireworks and celebrations go together, especially during the Fourth of July, but there are precautions parents can take to prevent these injuries. The best defense against kids suffering severe eye injuries and burns is to not let kids play with any fireworks.

Do not purchase, use or store fireworks of any type. Protect yourself, your family and your friends by avoiding fireworks. Attend only authorized public fireworks displays conducted by licensed operators, but be aware that even professional displays can be dangerous.

Prevent Blindness America supports the development and enforcement of bans on the importation, sale, and use of all fireworks, except those used in authorized public displays by licensed operators, as the only effective means of eliminating the social and economic impact of fireworks-related trauma and damage.

If an accident does occur, what can you do right away to minimize the damage to the eye?

These six steps can help save your child's sight.

- **Do not rub the eye.** Rubbing the eye may increase bleeding or make the injury worse.

- **Do not attempt to rinse out the eye.** This can be even more damaging than rubbing.

- **Do not apply pressure to the eye itself.** Holding or taping a foam cup or the bottom of a juice carton to the eye are just two tips. Protecting the eye from further contact with any item, including the child's hand, is the goal.

- **Do not stop for medicine!** Over-the-counter pain relievers will not do much to relieve pain. Aspirin (should never be given to children) and ibuprofen can thin the blood, increasing bleeding. Take the child to the emergency room at once—this is more important than stopping for a pain reliever.

- **Do not apply ointment.** Ointment, which may not be sterile, makes the area around the eye slippery and harder for the doctor to examine.

- **Do not let your child play with fireworks**, even if his/her friends are setting them off. Sparklers burn at 1,800 degrees Fahrenheit, and bottle rockets can stray off course or throw shrapnel when they explode.

Part Ten

Living with Low Vision or Blindness

Chapter 63

Going to a Low Vision Center: What You Should Know and What to Expect

For those who are going to a low vision center for the first time, it can be an overwhelming and misunderstood experience for both the patient and the family. This text explores some key points, which may help you in your expectations and in minimizing frustrations before going to a low vision center.

Unlike most eye appointments, a low vision appointment means you as a patient take an active role. That is, the more you can put into it, the more successful and satisfied you will be at the end of your experience.

What Do You Mean I Have to Put Something into It?

Low vision services are geared to help persons with vision loss maximize the vision they have now—it usually means not helping you to see better in general—it means helping you function better in your everyday life. For instance, if you were to make a list of all the tasks that frustrate you or that you have given up on, but would like to do again, this would be a great beginning of your "hard work" toward your successful out come. More on this later.

Another way to understand low vision services is to explain what it is not. For example, if you have one eye that has much worse vision than another, low vision services cannot "help the bad eye." Maximizing vision will almost always mean concentrating on the better seeing eye to help you accomplish things. Low vision is not medical services per se; so going for low vision does not mean you are going to get treatment to "fix" your vision. The low vision specialist will not be doing things for you—they will more accurately describe their role as someone who can work together with you and guide you as you work hard to achieve one goal, then another and another.

Low Vision—A Lifelong Process:

Low vision therefore is not to be seen as an appointment or two, but a beginning of a rehabilitation process that may continue (with or without professional help) for the rest of your life. As you regain the ability to read, your efforts may continue month after month so as to read faster and faster. Or, maybe reading short materials will be all that can be accomplished at first, increasing to magazines or books. Maybe it will mean starting with large print materials, and later reading normal print sizes.

Perhaps after accomplishing reading goals, you will want to learn about distant devices for watching TV, going to plays, or seeing a sporting event. Many people with low vision go far beyond what they ever dreamed could be accomplished, such as writing a book or using the computer. But, it all happens in steps, and you need the patience and the right expectations to succeed.

As stated earlier, a good starting point is to develop a list of specific tasks that you want to accomplish. Think of all the things you do in the course of a week—like reading the mail, reading magazines or books, adjusting the thermostat, writing checks and letters, personal grooming, cooking and so on. Work on the list for a week or so, so as to put down an entire range of tasks and not to forget any. (Again, many will not be able to be accomplished quickly, but you need to remember what they are.)

Next, try to rewrite the list in order of importance to you. This prioritizing can help you to be clear and to the point when you go for low vision service. In fact, if you have samples of reading materials such as a Bible, favorite magazine or work papers, bring them along to your low vision appointment. If you like sewing or crafts, this is also a good thing to bring along so that you can see what works best for you regardless of the task.

There will almost always be a lot of new information discussed during a low vision appointment, so you should consider bringing a small tape recorder. It is also advisable to have an interested family member or friend attend with you, so you can later discuss the points brought up during your appointment. Do not, however, depend solely on the family member or friend to help you—this is **your** recovery process. You will be slowly recovering the things you've lost and you want to take ownership of the process. When you do, you will also feel great at the end knowing it was difficult, but you did it.

Difficult—did I say difficult? Yes, I think learning to read a different way or learning to use any new device can be very difficult and taxing. It may be the most difficult thing you have ever done. Let's just say it will not be easy, so you must be prepared to take it slow, take it in bite size pieces and don't overdo it. You should expect it to be hard, and know this before attempting to go for an appointment. The idea that someone will give you glasses or a lens and you will begin to see and read again is a false expectation. You will be setting yourself up for disappointment. Just as a person with a hip or knee replacement does not go out dancing after their medical treatment— a person with vision deterioration also does not go out and read immediately after medical treatment. It takes time; it is a process (a rehabilitation process) yet many do not think of vision help as a slow, hard process. All our lives we went to the eye doctor and got glasses or contact lenses and walked away seeing fine. This old expectation is hard to break and we must realize our eyes have some permanent damage and we will have to develop new strategies to see.

Many people, however, do see some immediate gains during their first low vision appointment. Family members are often times very encouraged by how their family member can read. With the help of a low vision professional, the person with macular degeneration, or another eye condition, is able to spot tiny print or read a short amount of material from the newspaper during their appointment. Then, after returning home, the person realizes that what was accomplished for a short duration cannot be sustained at home. This realization can be discouraging, and some want to give up. They say, "If this is what I have to do in order to read, it's not worth it!"

This back and forth response is very normal. That is, in a rehabilitation process, a person will always show gains, followed by a setback. This type of progress, often called two steps forward and one back, can take plenty of energy. Family members and professionals can be a big help during this time when support and encouragement are needed. I have had many tell me, "If I didn't have much patience before, this is truly forcing me to get some!" This is true—that overcoming vision loss can be very slow. I often use the expression, it's not low vision, it's slow vision! Everything takes twice as long to accomplish as before. So, my advice is to not just think of this step-by-step process as regaining vision, think of it as also building your character.

Also, be kind to yourself. Many people push themselves too hard and cause irritation and frustration to themselves and to their eyes. Others also say negative things to themselves if they feel they are not progressing as they should. It is hard enough losing vision; negative messages only compound the problem. Give yourself encouragement instead.

Don't be afraid to try new things. If one or two or three low vision devices have been recommended for you, and some are not working for you, feel free to go back and try other options. Do not stick a device in the drawer and forget about it—give the low vision center a second or third chance to make it right for you. If not, you are only making it harder on you. Keep an open mind. Learn about the entire range of devices open to all. There are also new low vision products being developed all the time, so try to learn what new devices can help you.

There are a wide array of low vision devices on the market, from simple magnifiers to reading glasses and CCTV video magnifiers. Do not rule out any device at first—but give yourself the opportunity to try things. Some centers loan devices; other centers have clear return policies that give you a chance to learn how a particular device can work for you in your home.

If an optical magnifier is not working, try a CCTV video magnifier. These reading machines are still one of the most popular items around the world in helping persons with moderate or severe macular degeneration read and write independently.

Finally, do not be surprised when depression or anger returns. This is normal. Many people get discouraged thinking they are "over" this loss and then all the strong emotions return. Some people do take time out from their learning to read again to grieve the loss of sight. This loss or grieving period is different for all, but should be given its proper place in one's life. For some, the loss of vision also triggers other memories and losses. This too is normal.

To try to hurry the process along may have other consequences such as physical disease, alienation from others or poor coping mechanisms such as excessive drinking to name one.

Giving yourself a chance to grieve is actually a kind way to help yourself. After sorrow subsides, there will be plenty of time to learn new things. Regaining independence will come—but the timing is not the same for everyone. The best way for others may not be the best way for you. But, you must try to communicate clearly and often on what you need. This is your responsibility. Then, others around you will know how you feel and what is important for you as you go through this process. They cannot guess. You must try and be clear. Ask for what you need. Even though others may not seem to understand, try and put it into words for them. In the long run, you will then feel more in control of your situation and less of that "out of control" feeling will be evident. You will be in charge of your recovery—you will look back and feel good knowing you communicated with your head held high. This will bring a boost in self-esteem and help friends and family to best help you.

Also, don't sell yourself short. Many persons with macular degeneration have gone on to accomplish far beyond what they ever thought they could. Slowly over time, try new and different things. Push yourself to go beyond what you thought you could accomplish. Try new things—with each new trial you may need to return to a low vision center for guidance. Together with you, they will help you to learn that living with vision loss can be a rewarding and rich experience. Many have gone on to start a self-help group to guide others—no matter what you decide, you will be the beneficiary.

Chapter 64

How Will Life Change If You Have Vision Loss?

Chapter Contents

Section 64.1

Suggestions for People with Recent Vision Loss

How much will life change? It is not necessary for a person who has low vision to be helpless or dependent. With proper training, encouragement, and opportunities, that person can be active, self-sufficient, and productive.

The most important thing to do is to gather information about how to function effectively using some new approaches. This includes the use of daily living skills and work-related skills. Most alternative methods that people with low vision need are simple, commonsense methods. Not much special equipment is required. Some simple tools will be helpful, and there are expensive devices available also. Most of the appliances, tools, and equipment you have been using will still be what you need.

For example, some women whose vision has deteriorated have expressed concern about using their good dishes. You will learn to take reasonable precautions with breakable objects as you gain experience. You should guard against trying to do everything visually. If, for instance, you wish to place a serving dish in the middle of the dining room table put it on the corner first. Then use your hands to find a clear spot in the middle of the table. You may wish to fill the water glasses from a pitcher after the people are seated, or let them pour their own water. If you are serving dessert, no one should mind if you touch a shoulder in order to know exactly where to put the dessert plate in front of the person.

Another example would be lighting a match. You can hear it ignite and feel through the match itself when it touches a candle wick or hear the 'poof' when a gas stove burner is lit. An activity such as lighting a match may be frightening at first, but will become easier with practice. We give this as an example of when it is not desirable to get close to 'see' what you are doing. Most blind and visually impaired individuals continue to use matches safely.

You need to remember that you have a lifetime of experience to offer your family, friends, and the rest of the world. Just because you have lost some vision does not mean that you don't still have a lot to offer to other people. Some new techniques, such as those discussed here, are required. Learning to read and write Braille takes time and motivation. Using records and tapes instead of reading with your eyes takes some getting used to. Finding and learning to work with readers is a skill to be developed. Budgeting money to pay readers or finding volunteers is a new approach. Using public transportation and arranging for drivers are also changes.

These adjustments require an optimistic attitude, and this will make it possible to continue a variety of activities. You will come to understand that everyone has needs and that the needs of people with low vision are not necessarily greater than those of others. Most people find ways of giving to others, as well as getting others to help them. You will feel better about yourself with low vision when you realize that you still have a lot to offer to others. It is easy to become overwhelmed by your own needs and forget that the greatest need of all is to continue giving.

How can I read? When an individual begins to lose vision, the first thought is often to get a magnifying glass. Enlarging print is one way to read for a person with low vision. There are literally hundreds of different magnification devices on the market. Optometrists and ophthalmologists should know of some local sources. It is desirable to try magnifiers before purchasing, since personal preference will mean that not everyone will wish to use the same sort of device. Lighting is also important. For example, you may wish to exchange 60 watt bulbs for 100 watt bulbs. You will probably wish to place reading material directly under a good light. Some large magnifiers come with lights attached. Others require you to arrange your own lighting. It is generally desirable to keep glare to a minimum, but you will need to experiment with lighting and magnification.

CCTV: There are several other ways to read and write with low vision. CCTV (closed circuit TV enlarger) includes a moving platform on which reading material can be placed and a screen (like a television screen) on which words and numbers are displayed. As the platform underneath is moved side to side and front to back, the reader is able to read the part of the page he or she wishes to see on the screen. This device magnifies the print many times its original size. It is rather expensive, but many people with low vision use these machines very successfully.

These devices are especially useful for reading mail and paying bills. Books, magazines, and newspapers are generally available in other forms that will be preferable to most.

Many public libraries have begun to include large-print books as a part of their collections. Some also include a collection of books recorded on cassettes or CDs. These collections are generally small, but may be borrowed by anyone with a library card.

Regional libraries: In this country, there are regional libraries for the blind and physically handicapped. The books for the blind program at the Library of Congress produces books on tape and in Braille for distribution through this nationwide network of libraries which circulate books recorded on cassette tapes to individuals who are legally blind. They also lend a cassette player to readers. It is desirable to borrow this player from these libraries because the books they provide are recorded on four tracks per cassette instead of two as commercial cassettes are produced, and at a slower playing speed. This makes it possible to include much more reading material on each cassette. Many of these libraries also distribute large print books. Both recorded books and large print books may be mailed free of postage from the libraries to the readers and back again. Thus, this service is truly a free library service.

Religious materials: If you are interested in material published by your church, there may be quite a bit available on recorded tapes or in large print. You will need to inquire through your pastor or other church leaders. A limited number of translations of the Bible have been recorded, but they are available through your regional library and some other private providers. Many denominations have special publications for the blind and visually impaired.

Directory assistance: Directory assistance is the service offered by the phone companies for those who cannot use standard phone books. 1-[area code]-555-1212 will get directory assistance anywhere. There may be other local numbers in various towns and cities. You will need to fill out a form to become qualified to receive directory assistance without charge on your home phone. This form is available though your local phone company. This service is available to the blind because we do not read the phone book. The National Federation of the Blind demonstrated to the phone companies that the phone books are free to the sighted, so directory assistance should be free for those who cannot read the phone book.

NFB-NEWSLINE®: Newspapers may be read by the blind by telephone. This service is called NEWSLINE® and is described in the resource section of this booklet.

Any individual who can no longer read print will need to depend on other people for some reading. Often family members serve as readers for mail and bill paying. Sometimes it is possible to find a volunteer to help in this way. Some blind people hire readers to do a variety of reading. When working with a reader, it is helpful if the reader understands that he or she should be responsive to the needs and wishes of the blind person. If you wish to find information in a bill or magazine, it is not for your reader to tell you whether that is important or not.

The more you work with one individual, the better you work together. It is possible to have a reader describe items in a catalog and fill out the order form. It is possible to teach a reader to skim for you by telling him or her to jump to the next paragraph or next page if you wish to do so. Most readers try to do as asked. Since you have been reading print all your life, you can make intelligent guesses about what to tell your reader to look for. At first, working with a reader may seem awkward, but the more you do it, the easier it becomes.

It is respectable to be blind. You may choose to use the terms "low vision," "visually impaired," "sight impaired," "partially sighted," or something else. These are all appropriate terms. So is "blind." From time to time it will be necessary to explain to friends and associates what you can and cannot do, whatever language you use. Occasionally, people will think you are more dependent than you are until you explain that they have not totally understood your situation. Try to remember to smile when this occurs. As you know, a smile usually makes everyone more comfortable.

Whether you are telling others that most blind people have a little usable vision or that you have lost some sight, the end result is very similar. You still have the experience, knowledge, interests, skills, and goals that you have always had. The changes you make as your vision worsens are small changes. The more you are expecting to continue with your former activities, the more you will find ways to do so.

Who needs a white cane? A long white cane is a tool that a person with poor vision or no vision can use to find obstacles, landmarks, and general information about the sidewalk, corridors, and other areas where he or she is walking. Getting information is an important reason for carrying a white cane, but it is not the only one. The white cane helps to identify a person who is legally blind. It may increase courtesy and understanding of those who meet a blind person. It also may increase safety if drivers and others realize the person with a cane in hand does not see everything others see. If a person carrying a white cane does not respond to a hand signal or a wave, others generally realize that this person is not just ignoring those around him or her. Rather, we do not see them.

Where can you learn the best methods for using the white cane? A small book entitled *Care and Feeding of the Long White Cane* may be purchased in large print or on cassette from the NFB Independence Market. This book goes into much more detail about techniques for using the white cane. Most rehabilitation agencies for the blind employ teachers who should be able to teach cane travel techniques. It may also be possible to enroll in a full-time residential program of training to learn cane travel, Braille, use of computers with speech output, and much more. Three excellent facilities of this kind are operated by the National Federation of the Blind. For more information about them, contact your state or local president of the NFB.

If the cane is to be used for support, a white one still indicates poor vision. If you do not need a cane for support, you will probably choose a longer straight white cane. Long canes may be made of fiberglass, carbon fiber, or metal. Most people who depend on the cane prefer a rigid one, but folding canes are also available.

Certain techniques can be used to gather information. The cane is swung from side to side in front of the person using it. The width of the arc should be a little wider than the person's shoulders. Generally, it is desirable to tap the cane on the floor or pavement at the outside edge of each swing. It is possible to drag the cane one way when looking for grass, a sidewalk going to one side, a retaining wall, etc. There are other techniques to be used for ascending and descending stairs.

A person who still has some reliable vision may wish to vary the technique slightly depending on lighting, the density of a crowd, the speed with which he or she is walking, and other things. The length of the cane may also vary depending on the height of the person, the speed at which he or she travels, and personal preference. Some people feel more need for the white cane at night or in bright sunlight. White canes may be ordered from the NFB Independence Market.

Who can use a guide dog? Today it should be possible for anyone who wishes to use a guide dog to do so. However, many seniors do not choose to get a guide dog. Guide dogs are usually medium-sized dogs, such as German Shepherds or Labrador Retrievers. Therefore, it is also a good idea for the person using the dog to have enough strength to control the dog if discipline is necessary. Although guide dogs are associated with the blind, many people who have partial vision use them successfully.

The blind person is always in charge. The dog can provide information about an approaching flight of steps, the location of street crossings, and sometimes find an outside door. It is trained to go around obstacles. But perhaps the most important thing the dog learns is to stop and wait until the person determines the reason for the stop and instructs the dog to go forward. The dog may memorize a route, such as where a friend lives or the way to work, but the blind person may not always follow the same route, so the dog must take instructions. The blind person listens to traffic and decides when it is time to cross a street. The dog walks slightly in front of the blind person who holds the handle of the harness in his or her left hand.

Guide dogs are trained at special schools across the country. Any of these schools will provide information to an individual who is considering the acquisition of a guide dog. The school will be able to describe the training required by the person and the care required by the dog. Guide dogs are not pets, but there is generally a very close relationship between the guide dog user and the dog.

If you are considering a guide dog as a travel assistant, the president of your state affiliate will be able to tell you which schools are most commonly used by blind individuals in your area. Guide dog schools are generally financed with public funds, so there should be little or no charge for the dog or training to use it. Of course, dog food and veterinary care arc the dog owner's out-of-pocket expenses.

Who can learn Braille? Braille is a system of dots to be read with the fingertips. It is not more difficult to learn than print, just different. A child who learns to read using Braille picks it up at about the same rate of speed as a child learning to read print. When an adult loses vision, it is possible to learn Braille, but it may take a little longer to acquire a rapid reading speed.

Standard Braille is written with about 200 signs, but it is perfectly reasonable to write and read some Braille without these signs. The memory work is less if you simply learn the alphabet and the numbers. This makes it possible to keep phone numbers, addresses, recipes and other small notes in Braille. Braille is a convenience for anyone who knows it. If you are motivated to do so, the earlier you begin learning

Braille, the better you are likely to be at reading and writing. Some men and women who lose their vision late in life do not learn Braille. Whether this is desirable or not is a matter for debate. There is a card showing the Braille and print alphabets included in the Low Vision Resource Kit by the National Federation of the Blind.

When reading Braille, an individual needs to keep his or her fingers light on the dots. New Braille readers often feel as though they need to push down to feel the Braille better. To the contrary, pushing down makes it harder to feel the dots. Brushing the fingers lightly across the lines makes the Braille much clearer.

Braille can be written with the Braille Writer, which is expensive. Or it can be written with a slate and stylus, which consists of a frame as a guide and a punch which is used to push the dots down through the paper.

Hadley School for the Blind, 700 Elm St., Winnetka, IL 60093, 800-323-4238, offers a correspondence course in Braille reading and writing. Independent living programs at rehabilitation agencies may offer Braille instruction if it is requested. Braille instruction books are also available from the NFB Independence Market. Many members of the NFB are happy to provide some instruction in Braille for new readers.

Larger Braille cells can be produced for people who really do have impaired touch in their fingers. This is called Jumbo Braille. Some blind persons also keep notes on a cassette tape recorder.

How can I learn to use a computer? Your local chapter or state affiliate of the NFB should be able to put you in touch with someone who can help determine what hardware and software would be necessary to do the things you wish to do. Your rehabilitation agency may have staff who can provide similar information. If you purchase a program to enlarge the print on the screen, you may need some special instruction to learn to use it. If you purchase speech or Braille output, you may need to arrange for training from another visually impaired person or a special instructor. You will need to use the entire keyboard to operate a speech output program, and the commands are numerous. However, many, many blind and visually impaired individuals are proficient computer users.

Color is important: As you lose vision, you may lose much of your ability to discern colors. Still, you know which colors are attractive together, so you will wish to keep track of the colors of your clothing and other items. Be sure you know what the colors of new purchases are.

When sorting clothing, pay attention to identifying characteristics such as buttons, collars, and pleats. This author likes to knit. When I am purchasing yarn, I ask that each color be placed in a separate bag. If I cannot identify different colors by the feel of the skeins, I may tie the top of one bag or tear off one label. But I want to be able to keep these colors straight when there is no one around who can see it. I am planning to make a baby blanket of rainbow colors. I will use rubber bands, safety pins, stitch holders and whatever it takes to keep track of the seven colors plus white. I do not like to rip out my work, and I certainly am not willing to have the colors in the wrong order. Therefore, I must be creative.

Can I continue to sew and do handwork? In our Independence Market we have self-threading needles and a needle threader for sale. These items are also available in local fabric stores. To use the self-threading needle, hold the thread taut between your hands and pull it into the end of the needle which is divided. You will feel a small 'pop' when the thread goes in. Many individuals use self-threading needles for mending, sewing on buttons, and hemming.

Some blind and visually impaired individuals prefer to use the needle threader with a regular needle. You may find that large-eye needles are easier to use. Place the wire loop of the needle threader through the eye of the needle; then drop the thread through the wire loop and pull it through the needle. This draws the thread through the eye of the needle so you can tie it and proceed to sew.

Many blind individuals continue to sew, both by hand and with the sewing machine. It is possible to guide the fabric on the sewing machine by touching a seam guide or the presser foot. It is also possible to cut around the edge of a tissue paper pattern.

Many women and some men like to knit, crochet, do latch hook, and other handicrafts. Most of these can be done by touch very well. We recommend that you talk to other blind and visually impaired individuals if you have questions or interest in any of these hobbies. The president of the National Federation of the Blind in your state should be able to refer you to people whose interests correspond to yours.

Labeling foods and medications: Cupboards and freezers may be organized in a certain order. Labels may be made with black markers or Braille and attached with rubber bands. Braille labels for cans may be purchased also.

If you take several medications and need to mark bottles to tell them apart, you may use black markers or tactile markers. You may wish to put tape on the lid of one bottle and on the bottom of another. You could put a rubber band around a third bottle. Different locations may also be a way to know which bottle is which. Many seniors use containers divided into seven compartments (one for each day of the week) to pre-sort their medications. If necessary you may have one divided container for mornings and a second for evenings. Develop your own system, and stick to it.

Restaurants: When you go to a restaurant, relax and enjoy yourself. If you need to have your server read a menu or part of it, he or she should be glad to do so. Do not hesitate to ask if the restaurant has large print or Braille menus. Some do. If they do not, this will bring to the attention of the restaurant personnel that special menus would be used if available. You may also wish to ask your server to tell you when he or she places something in front of you. If drinks are placed in the middle of the table, you may not always be aware when this occurs. We tip servers for service, but we cannot expect them to know our needs if we do not say something.

Generally, you will not need to have your food served in a special way. If you wish to have the lettuce cut up in your salad, ask that this be done in the kitchen before it is served. Use your fork and knife to find the food on your plate. You can practice at home cutting meat and picking up vegetables with your fork without bright light. Most people with low vision find dimly lighted restaurants difficult if they do not practice eating in dim light anywhere else.

If you wish to go through the salad bar line, ask if someone has time to help you identify what is there.

How do I know it is clean? It is easy to feel dust on knickknacks and furniture. You can generally tell by touch when counters, sinks, tubs, etc. are clean. It may be desirable to have someone else check for stains occasionally. Many people with low vision like to vacuum the floor with bare feet to help check for dust. Systematic parallel strokes will help you know when you have covered the entire floor. You say you have cobwebs along the ceiling from time to time? Using a white cane and a cloth is a good way to knock them down.

Telephones: A touch-tone telephone is very easy to use by touch. You can also purchase large button phones. But you may find it less stressful not to have to look at all. Put three fingers across the top three buttons to push one, two, and three. Move them down a row when you wish to push four, five or six. Move down another row to push seven, eight, and nine. You may move down another row for zero or use your thumb. Those buttons are easy to feel. Be sure the phone is not at an angle when you are dialing, and a little practice will be all you need.

Where can I live? A blind or visually impaired person can live comfortably and safely almost anywhere he or she chooses. Certainly, the same choices about living quarters should be available to the blind and visually impaired as are available to sighted individuals. Landlords are required by law not to discriminate against tenants because of vision loss.

In recent years thousands of older citizens have found it desirable to move into senior citizens' villages, apartment buildings, mobile home parks, or clusters of houses reserved for retired people. Some of these include group dining rooms and recreation facilities, while others have very few special services. Undoubtedly, some people with low vision will find arrangements such as these desirable. Some will not. Blind and visually impaired people have the opportunity to live in these senior citizen villages along with everyone else. Assuming there are no health problems that make nursing home care necessary, elderly individuals with low vision should be able to learn alternative skills to care for themselves and live in whatever type of housing situation they prefer.

How to get around without driving? Sooner or later loss of vision makes it necessary to stop driving. No one wants to be unsafe as a driver, but driving is a convenience that may be hard to give up. Nevertheless, there are many other ways to go places, and it may actually save money not to maintain a car.

Most cities of 100,000 people or more have city buses and some smaller cities do also. The quality and quantity of bus service varies considerably from one city to the next. A person with poor vision or no vision can learn to use these buses if motivated and if he or she does not have other serious physical disabilities. A blind person waiting at a bus stop may not be able to read the sign on the front of the bus. Then, when the door opens, one simply steps up to it and asks the driver the number or name of the bus. Drivers are required to announce stops. It may be helpful to tell the driver ahead of time which stop you want to help insure that he or she does not forget to announce it.

There is an information number in most cities that can provide information about where each route goes and on what schedule. This information is also printed and can be mailed to interested persons, but it may be more convenient to call the general bus information number.

Bus service is called fixed route service. Most cities also provide dial-a-ride service. This is intended for persons who live on the bus routes and cannot use the fixed route service. Many seniors can qualify. One must become certified for this service and then order it ahead of time. Either the bus company or the mayor's office can tell you how to get in touch with this service. Many smaller towns and cities have only this dial-a-ride service.

Taxis are used by many blind and visually impaired people. They are more expensive than buses or dial-a-ride services, but may not cost as much as maintaining a car, especially if you do not need to use one too frequently. Paying for a taxi once or twice a week is certainly a bargain compared to owning and operating a car. In addition, taxicabs generally operate 24 hours a day seven days a week. This is not true of city buses or dial-a-ride systems. Some towns and cities provide a subsidy for disabled people and seniors to use with taxis. This may be called scrips or something else. You may learn about this subsidy by calling the mayor's office or services for the aging.

Many blind people who can afford to do so own cars and get friends, family members, or employees to drive them when needed. The insurance company will require you to name a primary driver, but this does not prevent other people from driving your car. Some blind people find that this system is more reliable than depending on other people's cars which sometimes are not available or may not always be in good repair. Of course, much depends on personal resources and preferences.

Many people with low vision ride bicycles, especially in good weather. It is important to be honest with yourself about when this is safe and when it is not. This depends on vision and traffic, but it is a personal decision and is not regulated in most places by rules or laws.

Of course many people with low vision walk more than they did before losing sight. The white cane can provide a great deal of information both to the person using it and to those he or she meets. Anyone who is legally blind is entitled to carry a white cane. For more information about how to use the cane, see the section, "Who needs a white cane?"

There are some special van services for seniors associated with senior activities and with some senior residences. These may be an important factor when choosing a place to live. These vans may provide transportation to doctors' offices, shopping, recreational activities, and other places a group of people wish to go.

Many people with low vision also find it important to choose an apartment or house located near a city bus route if bus travel is going to be used. Most individuals who do not drive find it best to use several different kinds of transportation. Some live where they still have access to Greyhound buses or trains. These are also good transportation alternatives for those who do not drive. Airports and airlines provide escorts if needed when going from gate to gate or from check-in to flight. These services should be offered, not required. It is up to the blind person or the person with low vision to decide which services are helpful to him or her, but it is very helpful that the airlines offer special consideration.

Those who live in rural areas may have fewer choices available when planning transportation. It may be necessary to rely on friends and neighbors for help in getting places that are too far from home to walk. Most people who find themselves in this situation learn to find things to do for those who help them. One woman goes grocery shopping with a neighbor and then treats the neighbor to lunch.

Many hire high school or college students for some help. Many people with low vision are fortunate to have family members who are able to assist with transportation to doctors' appointments or shopping, but it is best not to be totally dependent on friends and family.

Sorting money: Coins are easily sorted by touch. Dimes and quarters have rough edges, while nickels and pennies have smooth edges. Quarters are the largest; nickels somewhat smaller; and dimes and pennies are the smallest.

Paper money can be folded or sorted in separate compartments of the wallet. There is no wrong or right way to sort money. Each person should decide what to do and follow the same plan consistently. This writer folds ones and fives in fourths and keeps them in different compartments. Tens are folded lengthwise first and end to end second. Twenties are folded end to end first and then side to side. Anything larger than twenty is kept in a remote section. This is only an example of one approach, but each person will make variations.

You will find a check-writing guide in the Low Vision Resource Kit. You may also use it as a signature guide. Your handwriting will continue to be as legible as previously. You merely need a guide so that you write in the correct places. You may wish to keep your check register on a computer or a separate notebook. Some individuals with low vision use black markers for check registers. Some record this information on tape.

Many people, both blind and sighted, like to shop with friends. If you do, your friend will be glad to tell you prices and read other information about the products you are considering. If you prefer to shop on your own, sales clerks will, as they have time, read the same information. Of course, sales clerks also want to sell the products so you can't depend solely on them to decide what you need or like.

You may also need to ask directions to go from one department or store to another. Strangers are often uncomfortable giving a blind or visually impaired person directions. This is because they use visual landmarks to know where they are. You may need to suggest other pieces of information. For instance, "You mean I should turn left at the first aisle after the carpet ends?" Or "So the escalator is this way (motion with your hand), and I should go past it and turn right?" Thus, you are confirming directions that may not have been quite clear. The person you are talking with can affirm that you are correct or not. As with so many other things, you develop skill in this area with experience.

Can I get financial or medical assistance other than Social Security and Medicare? If you are sixty-five or older, you will not receive any additional money from Social Security just because you are blind. If you are under age 65, it is very important for the Social Security worker to know that you are legally blind. If you are eligible for Social Security Disability Insurance, you may continue to receive disability benefits (which may be higher) until you are age 65, at which time your payments will convert to Social Security Retirement based on the fact that you have attained age 65.

Medicare pays hospital and doctor expenses under certain rules and limitations, but if your income is very low and/or you have some large medical bills, you may be eligible for some other medical assistance through your state or local programs.

Depending on your financial circumstances, it may be possible to qualify for medical assistance through your State Department of Social Services. Most states also have what is called a "spend down program." If you are found eligible for this, you will pay a set amount of medical expenses for a six-month period of time, and the Department of Social Services will pay anything above this amount. Please check with your State Department of Social Services for further details. In a few states, rehabilitation agencies for the blind can provide financial assistance for medical treatments to prevent blindness. This may include treatment of diabetic retinopathy and wet macular degeneration.

There are university hospitals in most states which are teaching hospitals for medical students. They are often able to provide medical services at a reduced rate. Other hospitals which have been constructed with federal funds are sometimes required, at least for a number of years, to provide some assistance to low-income individuals. Please check with hospitals in your area for this type of program.

If you are a Medicare recipient, there are some doctors who will accept for payment the amount that Medicare will pay. Many hospitals have doctor referral services and can tell you which doctors will accept Medicare patients.

If you are 65 or older, a U.S. citizen or legal resident, and you do not have access to an ophthalmologist that you have seen in the past, you may be eligible for the National Eye Care Project. If you think you may be eligible, call 800-222-EYES (3937). Callers who meet the eligibility requirements are mailed the name of a participating ophthalmologist near their home. Participating doctors provide medical eye exams and treatment for conditions or diseases if necessary. Qualified callers will receive treatment at no out-of-pocket expense for the doctor's services. Eyeglasses, prescriptions, hospital services, and other medical services are not covered under the program. Doctors accept insurance assignment as payment in full.

It is the responsibility of the agency on aging in your state to act as a referral agency for older citizens. There is also a state rehabilitation agency for the blind in your state which should be able to give you information. There may be other state or local services for which you may be eligible.

Section 64.2

Understanding Low Vision Devices

"Low Vision FAQ: Resources," is from the National Eye Institute (NEI, www.nei.nih.gov), part of the National Institutes of Health, June 2007.

What resources and strategies can help people perform daily tasks at home? At home, people need devices that can help them read, write, and manage the tasks of daily living. These adaptive devices include adjustable lighting, prescription reading glasses, large-print publications, magnifying devices, and closed-circuit televisions.

People can place colored tape on the edges of steps to help them see the steps and prevent a fall. Dark-colored light switches and electrical outlets can provide contrast on light-colored walls. Motion lights that automatically turn on when someone enters a room are helpful. Telephones, clocks, and watches with large numbers can help people use those instruments more easily.

Visual devices can help people with low vision, such as reading glasses with high-powered lenses and reading prisms, telescopes and telescopic spectacles, and reversed telescopes for visual field defects. These devices must be prescribed by eye care professionals, and patients must be trained to use them properly.

Chapter 65

Emotional and Daily Living Considerations If You Have Vision Loss

Chapter Contents

Section 65.1

Vision Loss and Depression

A number of studies demonstrate that people experiencing vision loss are significantly more likely to suffer from clinical depression than the general population.

For example, in a recent study of vision loss, rehabilitation, and depression conducted by the Arlene R. Gordon Research Institute of Lighthouse International, one-third of visually impaired participants had clinically significant depressive symptoms. When we talk about clinical depression we do not mean occasional feelings of low mood, lack of motivation or anger. We talk of feeling clinically depressed when symptoms last for last two weeks or more, and are so severe that they interfere with daily living.

If people with vision loss experience depression this is likely to have a major impact on their families and friends, in particular on their partners. They also tend to be less open to rehabilitation thus prolonging the time it takes them to adjust to their vision loss.

This is therefore a problem that needs to be taken seriously. If somebody is given the diagnosis of Age-related macular degeneration they need to be prepared for the psychological impact of this condition. It is often people who experience gradual vision loss who are most at risk of depression since they live with the daily fear of waking up to a further deterioration of their sight. Most people who are grieving have feelings of sadness or unhappiness—but these feelings can lift. Some degree of depression is common in people who are coping with AMD, and it may make their vision seem worse that it is. But when you experience long lasting sadness or are having difficulty carrying out day-to-day activities, you may have clinical depression. Serious or clinical depression is a disorder that can be dealt with using a variety of treatments including medication, psychotherapy or counseling, or a combination of both. These therapies improve the quality of life and psychological condition of people with AMD and reduce their suffering, and may even improve their visual functioning. In a clinical depression, a person loses interest and pleasure in activities that were once satisfying, and these feelings persist for weeks. Other symptoms may include:

- persistent sad or "empty" mood almost every day for most of the day;
- significant weight loss or gain;
- feeling "slowed down" almost every day;
- fatigue, almost every day;
- insomnia, early waking, oversleeping, or other sleep disturbances;
- loss of appetite or overeating;
- difficulty concentrating, remembering, making decisions;
- feelings of guilt, worthlessness, helplessness;
- irritability;
- excessive crying;
- chronic aches and pains for no apparent reason; and
- thoughts of death or suicide, suicide attempts.

If these symptoms last for 2 weeks or longer, or are severe enough to interfere with normal functioning, it is important to get an evaluation for clinical depression by a qualified health or mental health professional.

Denial, anger, fear, grief, and even depression are all common emotions among people diagnosed with AMD. For many AMD patients, it is critical to get help coping.

Section 65.2

Adapting Your Home If You Have Vision Impairment or Loss

Whether you live in a house or an apartment, you want to feel comfortable, capable, and in charge of your surroundings—that is what transforms living quarters into a home. Here is some basic advice about making your environment safe and well organized. It is founded on five important principles:

- Increase lighting
- Eliminate hazards
- Create color contrasts
- Organize and label items
- Reduction of glare

Increase Lighting

- Use stronger light bulbs or 3-way bulbs to provide nonglare lighting.
- Put lamps in places where you do close work. For example, put a gooseneck lamp in your reading-writing area. Many companies make lighter light bulbs that simulate natural day light, which can be very helpful to someone with low vision.
- Install extra lights in the bedroom closet and other frequently used closets in other rooms.
- Put special lighting over all stairways—the places where accidents are most likely to occur.
- Make sure the lighting level is consistent throughout the house

so shadows and dangerous bright spots are eliminated. Install rheostats.

- Be certain you can easily reach light switches from doorways and from your bed.
- Use a night light in the bedroom, hallway, and bathroom.

Eliminate Hazards

- Mark thermostats with brightly colored fluorescent tape at settings you typically use.
- Use nonskid, nonglare wax to polish floors.
- Close closet and cupboard doors and drawers completely as soon as you've taken out what you need.
- Pick up shoes, clothing, books, and other items that you could trip over. In fact, put away an object when you are through using it—for the sake of safety and so you can find it easily again.
- Mop up spills as soon as they occur.

Create Color Contrasts

- Put light-colored objects against a dark background—a beige chair against a dark wood paneled wall, for example—and vice versa—a black switch plate on a white wall.
- Install doorknobs that contrast in color with the door for easy location.
- Avoid upholstery with patterns. Stripes, plaids, and checks can be visually confusing.

Organize and Label Items

- Keep items that are used together near each other—on the same shelf, in the same closet, or in the same box.
- Label each box using a broad-tipped black felt marker. Or write the contents on index cards and attach the cards to the boxes with rubber bands. Self-adhesive labels are also handy.

Reduce Glare

- Glare can be caused by sunlight or light from a lamp and can make it difficult for an individual with low vision to see when it hits shiny surfaces, such as a glass or highly polished table top, waxed floors, or the TV screen.

- Sunlight can fill the room with light without producing glare.

- Mini blinds are one of the best window coverings because they can be altered during the course of the day to eliminate the glare.

- Avoid using wax on the floor; use a flat finish.

- To make the television easier to see, simply turn the screen away from the sun or a lamp so the light source is behind the screen.

Learn more in *Prescriptions for Independence* [http://www.afb.org/store/product.asp?sku=0%2D89128%2D244%2D0&mscssid=0410HSK7UW7R9N1H6UPR20WFQ08R98G5], by Nora Griffin-Shirley, Ph.D., and Gerda Groff.

Section 65.3

Keep Track of Your Medications

"Keep Track of Your Medications" was provided courtesy of, and is copyrighted, by Lighthouse International, www.Lighthouse.org, a leading nonprofit organization that helps people of all ages overcome the challenge of vision loss. © 2007.

- Ask the pharmacist to explain the prescription. Inquire about the dose, best time to take the medication, and possible side effects. Record the information—along with any known drug allergies and refill instructions—in a medication log using a format you can access: braille, large print, or audiocassette. Include medical emergency contact phone numbers.

- Keep a print copy of your medication log. Always bring it with you when visiting a doctor or filling a prescription to guard against possible drug interactions.

- Label containers to differentiate among medicines and ensure proper use. Select a method that's easy to understand and remember. Use braille, large print, numbers, color coding, or tactile markings. You can purchase commercial-labeling products as well. Whatever system you choose, be consistent.

- Try to remember pills by their unique shape, size, and, if applicable, color, as a backup.

- Take advantage of medication organizers available in drug stores or specialty catalogs. They come in a variety of shapes, sizes, and contrasting colors. Or ask your pharmacist to use different size bottles when dispensing similar-shaped pills. And, should you need it, you can purchase eyedrop guides for help self-administering eye medications.

- Wrap rubber bands around the bottle equaling the number of daily doses. This will help you remember if you've taken the right amount. Remove one band each time you take the medication, and replace all of them for the following day. Or, consider a pill organizer with a beeping alarm to alert you that it's time for the next dose.

- Seek assistance if you're unsure of what to take and when.

Section 65.4

Fire Safety Tips for People with Visual Impairment

"The Visually Impaired" is from the U.S. Fire Administration (www.usfa.dhs.gov), December 28, 2006.

Over 10 million Americans are visually impaired. During a fire emergency, the senses that visually impaired persons rely upon have a high probability of being overpowered.

The United States Fire Administration (USFA) encourages the visually impaired population to practice the following precautionary steps to help protect themselves, their home, and their surroundings from the danger of fire.

Install and Maintain Smoke Alarms

- Make sure working smoke alarms are installed on each level of your home. You may want a family member or friend to assist you.

- Remember to test smoke alarms monthly and change the batteries at least once a year. You may want a family member or friend to assist you.

- Audible alarms should pause with a small window of silence between each successive cycle so that blind or visually impaired people can listen to instructions or voices of others.

Don't Isolate Yourself

It is important that older adults speak up—55% of the visually impaired population is over the age of 65.

- Speak to your family members, building manager, or neighbors about your fire safety plan and practice it with them.

- Ask emergency responders to keep your special needs information on file.

- Contact your local fire department's non-emergency line and explain your special needs. They will probably suggest escape plan ideas, and may perform a home fire safety inspection and offer suggestions about smoke alarm placement.

Live near an Exit and Plan Your Escape

You'll be safest on the ground floor if you live in an apartment building. If you live in a multi-story home, arrange to sleep on the first floor.

- Being on the ground floor and near an exit will make your escape easier.

- If necessary, have a ramp available for emergency exits.

- Unless instructed by the fire department, never use an elevator during a fire.

- If you encounter smoke, stay low to the ground to exit your home.

- Once out, stay out, and call 911 or your local emergency number from a neighbor's house.

Be Fire-Safe around the Home

- When cooking, never approach an open flame while wearing loose clothing and don't leave cooking unattended. Use a timer to remind you of food in the oven.

- Don't overload electrical outlets of extension cords.

- Never use the oven to heat your home. Properly maintain chimneys and space heaters.

- Keep a phone near your bed and be ready to call 911 or your local emergency number if a fire occurs.

Know Your Abilities

Remember, fire safety is your personal responsibility.

Section 65.5

Tips for Older Drivers

"Tips for Older Drivers" was provided courtesy of, and is copyrighted, by Lighthouse International, www.Lighthouse.org, a leading non-profit organization that helps people of all ages overcome the challenge of vision loss. © 2007.

The ability to drive a car and get around independently is essential for millions of people. While driving safely is a key concern for everyone, changes in the aging eye make it especially relevant for older adults.

If you are 60 years of age or over, you are driving with only about one third of the light you had when you were 20 years old. This is due to changes occurring within the eye (such as yellowing of the lens and decreasing pupil size), that most people don't even realize have occurred. Also, as an older driver, you cannot process and respond to visual information as quickly and efficiently as you could when you were younger.

The following tips can make the driving experience much safer for the older driver:

- Have regular eye check-ups to maintain eye health and to ensure that your ability to drive safely is not compromised by undetected vision loss.

- Be aware that driving under the influence of some medications can dramatically diminish your ability to react to unexpected road hazards. Ask your doctor about the side effects of any medications you're taking.

- Nighttime driving, which typically involves exposure to bright, fleeting glare, presents a particular challenge to older drivers. With this in mind, take extra caution regarding your decision to get behind a wheel at night.

- To minimize glare exposure when driving at night, do not look directly at the headlights of oncoming vehicles. Instead, direct your gaze down the road and toward the right side of the lane in which you're driving.

- Older drivers require more time to adjust to sudden changes in light level, such as when one enters a darkened tunnel from the bright afternoon sunlight. You can partially solve this problem with a pair of flip-up/down sunglasses. Look through the sunglasses for a few minutes while approaching a tunnel. Then flip them up and out of the way on entering the tunnel. You can also use wrap-around sunglasses that fit over the top of your prescription eyeglasses, but can be removed easily upon entering a tunnel or other light-altering situation.

- Cataracts can interfere seriously with driving performance, even though they may only produce a small decline in one's ability to read a chart in the doctor's office. If you're developing cataracts, check with your eye doctor about whether or not it's time to have them removed.

- Plan your travel to minimize the impact of any visual limitations. When possible, drive in familiar locations, and avoid driving at night, in bad weather and during busy rush hours.

- Familiarize yourself with the vision requirements for holding a driver's license where you live; the regulations vary greatly from state to state.

- Consider speaking to an eye care specialist, friend or family member about any concerns you may have related to driving.

If you're worried that a family member can no longer see well enough to drive, your first step should be to discuss the issue with the driver. In many instances, older drivers change their driving behaviors to compensate for vision changes—you may be relieved to learn that your family member is aware of the problem and is taking steps to ensure his or her safety. If your relative doesn't agree that there's a problem, try to convince him or her to discuss the issue with an eye doctor and, if it's acceptable, go along to the appointment yourself. Often, when both family members and a doctor express concern, a patient will heed the warning.

These tips are based on an established body of research and on original research conducted by the Arlene R. Gordon Research Institute of Lighthouse International.

Chapter 66

Know Your Employment Rights: State Vocational Rehabilitation Services

What is the State Vocational Rehabilitation (VR) Services Program?

Under the Rehabilitation Act of 1973, as amended, federal grants are awarded to assist states in operating a comprehensive vocational rehabilitation program. This program provides VR services to eligible individuals with disabilities, consistent with their strengths, resources, priorities, concerns, abilities, and capabilities, so that such individuals may prepare for and engage in gainful, competitive employment.

Who is eligible for VR services?

To be eligible for VR services, an individual must:

* have a physical or mental impairment that is a substantial impediment to employment;

* be able to benefit in terms of employment from VR services; and

* require VR services to prepare for, enter, engage in, or retain gainful employment that is consistent with the individual's strengths, resources, priorities, concerns, abilities, capabilities, and informed choice.

How does an eligible individual receive VR services?

A VR counselor is assigned to each eligible individual. The counselor gathers as much information as possible about the individual's work history, education and training, abilities and interests, rehabilitation needs, and possible career goals. Together, the counselor and the individual develop an Individualized Written Rehabilitation Program (IWRP) that identifies the individual's long-term vocational goals.

The IWRP lists the steps necessary to achieve the individual's goals, the services required to help the individual reach those goals, and evaluation criteria used to determine whether goals have been achieved. The IWRP also contains a description of how the individual was involved in choosing among alternative goals, objectives, services, and service providers.

The state VR counselor provides some services directly to the eligible individual and arranges for and/or purchases other services from providers in the community.

What are the VR services an eligible individual may receive?

VR services are those services that an eligible individual may need in order to achieve his/her vocational goal. These include, but are not limited to:

- an assessment to determine eligibility and VR needs;
- vocational counseling, guidance, and referral services;
- physical and mental restoration services;
- vocational and other training, including on-the-job training;
- maintenance for additional costs incurred while the individual is receiving certain VR services;
- transportation related to other VR services;
- interpreter services for individuals who are deaf;
- reader services for individuals who are blind;
- services to assist students with disabilities to transition from school to work;
- personal assistance services (including training in managing, supervising, and directing personal assistance services) while an individual is receiving VR services;

- rehabilitation technology services and devices; and

- supported-employment and job-placement services.

Does every eligible individual receive VR services?

If a state VR agency is unable to serve all eligible individuals with the resources available for the VR program, it must establish an order of selection for services, serving first those individuals with the most severe disabilities. Individuals who cannot be selected immediately for services are placed on a waiting list.

Does the eligible individual ever have to pay for VR services?

Based on the individual's available financial resources, the state VR agency may require an eligible individual to help pay for services. However, all eligible individuals who are accepted have access to the following at no cost to them:

- assessments to determine eligibility and VR needs;

- vocational counseling, guidance, and referral services; and

- job-placement services.

What are comparable services and benefits?

Before providing certain services, the VR counselor must consider the availability of comparable services and benefits for which the individual is eligible through other sources, such as private insurance, Medicaid, and so on. A counselor is not required to consider the availability of comparable services and benefits, however, when such consideration would delay the provision of services to an eligible individual who is at extreme medical risk or whose job placement might be lost as a result of a delay in services.

What is the earnings status of rehabilitated persons in the years after case closure compared to persons who were not rehabilitated?

Based on data from the Rehabilitation Services Administration, rehabilitated persons were more likely than those not rehabilitated to have had earnings five years after closure. The likelihood of having earnings was more nearly equal in the years before rehabilitation services. Rehabilitated persons were more likely than persons not rehabilitated to have had earnings the fifth year after closure, but only 6% were more likely to have had earnings the fifth year before closure. Rehabilitated persons were 44% more likely than persons not rehabilitated to have had earnings the fifth year after closure, but only 6% were more likely to have had earnings the fifth year before closure.

After the delivery of rehabilitation services, the gap in average annual earnings favoring rehabilitated workers over those not rehabilitated rose to about $2,200. Prior to rehabilitation services, the difference in average annual earnings between the two groups of workers was consistently below $1,000.

In the last five post-closure years for which data were available (1984 to 1988), the average earnings differential in earnings favoring rehabilitated workers widened steadily each year reaching $2,630 in 1988. Rehabilitated workers averaged 31% more in annual earnings than workers not rehabilitated. For each case, the typical rehabilitated person (including nonwage earners) amassed $46,684 on the eight post-closure years, nearly twice the per case, or per capita, accumulation of $24,307 for persons who were not rehabilitated. On a per capita basis, rehabilitated persons averaged 87% more in annual earnings than persons not rehabilitated.

What is the impact on individuals with disabilities?

Sixteen million individuals with disabilities have been assisted in acquiring gainful employment over the 75-year history of the state vocational rehabilitation (VR) program. In fiscal year 1994 alone, this program assisted 202,000 individuals with disabilities in obtaining employment, making them taxpaying members of society. On average, it is estimated that only four years are required for a person rehabilitated by the VR program to pay back costs incurred during his/her rehabilitation in the form of federal and state income and sales taxes and reductions in the cost of dependency.

What is the uniqueness of the VR program?

Well-trained professional staff are the key. At the core of the VR program is the relationship between a well-trained counselor and an individual with a disability. The counselor and the individual with a disability forge a partnership whereby a plan is developed and designed to provide those services necessary to achieve the individual's vocational goal consistent with her/his abilities, needs, and informed choices. In this context, the counselor provides the individual with information and guidance about trends in the job market, how the individual's abilities might be best utilized, reasonable accommodations available, training options available, and other services needed to help the individual prepare for and secure work.

State/Private Partnership

Many VR services are purchased through local service providers such as community-based rehabilitation programs, traditional rehabilitation facilities such as those run by the local affiliates of national organizations, hospitals, physicians, colleges, technical schools, and a wide range of other nonprofit and for-profit sources. For example, rehabilitation technology and transportation services can be purchased to assist clients as part of their rehabilitation programs.

These vendor relationships are well established and are typically based on the knowledge of the counselor and the state agencies regarding long-term histories of success and performance with clients with various types of disabilities.

Established Program Linkage

The VR program has a long and impressive history of cooperation with other federal and state programs. For instance, state VR agencies have developed strong relationships with education agencies at both the state and local levels to coordinate services for students with disabilities transition from school to employment-related activities. Without this seamless transitioning, many such students lose the employment-related skills they have gained while in school. The VR program has a long history of cooperation with other programs. For instance, a unique relationship exists between this program and the Social Security Administration to enable recipients of Social Security Disability Insurance (SSDI) and Supplemental Security Income (SSI) to become employed and decrease their reliance on these entitlement programs. The VR program also has a strong relationship with other employment programs (e.g., programs administered by the Department of Veterans Affairs, programs under the Job Training Partnership Act, etc.).

Chapter 67

Tips for Contacting Social Security If You Are Blind or Have Low Vision

If You Are Blind

If you are blind, the Social Security Administration (SSA) has special rules that allow you to receive benefits when you are unable to work.

The SSA pays benefits to people who are blind under two programs: the Social Security disability insurance program and the Supplemental Security Income (SSI) program. The medical rules they use to decide whether you are blind are the same for each program. Other rules are different.

You Can Get Disability Benefits If You Are Legally Blind

You may qualify for Social Security or SSI disability benefits if you are considered "legally blind." The SSA considers you to be legally blind if your vision cannot be corrected to better than 20/200 in your better eye, or if your visual field is 20 degrees or less in your better eye.

You Can Get Disability Benefits Even If You Are Not Legally Blind

If your vision does not meet the legal definition of blindness, you may still qualify for disability benefits if your vision problems alone

Excerpted from "If You Are Blind or Have Low Vision—How We Can Help," by the Social Security Administration (SSA, www.ssa.gov), SSA Publication No. 05-10052, January 2007.

or combined with other health problems prevent you from working. For Social Security disability benefits, you also must have worked long enough in a job where you paid Social Security taxes. For SSI payments based on disability and blindness, you need not have worked, but your income and resources must be under certain dollar limits.

How You Qualify for Social Security Disability Benefits

When you work and pay Social Security taxes, you earn credits that count toward future Social Security benefits.

If you are legally blind, you can earn credits anytime during your working years. Credits for your work after you become blind can be used to qualify you for benefits if you do not have enough credits at the time you become blind.

Also, if you do not have enough credits to get Social Security disability benefits based on your own earnings, you may be able to get benefits based on the earnings of one of your parents or your spouse.

Disability Freeze

There is a special rule that may help you get higher retirement or disability benefits some day. You can use this rule if you are legally blind but are not getting disability benefits now because you are still working. If your earnings are lower because of your blindness, the SSA can exclude those years when they calculate your Social Security retirement or disability benefit in the future. Because Social Security benefits are based on your average lifetime earnings, your benefit will be higher if they do not count those years. They call this rule a disability freeze. Contact the SSA if you want to file for this freeze.

You Can Get SSI Disability Payments

SSI payments are based on need. Your income and resources must be less than certain dollar limits. The income limits vary from one state to another. You need not have worked under Social Security to qualify for SSI. Ask your local Social Security office about the income limits in your state and contact them for Supplemental Security Income (SSI).

You Can Work While Receiving Benefits

A number of rules make it easier for people receiving disability benefits to work. These rules are called work incentives.

People getting Social Security disability benefits can continue to receive their benefits when they work as long as their earnings are not more than an amount set by law.

If you are receiving Social Security disability benefits and you are legally blind, you can earn as much as $1,500 a month in 2007. This is higher than the earnings limit of $900 a month that applies to disabled workers who are not blind. The earnings limits change each year.

Additionally, if you are blind and self-employed, the SSA does not evaluate the time you spend working in your business as they do for people who are not blind. This means you can be doing a lot of work for your business, but still receive disability benefits, as long as your net profit averages $1,500 or less a month in 2007.

Work Figured Differently after Age 55

If you are age 55 or older and legally blind, the SSA determines your ability to work differently than they do for people who are not blind. After age 55, even if your earnings exceed $1,500 a month in 2007, benefits are only suspended, not terminated, if the work you are doing requires a lower level of skill and ability than what you did before you reached 55. They will pay you disability benefits for any month your earnings fall below this limit.

Different work incentives apply to people getting SSI.

Special Services for People Who Are Blind

There are a number of services and products specifically designed for people who are blind.

Social Security Letters

You can choose to receive letters from the SSA in several ways. Just let them know which option you prefer. You can receive your letters:

- by regular mail only;
- by regular mail followed by a telephone call to explain the information in the letter; or
- by certified mail.

If you have a question about a Social Security letter, you may call their toll-free number (see below for the number), or call or visit your local Social Security office to ask for the letter to be read or explained to you.

Radio Reading Service

The SSA provides special tapes of their publications to local radio stations that offer reading services for their blind and low-vision listeners. To find out which stations in your area provide radio reading services, you should call your local Social Security office.

Publications Available in Braille

Many of the SSA publications are available in Braille, audio cassette tapes, compact disks, or in enlarged print for people who are blind or visually impaired.

To request copies of publications in alternative formats such as Braille, you can go to the SSA website, www.socialsecurity.gov/pubs/alt-pubs.html, or call the Social Security Administration at 800-772-1213 or 800-325-0778 (TTY).

Chapter 68

Caring for Someone with Vision Problems

All of us recognize the importance of being able to see properly. But our eyes do change with age. It is important that you as a caregiver follow guidelines for disease prevention and treatment so your family member maintains the highest visual acuity possible.

First, make sure your family member receives regular checkups. Following are some suggestions to ensure your loved one's visual health is receiving appropriate care.

- Schedule regular visits with the person's physician to check for such diseases as diabetes, which can cause severe vision problems.

- Take your loved one for a complete eye exam every year or two. The eye specialist should dilate your family member's eyes to check for certain eye diseases, test his/her vision, check the eyeglasses prescription, test the eye muscles, and check for glaucoma.

There Are Many Problems That Can Affect Our Vision

- Floaters (spots that float across the field of vision): These are not uncommon but if they happen with flashes, have the ophthalmologist check for retinal detachment.

- Dry eyes cause itching, burning, or even impaired vision: Keep your family member's home well humidified and ask the eye doctor to recommend special eyedrops.

From "Caregiver Handbook," © 2005 Denver Regional Council of Governments. Reprinted with permission.

- Excessive tearing can result from light, wind or temperature sensitivity, but it may also indicate a blocked tear duct or eye infection: Consult your family member's eye doctor.

- Presbyopia occurs in most individuals at about age 40, gradually reducing our ability to see close objects or small print: It can generally be corrected with eyeglasses.

- Cataracts form in all or part of the eye lens, causing loss of eyesight: If they become large or thick, cataract surgery is recommended to improve your family member's vision.

- Glaucoma, the consequence of too much fluid pressure inside the eye, is a very serious condition causing vision loss or blindness: It can be treated, however, if caught in time via eyedrops, medications, or surgery.

- Retinal disorders include macular degeneration, diabetic retinopathy, and retinal detachment, impairing vision or resulting in total blindness: Sometimes surgery or treatment can bring back all or part of the lost eyesight, but early detection is essential to increase the likelihood that your family member's vision can be saved.

- Conjunctivitis involves inflammation of the cornea: It is caused by infection or allergies and can generally be treated.

How Can You Recognize Vision Loss in an Older Person?

Watch for the following signs:

- changes in how a person reads, drives, walks, or watches television;

- squinting or tilting of the head from side to side to focus;

- difficulty identifying people or items;

- cannot locate things even in a familiar environment;

- wearing clothes with unusual color combinations;

- no longer wanting to read or holding reading material close to the face/at an angle;

- writing illegibly;

- running into objects, the door frame, or walls when walking;

- demonstrating difficulty getting food on a fork or cutting his/her food; or

- knocking over glasses frequently while dining at the table.

If you observe several of these warning symptoms, schedule an eye exam with an ophthalmologist.

Several other, largely correctable, factors affect vision, especially for older adults.

- **The need for more light:** On average, someone 80 years of age requires 10 times as much light as someone who is 25 years old. To correct, have more than one light source in the room, use higher watt bulbs, and direct the light source to the reading material.

- **Difficulty with glare:** If too much bright light shines directly or reflects into the eye, the older individual will not be able to see clearly. To address this problem, reduce the shiny surfaces in the home (high-gloss floors, mirrors, windows without curtains) and get reading materials that are not on high-gloss paper. Use incandescent rather than fluorescent bulbs for close-work tasks (reading, sewing).

- **Problems accommodating between light and darkness:** An older person's eyes do not adapt as quickly as a younger person's eyes. Don't rush your family member when walking from an enclosure into the sunshine outdoors. Encourage him/her to rely on your arm, especially if entering or leaving a darkened room such as a movie theatre.

- **Reduction in contrast sensitivity and color perception:** Differences in contrasts of colors make objects easier to see. Even identifying faces involves the ability to see contrasts, textures, and patterns. Use as much color contrast as possible to help the person distinguish objects in his/her environment. For example, consider painting the door frame a dark color if you have white walls or vice versa. Try to obtain reading materials with crisp black letters on white or pale yellow paper. Avoid using colors that are close to one another on the hue circle, such as blue and green or red and orange.

- **Depth perception reduction:** Loss of depth perception greatly increases a person's risk for falling since s/he will have trouble determining how close or far objects are and where curbs or stairs begin and end (e.g., place a different color tape or paint at the edge of each stairstep). Make sure your family member's home has adequate lighting, reduce glare where possible, and use color contrasts to help with depth perception.

General Tips to Improve Visual Capabilities

- Ensure that eyeglasses are clean, easy to locate, and worn at all times except in bed.

- Have your family member wear sunglasses when in the sun to reduce glare and help prevent the development of cataracts.

- Provide an easy-to-turn-on reading lamp behind your loved one's shoulder but focused toward the reading or sewing materials.

- Find large-print reading materials.

- Avoid moving furniture in the family member's environment to avoid confusion regarding where things are located when walking.

- Leave night lights on in darker areas of the home.

- Purchase a telephone with large numbers.

Vision and Driving

If your loved one still drives a car, it is imperative that you make sure his/her vision has not deteriorated so that driving becomes a serious risk for your family member or others on the road. Drivers age 65 and older rank second only to 16- to 24-year-olds in the number of accidents per vehicle-mile traveled. This is particularly problematic because older drivers are frequently more seriously hurt in accidents due to having frailer bones and more easily injured muscles/tissues. Adhere to the following suggestions to reduce driving risks.

- Try to avoid having your family member drive at night. Night blindness becomes an increasing problem with age.

- Ask your family member's eye doctor to evaluate driving abilities during annual eye exams.

- Encourage your loved one to avoid driving at peak traffic hours.

- Suggest to your family member that s/he should keep away from busy intersections by taking back streets to get to his/her destination.

- If glare appears to be a problem, purchase glasses with special antireflective coating.

- Suggest that your family member take the AARP [American Association of Retired Persons] course, 55 Alive, which helps teach road and driving safety measures for older adults.

Part Eleven

Additional Help
and Information

Chapter 69

Glossary of Terms Related to the Eyes and Vision

age-related macular degeneration (AMD): A disease associated with aging that gradually destroys sharp, central vision. Central vision is needed for seeing objects clearly and for common daily tasks such as reading and driving. AMD is the leading cause of vision loss in older Americans.

amblyopia: The medical term used when the vision in one of the eyes is reduced because the eye and the brain are not working together properly. This condition is also sometimes called lazy eye.

Amsler grid: A grid with a pattern resembling a checkerboard that is used to check for signs of age-related macular degeneration.

anophthalmia: The absence of one or both eyes.

Age-Related Eye Disease Study (AREDS) formulation: A specific high-dose formulation of antioxidants and zinc shown to significantly reduce the risk of advanced age-related macular degeneration and its associated vision loss.

astigmatism: A condition in which the uneven curvature of the cornea blurs and distorts both distant and near objects.

Behçet disease: Behçet disease is an autoimmune disease that results from damage to blood vessels throughout the body, particularly veins.

This glossary contains terms excerpted from glossaries and documents produced by the following government agencies: National Eye Institute (NEI); National Institute of Neurological Disorders and Stroke (NINDS); National Institutes of Health (NIH); and the U.S. Food and Drug Administration (FDA).

Bietti crystalline dystrophy (BCD): An inherited eye disease that tends to lead to progressive night blindness and visual field constriction.

blepharitis: A common condition that causes inflammation of the eyelids.

blepharospasm: An abnormal, involuntary blinking or spasm of the eyelids.

Bowman layer: A transparent sheet of tissue in the eye that is composed of strong layered protein fibers called collagen.

cataract: A clouding of the lens. People with cataracts see through a haze. In a usually safe and successful surgery, the cloudy lens can be replaced with a plastic lens.

chalazion: This condition can follow the development of a stye. It is a usually painless firm lump caused by inflammation of the oil glands of the eyelid.

choroid: A layer of blood vessels that provides blood and nutrients to the retina.

color blindness: A hereditary trait that results in the inability to tell apart shades of color, such as red and green.

corneal dystrophy: A corneal dystrophy is a condition in which one or more parts of the cornea lose their normal clarity due to a buildup of cloudy material.

corneal transplant: A corneal transplant involves replacing a diseased or scarred cornea with a new one.

Descemet membrane: A thin but strong sheet of tissue in the eye that serves as a protective barrier against infection and injuries.

diabetes: Diabetes is a chronic disease in which blood sugar levels are above normal. Complications may lead to vision loss.

diabetic eye disease: A group of eye problems that people with diabetes may face as a complication of diabetes.

diabetic retinopathy: Damage to the blood vessels in the retina due to diabetes.

dilated eye exam: An eye examination where drops are placed in your eyes to widen, or dilate, the pupils. The eye care professional uses a special magnifying lens to examine the retina and optic nerve for signs of damage and other eye problems. After the exam, your close vision may remain blurred for several hours.

drusen: Drusen are yellow deposits under the retina. They often are found in people over age 60.

endothelium: The extremely thin, innermost layer of the cornea. Endothelial cells are essential in keeping the cornea clear.

epithelium: The cornea's outermost region, comprising about 10 percent of the tissue's thickness.

excimer laser: One of the technologies developed to treat corneal disease. This device emits pulses of ultraviolet light—a laser beam—to etch away surface irregularities of corneal tissue.

eye care professional: An optometrist or ophthalmologist.

floaters: Floaters are little cobwebs or specks that float about in your field of vision.

focal laser treatment: A laser surgery treatment where an ophthalmologist places up to several hundred small laser burns in the areas of retinal leakage surrounding the macula.

fovea: The center of the macula; it gives the sharpest vision.

glaucoma: An eye disease, related to high pressure inside the eye, which damages the optic nerve and leads to vision loss. Glaucoma affects peripheral, or side, vision.

histoplasmosis: A disease caused when airborne spores of the fungus *Histoplasma capsulatum* are inhaled into the lungs. Histoplasmosis can later cause a serious eye disease called ocular histoplasmosis syndrome (OHS), a leading cause of vision loss in Americans ages 20 to 40.

hyperopia (farsightedness): The opposite of myopia. With hyperopia, images focus on a point beyond the retina. Hyperopia results from an eye that is too short.

iris: The colored part of the eye that regulates the amount of light entering the eye.

keratoconus: A progressive thinning of the cornea that arises when the middle of the cornea thins and gradually bulges outward, forming a rounded cone shape.

lacrimal gland: The gland in the eye that secretes tears.

laser trabeculoplasty: A surgical procedure that helps open up the drainage angle to allow more fluid to pass out of the eye.

laser-assisted in situ keratomileusis(LASIK): Eye surgery done with a laser to help people see better. The laser makes tiny cuts that change the shape of the cornea. If done right, it can reduce a person's need for glasses or contact lenses.

lens: The lens is a clear part of the eye that helps to focus light, or an image, on the retina.

low vision: A visual impairment, not corrected by standard eyeglasses, contact lenses, medication, or surgery, that interferes with the ability to perform everyday activities.

macula: Small central area of the retina; area of acute central vision.

macular edema: When fluid leaks into the center of the macula, the part of the eye where sharp, straight-ahead vision occurs. The fluid makes the macula swell, blurring vision.

macular hole: A small break in the macula, located in the center of the eye's light-sensitive tissue called the retina. A macular hole can cause blurred and distorted central vision.

macular pucker: Scar tissue that has formed on the eye's macula, located in the center of the eye's light-sensitive tissue called the retina. A macular pucker can cause blurred and distorted central vision.

microphthalmia: Microphthalmia is a disorder in which one or both eyes are abnormally small.

myopia (nearsightedness): Myopia is when the cornea is curved too much. Faraway objects will appear blurry because they are focused in front of the retina.

ocular herpes: Herpes of the eye, or ocular herpes, is a recurrent viral infection that is caused by the herpes simplex virus and is the most common infectious cause of corneal blindness in the United States.

ophthalmologist: A medical doctor who diagnoses and treats all diseases and disorders of the eye, and can prescribe glasses and contact lenses.

optic nerve: Largest sensory nerve of the eye; carries impulses for sight from the retina to the brain.

optician: A trained professional who grinds, fits, and dispenses glasses by prescription from an optometrist or ophthalmologist.

optometrist: A primary eye care provider who prescribes glasses and contact lenses, and diagnoses and treats certain conditions and diseases of the eye.

orientation and mobility specialist: A person who trains people with low vision to move about safely in the home and travel by themselves.

phakic intraocular lenses: Lenses made of plastic or silicone that are implanted into the eye permanently to reduce a person's need for glasses or contact lenses.

presbyopia: The loss of the ability to focus up close that occurs with aging.

pterygium: A pinkish, triangular-shaped tissue growth on the cornea.

pupil: The opening at the center of the iris.

refractive errors: Vision problems that occur when the curve of the cornea is irregularly shaped. When the curve of the cornea is irregularly shaped, the cornea bends light imperfectly on the retina. This affects good vision. Refractive errors are usually corrected by eyeglasses or contact lenses.

retina: The light-sensitive tissue at the back of the eye.

retinal detachment: When the retina is lifted or pulled from its normal position. If not promptly treated, retinal detachment can cause permanent vision loss.

retinoblastoma: A type of cancer that forms in the retina. The disease usually occurs in children younger than 5 years and may be in one eye or in both eyes. In some cases the disease is inherited from a parent.

retinopathy of prematurity (ROP): A potentially blinding eye disorder that primarily affects premature infants weighing about 2 3/4 pounds (1250 grams) or less that are born before 31 weeks of gestation.

scatter laser surgery: A laser surgery treatment where an ophthalmologist places 1,000 to 2,000 laser burns in the areas of the retina away from the macula, causing the abnormal blood vessels to shrink.

sclera: A protective physical barrier that shields the inner eye from the external environment.

Sjögren syndrome: An autoimmune disorder in which immune cells attack and destroy the glands that produce tears and saliva.

specialist in low vision: An ophthalmologist or optometrist who specializes in the evaluation of low vision. This person can prescribe visual devices and teach people how to use them.

strabismus: Misalignment of the eyes, which creates two discordant images that the brain must reconcile.

stroma: A layer of the cornea that comprises about 90 percent of the cornea's thickness.

stye: A red tender bump on the eyelid that is caused by an acute infection of the oil glands of the eyelid.

tear film: The liquid tear layer bathing the cornea and conjunctiva that performs optical, protective, and lubricative functions.

tonometry: An instrument that measures the pressure inside your eye. Numbing drops may be applied to your eye during this test.

Usher syndrome: An inherited condition that causes serious hearing loss that is usually present at birth or shortly thereafter and progressive vision loss caused by retinitis pigmentosa.

uveitis: A condition in which tissues in the eye become inflamed. If not properly treated, chronic inflammation causes scarring and leads to irreversible vision loss.

vision rehabilitation teacher: A person who trains people with low vision to use optical and nonoptical devices, adaptive techniques, and community resources.

visual acuity test: An eye chart test that measures how well you see at various distances.

visual and adaptive devices: Prescription and nonprescription devices that help people with low vision enhance their remaining vision. Some examples include magnifiers, large print books, check-writing guides, white canes, and telescopic lenses.

vitrectomy: A surgical treatment where an ophthalmologist removes the vitreous gel and replaces it with a salt solution.

vitreous detachment: When the fibers of the vitreous break, allowing the vitreous to separate and shrink from the retina. In most cases, a vitreous detachment is not sight-threatening and requires no treatment.

vitreous gel: Transparent, colorless mass that fills the rear two thirds of the eyeball, between the lens and the retina.

Chapter 70

Frequently Asked Questions about Eye Donation

What is a cornea and how do cornea transplants restore sight?

The cornea is a clear dime-sized tissue that covers the front of the eye. If the cornea becomes clouded through disease or injury, vision is impaired and sometimes lost entirely.

The only substitute for a human cornea is another human cornea donated at death by someone who thus leaves a living legacy.

Who can donate eyes?

Almost everyone can donate his or her eyes. Donor tissue that can't be used for transplant can, with consent, be used for medical education and research purposes.

How can I donate my eyes?

There are two important steps you must take to become a donor. First, enroll in a donor registry or sign your driver's license. Second, talk to your family. You must let your family members know that you wish to be an eye donor so they can make sure your wishes are carried out. Having a discussion about donation with your family is the first step in the effort to restore sight and save lives.

Is there a cost to donate?

There is no cost to donate. Transplant agencies pay any costs associated with recovery of organs and tissues from donors.

Would donating delay funeral arrangements?

Donating should not delay funeral arrangements. It may take additional time, usually no more than four hours, to coordinate the donation process with the funeral home, and for any extra efforts taken to prepare the body for presentation.

Can we have an open casket?

Eye donation should not prevent having an open casket service.

Does my religion support eye, organ, and tissue donation?

All major religions support donation. However, if you have concerns about your religion's position, please get in touch with your religious leader/representative.

Is cancer a rule-out for donation?

No, cancer does not automatically prohibit eye donation.

If I wear glasses can I still donate?

Yes, you can! People who have poor vision and wear glasses, or have had previous eye diseases or surgery can still donate, since these conditions may not affect the cornea. Eyes donated to The Eye-Bank that are not medically suitable for transplant may be used for medical research and education. For example, if you have had LASIK surgery you can donate for research and medical education purposes.

Are families told who will receive the donation?

It is Eye-Bank policy to keep donor and recipient identities completely confidential. However, certain information can be shared and The Eye-Bank offers to conduct correspondence between donor families and recipients as long as identities are kept anonymous. Recipients especially are encouraged to send thank-you notes to their donor families through The Eye-Bank.

Can the family designate a recipient?

It is possible to designate a recipient although it is fairly unlikely that a donation would occur in a timely manner to facilitate a needed transplant. However, if at the time of death a family member is in need of a cornea transplant then The Eye-Bank will make every effort to match the donor tissue with that person.

What kind of research is done with eye donations?

Research into diseases such as cataracts, glaucoma, and diseases of the retina are advanced through eye donation.

How long do recipients usually wait for a cornea?

Cornea transplant surgery is typically an elective procedure allowing the surgeon and patient to choose the most convenient day for the surgery to take place. The need for emergency tissue is met within 24 hours.

How long can a cornea be stored?

The Eye-Bank does keep a "bank" of tissue in its laboratory. Fortunately, cornea tissue can be preserved and stored for several days before it must be used for transplant. However, since demand for ocular tissue is so great most donor tissue is distributed within a day or two after its arrival.

What happens to unused tissue?

Tissue not used for transplantation or research is disposed of in an ethical manner.

Chapter 71

Directory of State Libraries for People with Vision Problems

Alabama

Alabama Regional Library for the Blind and Physically Handicapped
6030 Monticello Drive
Montgomery, AL 36130
Toll-Free: 800-392-5671
Phone: 334-213-3906

Alaska

Alaska State Library
Talking Book Center
344 West 3rd Avenue
Suite 125
Anchorage, AK 99501
Phone: 907-269-6575

Arizona

Arizona State Braille and Talking Book Library
1030 North 32nd Street
Phoenix, AZ 85008
Toll-Free: 800-255-5578
Phone: 602-255-5578

Arkansas

Library for the Blind and Physically Handicapped
One Capitol Mall
Little Rock, AR 72201-1081
Phone: 501-682-1155

"Directory of State Libraries for Persons with Print Disabilities" is from the American Foundation for the Blind, www.afb.org, 2005. All contact information was verified and updated in August 2007.

California (Northern)

California State Library
Braille and Talking Book
Services
P.O. Box 942837
Sacramento, CA 94237-0001
Toll-Free: 800-952-5666
Phone: 916-654-0640

California (Southern)

**Braille Institute Library
Services**
741 North Vermont Avenue
Los Angeles, CA 90029
Toll-Free: 800-808-2555
Phone: 213-663-1111 ext. 358

Colorado

**Colorado Talking Book
Library**
180 Sheridan Boulevard
Denver, CO 80226
Toll-Free: 800-685-2136
Phone: 303-727-9277

Connecticut

Connecticut State Library
Library for the Blind and
Physically Handicapped
198 West Street
Rocky Hill, CT 06067
Phone: 860-721-2020

Delaware

**Library for the Blind and
Physically Handicapped**
Delaware Division of Libraries
43 South DuPont Highway
Dover, DE 19901
Toll-Free: 800-282-8676
Phone: 302-739-4748

District of Columbia

**District of Columbia
Library for the Blind and
Physically Handicapped**
901 G Street, N.W., Room 215
Washington, DC 20001
Phone: 202-727-2142

**The National Library
Service for the Blind and
Physically Handicapped**
Library of Congress
1291 Taylor Street, N.W.
Washington, DC 20542
Toll-Free: 800-424-8567
Phone: 202-707-5100

Florida

**Bureau of Braille and
Talking Book Services**
420 Platt Street
Daytona Beach, FL 32114
Toll-Free: 800-226-6075
Phone: 386-239-6000

Georgia

Georgia Regional Library for the Blind and Physically Handicapped
Georgia Department of Technical and Adult Education
1150 Murphy Avenue Southwest
Atlanta, GA 30310
Phone: 404-756-4619

Guam

Guam Public Library for the Blind and Physically Handicapped
254 Martyr Street
Agana, Guam 96910
Phone: 671-475-4753

Hawaii

Hawaii Library for the Blind and Physically Handicapped
402 Kapahulu Avenue
Honolulu, HI 96815
Phone: 808-733-8444

Idaho

Idaho State Library
Services for Blind and Physically Handicapped
325 West State Street
Boise, ID 83702
Toll-Free: 800-233-4931
Phone: 208-334-2117

Illinois

Chicago Public Library
Illinois Regional Library
for the Blind and Physically
Handicapped
1055 West Roosevelt Road
Chicago, IL 60608
Phone: 312-746-9210

Indiana

Indiana State Library
Special Services Division
140 North Senate
Indianapolis, IN 46204
Toll-Free: 800-622-4970
Phone: 317-232-3684

Iowa

Iowa Library for the Blind and Physically Handicapped
Iowa Department for the Blind
524 4th Street, 4th Floor
Des Moines, IA 50309-2364
Toll-Free: 800-362-2587
Phone: 515-281-1333

Kansas

Kansas Talking Book Services
Kansas State Library
Emporia State University
Memorial Union
1200 Commercial
Emporia, KS 66801
Toll-Free: 800-362-0699
Phone: 316-343-7124

Kentucky

Kentucky Library for the Blind and Physically Handicapped
P.O. Box 537
Frankfort, KY 40602
Toll-Free: 800-372-2968
Phone: 502-564-8300

Louisiana

Louisiana State Library
Section for the Blind and
Physically Handicapped
260 North 3rd Street
Baton Rouge, LA 70802-5232
Phone: 504-342-4944

Maine

Maine State Library
Library Services for the Blind
and Physically Handicapped
State House Station Number 64
Augusta, ME 04333
Toll-Free: 800-762-7106
Phone: 207-287-5650

Maryland

Maryland State Library for the Blind and Physically Handicapped
415 Park Avenue
Baltimore, MD 21201
Toll-Free: 800-964-9209
Phone: 410-230-2424

Massachusetts

Massachusetts Braille and Talking Book Library
Perkins School for the Blind
175 North Beacon Street
Watertown, MA 021720
Toll-Free: 800-852-3133
Phone: 617-924-3434 ext. 240
Phone: 617-972-7240

Michigan (except Wayne County)

Library of Michigan
Services for the Blind and
Physically Handicapped
P.O. Box 30007
Lansing, MI 48909
Phone: 517-373-5614

Michigan (Wayne County only)

Wayne County Regional Library for the Blind and Physically Handicapped
30555 Michigan Avenue
Westland, MI 48186-5310
Toll-Free: 888-968-2737
Phone: 734-727-7300

Minnesota

Minnesota Library for the Blind and Physically Handicapped
388 South East 6th Avenue
Faribault, MN 55021
Toll-Free: 800-722-0550
Phone: 507-333-4828

Missouri

Wolfner Library for the Blind and Physically Handicapped
600 West Main
P.O. Box 387
Jefferson City, MO 65101
Toll-Free: 800-392-2614
Phone: 573-751-8720

Montana

Montana Talking Books Library
1515 East 6th Avenue
Helena, MT 59620
Toll-Free: 800-332-3400
Phone: 406-444-2064

Nebraska

Talking Book and Braille Service
The Atrium
1200 N Street, Suite 120
Lincoln, NE 68508-2023
Toll-Free: 800-742-7691
Phone: 402-471-2045

Nevada

Nevada State Library and Archives
Regional Library for the Blind
Talking Book Program
100 North Stewart Street
Carson City, NV 89701
Toll-Free: 800-922-9334

New Hampshire

New Hampshire State Library
Library Services to the
Handicapped Division
117 Pleasant Street
Concord, NH 03301
Toll-Free: 800-491-4200
Phone: 603-271-3429

New Jersey

New Jersey Library for the Blind and Handicapped
2300 Stuyvesant Avenue
Trenton, NJ 08618
Toll-Free: 800-792-8322

New Mexico

New Mexico State Library for the Blind and Physically Handicapped
325 Don Gaspar Street
Santa Fe, NM 87501
Toll-Free: 800-456-5515
Phone: 505-827-3830

New York (except New York City and Long Island)

New York State Talking Book and Braille Library
Cultural Education Center
Empire State Plaza
Albany, NY 12230
Toll-Free: 800-342-3688
Phone: 518-474-5935

New York (New York City and Long Island only)

Andrew Heiskell Library for the Blind and Physically Handicapped
New York Public Library
40 West 20th Street
New York, NY 10011
Phone: 212-206-5400

North Carolina

North Carolina Library for the Blind and Physically Handicapped
North Carolina State Library
1811 Capital Boulevard
Raleigh, NC 27635
Toll-Free: 888-388-2460
Phone: 919-733-4376

North Dakota

North Dakota State Library Services for the Disabled
604 East Boulevard
Bismarck, ND 58505-0800
Phone: 701-328-1477

Ohio (Northern)

Cleveland Public Library
Library for the Blind and Physically Handicapped
17121 Lake Shore Boulevard
Cleveland, OH 44110-4006
Toll-Free: 800-362-1262
Phone: 216-623-2911

Ohio (Southern)

Public Library of Cincinnati and Hamilton County
Library for the Blind and Physically Handicapped
800 Vine Street
Cincinnati, OH 45202-2002
Toll-Free: 800-582-0335
Phone: 513-369-6999

Oklahoma

Oklahoma Library for the Blind and Physically Handicapped
300 Northeast 18th Street
Oklahoma City, OK 73105
Toll-Free: 800-523-0288
Phone: 405-521-3514

Oregon

Oregon State Library
Talking Book and Braille Services
250 Winter Street Northeast
Salem, OR 97310
Phone: 503-378-3849

Pennsylvania (Eastern)

Free Library of Philadelphia
Library for the Blind and Physically Handicapped
919 Walnut Street
Philadelphia, PA 19107
Toll-Free: 800-222-1754
Phone: 215-683-3213

Pennsylvania (Western)

Carnegie Library of Pittsburgh
Library for the Blind and
Physically Handicapped
The Leonard C. Staisey Building
4724 Baum Boulevard
Pittsburgh, PA 15213
Toll-Free: 800-242-0586
Phone: 412-687-2440

Puerto Rico

Puerto Rico Regional Library for the Blind and Physically Handicapped
520 Ponce de Leon Avenue,
Suite 2
San Juan, PR 00901
Toll-Free: 800-981-8008
Phone: 787-723-2519

Rhode Island

Rhode Island Regional Library for the Blind and Physically Handicapped
300 Richmond Street
Providence, RI 02903
Phone: 401-277-2726

South Carolina

South Carolina State Library
Department for the Blind and
Physically Handicapped
1430 Senate Street
P.O. Box 821
Columbia, SC 29201
Toll-Free: 800-922-7818

South Dakota

South Dakota Library for the Handicapped
800 Governors Drive
Pierre, SD 57501-2294
Toll-Free: 800-423-6665
Phone: 605-773-3131

Tennessee

Tennessee Library for the Blind and Physically Handicapped
403 7th Avenue North
Nashville, TN 37243-0313
Toll-Free: 800-342-3308
Phone: 615-741-3915

Texas

Texas State Library
Talking Book Program
Capitol Station
P.O. Box 12927
Austin, TX 78711
Toll-Free: 800-252-9605
Phone: 512-463-5458

Utah

Utah State Library
Division for the Blind and
Physically Handicapped
2500 North 1950 West
Suite A
Salt Lake City, UT 84116
Toll-Free: 800-662-5540
Toll-Free: 800-453-4293
(outside Utah)
Phone: 801-715-6789

Vermont

Vermont Department of Libraries
Special Services Unit
578 Paine Turnpike North
Berlin, VT 05602
Toll-Free: 800-479-1711
Phone: 802-828-3273

Virginia

Library and Resource Center
Virginia Department for the
Visually Handicapped
395 Azalea Avenue
Richmond, VA 23227
Toll-Free: 800-552-7015
Phone: 804-371-3661

Virgin Islands

Virgin Islands Regional Library for the Visually and Physically Handicapped
3012 Golden Rock
Christiansted
St. Croix, Virgin Islands 00820
Phone: 340-772-2250

Washington

Washington Library for the Blind and Physically Handicapped
821 Lenora Street
Seattle, WA 98129
Toll-Free: 800-542-0866

West Virginia

West Virginia Library
Commission of Services for
the Blind and Physically
Handicapped
Science and Culture Center
1900 Kanawha Boulevard East
Charleston, WV 25305
Toll-Free: 800-642-8674
Phone: 304-558-4061

Wisconsin

Wisconsin Regional Library for the Blind and Physically Handicapped
813 West Wells Street
Milwaukee, WI 53233
Toll-Free: 800-242-8822
Phone: 414-286-3045

Wyoming

Book Lending: Utah State Library
Division for the Blind and
Physically Handicapped
2500 North 1950 West, Suite A
Salt Lake City, UT 84116
Toll-Free: 800-662-5540
Toll-Free: 800-453-4293
(outside Utah)
Phone: 801-715-6789

Machine Lending: Services for the Visually Impaired
Wyoming Dept. of Education
2300 Capitol Avenue
Hathaway Building, Room 144
Cheyenne, WY 82002-0050
Phone: 307-777-7256

Chapter 72

Directory of Government and Private Organizations That Provide Information about Eye Care or Vision Disorders

Government Agencies That Provide Information about Eye Care or Vision Disorders

Centers for Disease Control and Prevention
1600 Clifton Road
Atlanta, GA 30333
Toll-Free: 800-311-3435
Phone: 404-639-3311
Website: www.cdc.gov
E-mail: cdcinfo@cdc.gov

Healthfinder®
National Health Information Center
P.O. Box 1133
Washington, DC 20013-1133
Toll-Free: 800-336-4797
Phone: 301-565-4167
Fax: 301-984-4256
Website: www.healthfinder.gov
E-mail: healthfinder@nhic.org

National Cancer Institute
Cancer Information Service
6116 Executive Boulevard
Room 3036A
Bethesda, MD 20892-8322
Toll-Free: 800-4-CANCER
(422-6237)
TTY Toll-Free: 800-332-8615
Website: www.cancer.gov
E-mail: cancergovstaff@mail.nih
.gov

Resources in this chapter were compiled from several sources deemed reliable; all contact information was verified and updated in July 2007.

National Center for Complementary and Alternative Medicine
NCCAM Clearinghouse
P.O. Box 7923
Gaithersburg, MD 20898-7923
Toll-Free: 888-644-6226
Phone: 301-519-3153
TTY: 866-464-3615
Fax: 866-464-3616
Website: nccam.nih.gov
E-mail: info@nccam.nih.gov

National Center for Health Statistics
3311 Toledo Road
Hyattsville, MD 20782
Toll-Free: 866-441-NCHS
(441-6247)
Phone: 301-458-4000
Phone: 301-458-4636
Website: www.cdc.gov/nchs
E-mail: nchsquery@cdc.gov

National Digestive Diseases Information Clearinghouse
2 Information Way
Bethesda, MD 20892-3570
Toll-Free: 800-891-5389
Fax: 703-738-4929
Website: digestive.niddk.nih.gov
E-mail: nddic@info.niddk.nih.gov

National Eye Institute
31 Center Drive MSC 2510
Bethesda, MD 20892-2510
Phone: 301-496-5248
Website: www.nei.nih.gov
E-mail: 2020@nei.nih.gov

National Human Genome Research Institute
National Institutes of Health
31 Center Drive
Bethesda, MD 20892-2152
Phone: 301-402-0911
Fax: 301-402-4831
Website: www.genome.gov

National Institute of Allergy and Infectious Diseases (NIAID)
6610 Rockledge Drive, MSC 6612
Bethesda, MD 20892-6612
Phone: 301-496-5717
TDD: 800-877-8339
Fax: 301-402-3573
Website: www.niaid.nih.gov

National Institute of Arthritis and Musculoskeletal and Skin Diseases
1 AMS Circle
Bethesda, MD 20892-3675
Phone: 301-495-4484
Toll-Free: 877-22-NIAMS
(226-4267)
TTY: 301-565-2966
Fax: 301-718-6366
Website: www.niams.nih.gov
E-mail: niamsinfo@mail.nih.gov

National Institute of Neurological Disorders and Stroke
NIH Neurological Institute
P.O. Box 5801
Bethesda, MD 20824
Toll-Free: 800-352-9424
Phone: 301-496-5751
TTY: 301-468-5981
Website: www.ninds.nih.gov
E-mail: braininfo@ninds.nih.gov

National Institute on Aging
P.O. Box 5801
Bethesda, MD 20824
Publications
Toll-Free: 800-222-2225
Phone: 301-496-1752
TTY: 800-222-4225
Fax: 301-496-1072
Websites: www.nia.nih.gov
Publications Website:
www.niapublications.org
E-mail: niainfo@nia.nih.gov

National Institutes of Health
9000 Rockville Pike
Bethesda, MD 20892
Phone: 301-496-4000
TTY: 301-402-9612
Website: www.nih.gov
E-mail: NIHinfo@od.nih.gov

U.S. Department of Health and Human Services
5600 Fisher Lane
Rockville MD 20857
Toll-Free: 877-696-6775
Phone: 202-619-0257
Website: www.hhs.gov

U.S. Food and Drug Administration
5600 Fishers Lane, HFE-50
Rockville, MD 20857-0001
Toll-Free: 888-463-6332
Phone: 301-827-4420
Fax: 301-443-9767
Website: www.fda.gov

U.S. National Library of Medicine
8600 Rockville Pike
Bethesda, MD 20894
Toll-Free: 888-346-3656
Phone: 301-594-5983
Fax: 301-402-1384
TDD: 800-735-2258
Website: www.nlm.nih.gov
E-mail: custserv@nlm.nih.gov

Private Agencies That Provide Information about Eye Care or Vision Disorders

AllAboutVision.com
Access Media Group, LLC
7590 Fay Avenue, Suite 302
La Jolla, CA 92037
Website: www.allaboutvision.com

AMD Alliance International
1929 Bayview Avenue
Toronto, Ontario M4G 3E8
CANADA
Toll-Free: 877-263-7171
Phone: 416-486-2500 ext. 7505
Fax: 416-486-8574
Website: www.amdalliance.org
E-mail: info@amdalliance.org

American Academy of Allergy, Asthma, and Immunology
555 East Wells Street
Suite 1100
Milwaukee, WI 53202-3823
Patient Information and Physician Referral: 800-822-2762
Phone: 414-272-6071
Fax: 414-272-6070
Website: www.aaaai.org
E-mail: info@aaaai.org

American Academy of Family Physicians
P.O. Box 11210
Shawnee Mission, KS 66207-1210
Toll-Free: 800-274-2237
Phone: 913-906-6000
Website: www.aafp.org
E-mail: fp@aafp.org

American Academy of Ophthalmology
P.O. Box 7424
San Francisco, CA 94120-7424
Phone: 415-561-8500
Fax: 415-561-8533
Website: www.aao.org
EyeCare America:
www.eyecareamerica.org

American Academy of Pediatrics
141 Northwest Point Boulevard
Elk Grove Village, IL, 60007
Phone: 847-434-4000
Fax: 847-434-8000
Website: www.aap.org
E-mail: kidsdocs@aap.org

American Association for Pediatric Ophthalmology and Strabismus
P.O. Box 193832
San Francisco, CA 94119-3832
Phone: 415-561-8505
Fax: 415-561-8531
Website: www.aapos.org
E-mail: aapos@aao.org

American Board of Ophthalmology
111 Presidential Boulevard,
Suite 241
Bala Cynwyd, PA 19004-1075
Phone: 610-664-1175
Fax: 610-664-6503
Website: www.abop.org
E-mail: info@abop.org

American College of Eye Surgeons
334 East Lake Road, #135
Palm Harbor, FL 34685-2427
Phone: 727-366-1487
Fax: 727-836-9783
Website: www.aces-abes.org
E-mail: quality@aces-abes.org

American Council of the Blind
1155 15th Street NW
Suite 1004
Washington, DC 20005
Toll-Free: 800-424-8666
Phone: 202-467-5081
Fax: 202-467-5085
Website: www.acb.org

American Foundation for the Blind
11 Penn Plaza, Suite 300
New York, NY 10001
Toll-Free: 800-232-5463
Website: www.afb.org
E-mail: afbinfo@afb.net

American Glaucoma Society
P.O. Box 193940
San Francisco, CA 94119
Phone: 415-561-8587
Fax: 415-561-8531
Website: www.glaucomaweb.org
E-mail: ags@aao.org

American Medical Association/Medem
100 Pine Street, 3rd Floor
San Francisco, CA 94111
Toll-Free: 877-926-3336
Phone: 415-644-3800
Fax: 415-644-3950
Website: www.medem.com
E-mail: info@medem.com

American Optometric Association
243 N. Lindbergh Boulevard
St. Louis, MO 63141
Toll-Free: 800-365-2219
Phone: 314-991-4100
Website: www.aoa.org

American Osteopathic Association
142 East Ontario Street
Chicago, IL 60611
Toll-Free: 800-621-1773
Phone: 312-202-8000
Fax: 312-202-8200
Website: www.osteopathic.org

American Society of Ophthalmic Plastic and Reconstructive Surgery
5841 Cedar Lake Road
Suite 204
Minneapolis, MN 55416
Phone: 952-646-2038
Fax: 952-545-6073
Website: www.asoprs.org

Association for Retinopathy of Prematurity and Related Diseases
P.O. Box 250425
Franklin, MI 48025
Toll-Free: 800-788-2020
Website: ropard.org
E-mail: ropard@yahoo.com

Cleveland Clinic
9500 Euclid Avenue
Cleveland, OH 44195
Toll-Free: 800-223-2273
Phone: 216-444-2200
TTY: 216-444-0261
Website:
www.clevelandclinic.org

Contact Lens Association of America
2025 Woodlane Drive
St. Paul, MN 55125
Phone: 877-501-3937
Fax: 651-731-0410
Website: www.clao.org
E-mail: eyes@clao.org

Eye Bank Association of America
1015 Eighteenth Street NW, Suite 1010
Washington, DC 20036
Phone: 202-775-4999
Fax: 202-429-6036
Website: www.restoresight.org
E-mail: info@restoresight.org

Eye-Bank for Sight Restoration
120 Wall Street, 3rd Floor
New York, NY 10005-3902
Phone: 212-742-9000
Fax: 212-269-3139
Website: www.eyedonation.org
E-mail: info@ebsr.org

Eye Surgery Education Council
4000 Legato Road, Suite 700
Fairfax, VA 22033
Phone: 703-591-2220
Website:
www.eyesurgeryeducation.com

Foundation Fighting Blindness
11435 Cronhill Drive
Owings Mills, MD 21117-2220
Toll-Free: 800-683-5555
Phone: 410-568-0150
TDD: 800-683-5551
Website: www.blindness.org
E-mail: info@FightBlindness.org

Glaucoma Foundation
80 Maiden Lane, Suite 1206
New York, NY 10038
Phone: 212-285-0080
Website:
www.glaucomafoundation.org
E-mail:
info@glaucomafoundation.org

Glaucoma Research Foundation
251 Post Street, Suite 600
San Francisco, CA 94108
Toll-Free: 800-826-6693
Phone: 415-986-3162
Website: www.glaucoma.org

Helen Keller International
352 Park Avenue South
12th Floor
New York, NY 10010
Toll-Free: 877-535-5374
Phone: 212-532-0544
Fax: 212-532-6014
Website: www.hki.org
E-mail: info@hki.org

International Society of Refractive Surgery
655 Beach Street
P.O. Box 7424
San Francisco, CA 94109-7424
Website: www.aao.org/isrs

Knights Templar Eye Foundation, Inc.
1000 East State Parkway
Suite I
Schaumburg, IL 60173-4592
Phone: 847-490-3838
Fax: 847-490-3777
Website:
www.knightstemplar.org/ktef
E-mail: ktefofc@ix.netcom.com

Lighthouse International
The Sol and Lillian Goldman Building
111 East 59th Street
New York, NY 10022-1202
Toll-Free: 800-829-0500
Phone: 212-821-9200
TTY: 212-821-9713
Fax: 212-821-9707
Website: www.lighthouse.org
E-mail: info@lighthouse.org

Low Vision Centers of Indiana
Phone: 765-348-2020
Website: www.eyeassociates.com
E-mail:
drlaura@eyeassociates.com

Macular Degeneration Partnership
8733 Beverly Boulevard
Rm. # 201
Los Angeles, CA 90048
Toll-Free: 888-430-9898
Fax: 310-623-1837
Website: www.amd.org

Mayo Foundation for Medical Education and Research
200 First Street SW
Rochester, MN 55905
Website: www.mayoclinic.com
E-mail:
comments@mayoclinic.com

National Association for Visually Handicapped
22 West 21st Street
6th Floor
New York, NY 10010
Phone: 212-889-3141
Fax: 212-727-2931
Website: www.navh.org
E-mail: navh@navh.org

National Federation of the Blind
1800 Johnson Street
Baltimore, MD 21230
Phone: 410-659-9314
Fax: 410-685-5653
Website: www.nfb.org
E-mail: pmaurer@nfb.org

National Keratoconus Foundation

8733 Beverly Boulevard
Suite 201
Los Angeles, CA 90048
Toll-Free: 800-521-2524
Website: www.nkcf.org
E-mail: info@nkcf.org

Nemours Foundation Center for Children's Health Media

1600 Rockland Road
Wilmington, DE 19803
Phone: 302-651-4000
Fax: 302-651-4055
Website: www.kidshealth.org
E-mail: info@kidshealth.org

Prevent Blindness America

211 West Wacker Drive
Suite 1700
Chicago, IL 60606
Toll-Free: 800-331-2020
Website:
www.preventblindness.org
E-mail:
info@preventblindness.org

Research to Prevent Blindness

645 Madison Avenue, Floor 21
New York, NY 10022-1010
Toll-Free: 800-621-0026
Phone: 212-752-4333
Website: www.rpbusa.org

Retina Society

P.O. Box 8429
Boston, MA 02114
Phone: 617-227-8767
Fax: 617-367-4908
Website: www.retinasociety.org
E-mail: info@retinasociety.org

Social Security Administration

Office of Public Inquiries
Windsor Park Building
6401 Security Boulevard
Baltimore, MD 21235
Toll-Free: 800-772-1213
Website: www.ssa.gov

Sjögren's Syndrome Foundation

6707 Democracy Boulevard,
Suite 325
Bethesda, MD 20817
Toll-Free: 800-475-6473
Fax: 301-530-4415
Website: www.sjogrens.org

University of Illinois Eye and Ear Infirmary

Department of Ophthalmology
and Visual Sciences
1855 West Taylor Street
Room 3.138
Chicago, IL 60612
Phone: 312-996-6590
Fax: 312-996-7770
Website: www.uic.edu/com/eye
E-mail: eyeweb@uic.edu

Index

Index

623

Health Reference Series
COMPLETE CATALOG
List price $87 per volume. **School and library price $78 per volume.**

Adolescent Health Sourcebook, 2nd Edition

Basic Consumer Health Information about the Physical, Mental, and Emotional Growth and Development of Adolescents, Including Medical Care, Nutritional and Physical Activity Requirements, Puberty, Sexual Activity, Acne, Tanning, Body Piercing, Common Physical Illnesses and Disorders, Eating Disorders, Attention Deficit Hyperactivity Disorder, Depression, Bullying, Hazing, and Adolescent Injuries Related to Sports, Driving, and Work

Along with Substance Abuse Information about Nicotine, Alcohol, and Drug Use, a Glossary, and Directory of Additional Resources

Edited by Joyce Brennfleck Shannon. 683 pages. 2006. 978-0-7808-0943-7.

"It is written in clear, nontechnical language aimed at general readers. . . . Recommended for public libraries, community colleges, and other agencies serving health care consumers."
— *American Reference Books Annual, 2003*

"Recommended for school and public libraries. Parents and professionals dealing with teens will appreciate the easy-to-follow format and the clearly written text. This could become a 'must have' for every high school teacher." — *E-Streams, Jan '03*

"A good starting point for information related to common medical, mental, and emotional concerns of adolescents." — *School Library Journal, Nov '02*

"This book provides accurate information in an easy to access format. It addresses topics that parents and caregivers might not be aware of and provides practical, useable information."
— *Doody's Health Sciences Book Review Journal, Sep-Oct '02*

"Recommended reference source."
— *Booklist, American Library Association, Sep '02*

AIDS Sourcebook, 3rd Edition

Basic Consumer Health Information about Acquired Immune Deficiency Syndrome (AIDS) and Human Immunodeficiency Virus (HIV) Infection, Including Facts about Transmission, Prevention, Diagnosis, Treatment, Opportunistic Infections, and Other Complications, with a Section for Women and Children, Including Details about Associated Gynecological Concerns, Pregnancy, and Pediatric Care

Along with Updated Statistical Information, Reports on Current Research Initiatives, a Glossary, and Directories of Internet, Hotline, and Other Resources

Edited by Dawn D. Matthews. 664 pages. 2003. 978-0-7808-0631-3.

"The 3rd edition of the *AIDS Sourcebook*, part of Omnigraphics' *Health Reference Series,* is a welcome update. . . . This resource is highly recommended for academic and public libraries."
— *American Reference Books Annual, 2004*

"Excellent sourcebook. This continues to be a highly recommended book. There is no other book that provides as much information as this book provides."
— *AIDS Book Review Journal, Dec-Jan '00*

"Recommended reference source."
— *Booklist, American Library Association, Dec '99*

Alcoholism Sourcebook, 2nd Edition

Basic Consumer Health Information about Alcohol Use, Abuse, and Dependence, Featuring Facts about the Physical, Mental, and Social Health Effects of Alcohol Addiction, Including Alcoholic Liver Disease, Pancreatic Disease, Cardiovascular Disease, Neurological Disorders, and the Effects of Drinking during Pregnancy

Along with Information about Alcohol Treatment, Medications, and Recovery Programs, in Addition to Tips for Reducing the Prevalence of Underage Drinking, Statistics about Alcohol Use, a Glossary of Related Terms, and Directories of Resources for More Help and Information

Edited by Amy L. Sutton. 653 pages. 2006. 978-0-7808-0942-0.

"This title is one of the few reference works on alcoholism for general readers. For some readers this will be a welcome complement to the many self-help books on the market. Recommended for collections serving general readers and consumer health collections."
— *E-Streams, Mar '01*

"This book is an excellent choice for public and academic libraries."
— *American Reference Books Annual, 2001*

"Recommended reference source."
— *Booklist, American Library Association, Dec '00*

"Presents a wealth of information on alcohol use and abuse and its effects on the body and mind, treatment, and prevention." — *SciTech Book News, Dec '00*

"Important new health guide which packs in the latest consumer information about the problems of alcoholism." — *Reviewer's Bookwatch, Nov '00*

SEE ALSO Drug Abuse Sourcebook

Allergies Sourcebook, 3rd Edition

Basic Consumer Health Information about Allergic Disorders, Such as Anaphylaxis, Hives, Eczema, Rhinitis, Sinusitis, and Conjunctivitis, and Their Triggers, Including Pollen, Mold, Dust Mites, Animal Dander, Insects, Chemicals, Food, Food Additives, and Medications;

Along with Advice about the Diagnosis and Treatment of Allergy Symptoms, a Glossary of Related Terms, a Directory of Resources for Help and Information, and Suggestions for Additional Reading

Edited by Amy L. Sutton. 598 pages. 2007. 978-0-7808-0950-5.

"This book brings a great deal of useful material together. . . . This is an excellent addition to public and consumer health library collections."
— *American Reference Books Annual, 2003*

"This second edition would be useful to laypersons with little or advanced knowledge of the subject matter. This book would also serve as a resource for nursing and other health care professions students. It would be useful in public, academic, and hospital libraries with consumer health collections." — *E-Streams, Jul '02*

■

Alternative Medicine Sourcebook

SEE Complementary & Alternative Medicine Sourcebook

■

Alzheimer's Disease Sourcebook, 3rd Edition

Basic Consumer Health Information about Alzheimer's Disease, Other Dementias, and Related Disorders, Including Multi-Infarct Dementia, AIDS Dementia Complex, Dementia with Lewy Bodies, Huntington's Disease, Wernicke-Korsakoff Syndrome (Alcohol-Related Dementia), Delirium, and Confusional States

Along with Information for People Newly Diagnosed with Alzheimer's Disease and Caregivers, Reports Detailing Current Research Efforts in Prevention, Diagnosis, and Treatment, Facts about Long-Term Care Issues, and Listings of Sources for Additional Information

Edited by Karen Bellenir. 645 pages. 2003. 978-0-7808-0666-5.

"This very informative and valuable tool will be a great addition to any library serving consumers, students and health care workers."
— *American Reference Books Annual, 2004*

"This is a valuable resource for people affected by dementias such as Alzheimer's. It is easy to navigate and includes important information and resources."
— *Doody's Review Service, Feb '04*

"Recommended reference source."
— *Booklist, American Library Association, Oct '99*

SEE ALSO *Brain Disorders Sourcebook*

Arthritis Sourcebook, 2nd Edition

Basic Consumer Health Information about Osteoarthritis, Rheumatoid Arthritis, Other Rheumatic Disorders, Infectious Forms of Arthritis, and Diseases with Symptoms Linked to Arthritis, Featuring Facts about Diagnosis, Pain Management, and Surgical Therapies

Along with Coping Strategies, Research Updates, a Glossary, and Resources for Additional Help and Information

Edited by Amy L. Sutton. 593 pages. 2004. 978-0-7808-0667-2.

"This easy-to-read volume is recommended for consumer health collections within public or academic libraries." — *E-Streams, May '05*

"As expected, this updated edition continues the excellent reputation of this series in providing sound, usable health information. . . . Highly recommended."
— *American Reference Books Annual, 2005*

"Excellent reference." — *The Bookwatch, Jan '05*

■

Asthma Sourcebook, 2nd Edition

Basic Consumer Health Information about the Causes, Symptoms, Diagnosis, and Treatment of Asthma in Infants, Children, Teenagers, and Adults, Including Facts about Different Types of Asthma, Common Co-Occurring Conditions, Asthma Management Plans, Triggers, Medications, and Medication Delivery Devices

Along with Asthma Statistics, Research Updates, a Glossary, a Directory of Asthma-Related Resources, and More

Edited by Karen Bellenir. 609 pages. 2006. 978-0-7808-0866-9.

"A worthwhile reference acquisition for public libraries and academic medical libraries whose readers desire a quick introduction to the wide range of asthma information." — *Choice, Association of College & Research Libraries, Jun '01*

"Recommended reference source."
— *Booklist, American Library Association, Feb '01*

"Highly recommended." — *The Bookwatch, Jan '01*

"There is much good information for patients and their families who deal with asthma daily."
— *American Medical Writers Association Journal, Winter '01*

"This informative text is recommended for consumer health collections in public, secondary school, and community college libraries and the libraries of universities with a large undergraduate population."
— *American Reference Books Annual, 2001*

■

Attention Deficit Disorder Sourcebook

Basic Consumer Health Information about Attention Deficit/Hyperactivity Disorder in Children and Adults,

Including Facts about Causes, Symptoms, Diagnostic Criteria, and Treatment Options Such as Medications, Behavior Therapy, Coaching, and Homeopathy

Along with Reports on Current Research Initiatives, Legal Issues, and Government Regulations, and Featuring a Glossary of Related Terms, Internet Resources, and a List of Additional Reading Material

Edited by Dawn D. Matthews. 470 pages. 2002. 978-0-7808-0624-5.

"Recommended reference source."
— Booklist, American Library Association, Jan '03

"This book is recommended for all school libraries and the reference or consumer health sections of public libraries." — American Reference Books Annual, 2003

■

Back & Neck Sourcebook, 2nd Edition

Basic Consumer Health Information about Spinal Pain, Spinal Cord Injuries, and Related Disorders, Such as Degenerative Disk Disease, Osteoarthritis, Scoliosis, Sciatica, Spina Bifida, and Spinal Stenosis, and Featuring Facts about Maintaining Spinal Health, Self-Care, Pain Management, Rehabilitative Care, Chiropractic Care, Spinal Surgeries, and Complementary Therapies

Along with Suggestions for Preventing Back and Neck Pain, a Glossary of Related Terms, and a Directory of Resources

Edited by Amy L. Sutton. 633 pages. 2004. 978-0-7808-0738-9.

"Recommended . . . an easy to use, comprehensive medical reference book." — E-Streams, Sep '05

"The strength of this work is its basic, easy-to-read format. Recommended." — Reference and User Services Quarterly, American Library Association, Winter '97

■

Blood & Circulatory Disorders Sourcebook, 2nd Edition

Basic Consumer Health Information about the Blood and Circulatory System and Related Disorders, Such as Anemia and Other Hemoglobin Diseases, Cancer of the Blood and Associated Bone Marrow Disorders, Clotting and Bleeding Problems, and Conditions That Affect the Veins, Blood Vessels, and Arteries, Including Facts about the Donation and Transplantation of Bone Marrow, Stem Cells, and Blood and Tips for Keeping the Blood and Circulatory System Healthy

Along with a Glossary of Related Terms and Resources for Additional Help and Information

Edited by Amy L. Sutton. 659 pages. 2005. 978-0-7808-0746-4.

"Highly recommended pick for basic consumer health reference holdings at all levels."
— The Bookwatch, Aug '05

"Recommended reference source."
— Booklist, American Library Association, Feb '99

"An important reference sourcebook written in simple language for everyday, non-technical users."
— Reviewer's Bookwatch, Jan '99

Brain Disorders Sourcebook, 2nd Edition

Basic Consumer Health Information about Acquired and Traumatic Brain Injuries, Infections of the Brain, Epilepsy and Seizure Disorders, Cerebral Palsy, and Degenerative Neurological Disorders, Including Amyotrophic Lateral Sclerosis (ALS), Dementias, Multiple Sclerosis, and More

Along with Information on the Brain's Structure and Function, Treatment and Rehabilitation Options, Reports on Current Research Initiatives, a Glossary of Terms Related to Brain Disorders and Injuries, and a Directory of Sources for Further Help and Information

Edited by Sandra J. Judd. 625 pages. 2005. 978-0-7808-0744-0.

"Highly recommended pick for basic consumer health reference holdings at all levels."
— The Bookwatch, Aug '05

"Belongs on the shelves of any library with a consumer health collection." — E-Streams, Mar '00

"Recommended reference source."
— Booklist, American Library Association, Oct '99

SEE ALSO Alzheimer's Disease Sourcebook

■

Breast Cancer Sourcebook, 2nd Edition

Basic Consumer Health Information about Breast Cancer, Including Facts about Risk Factors, Prevention, Screening and Diagnostic Methods, Treatment Options, Complementary and Alternative Therapies, Post-Treatment Concerns, Clinical Trials, Special Risk Populations, and New Developments in Breast Cancer Research

Along with Breast Cancer Statistics, a Glossary of Related Terms, and a Directory of Resources for Additional Help and Information

Edited by Sandra J. Judd. 595 pages. 2004. 978-0-7808-0668-9.

"This book will be an excellent addition to public, community college, medical, and academic libraries."
— American Reference Books Annual, 2006

"It would be a useful reference book in a library or on loan to women in a support group."
— Cancer Forum, Mar '03

"Recommended reference source."
— Booklist, American Library Association, Jan '02

"This reference source is highly recommended. It is quite informative, comprehensive and detailed in nature, and yet it offers practical advice in easy-to-read language. It could be thought of as the 'bible' of breast cancer for the consumer." *— E-Streams, Jan '02*

"From the pros and cons of different screening methods and results to treatment options, **Breast Cancer Sourcebook** provides the latest information on the subject."
— Library Bookwatch, Dec '01

"This thoroughgoing, very readable reference covers all aspects of breast health and cancer. . . . Readers will find much to consider here. Recommended for all public and patient health collections."
— Library Journal, Sep '01

SEE ALSO *Cancer Sourcebook for Women, Women's Health Concerns Sourcebook*

■

Breastfeeding Sourcebook

Basic Consumer Health Information about the Benefits of Breastmilk, Preparing to Breastfeed, Breastfeeding as a Baby Grows, Nutrition, and More, Including Information on Special Situations and Concerns Such as Mastitis, Illness, Medications, Allergies, Multiple Births, Prematurity, Special Needs, and Adoption

Along with a Glossary and Resources for Additional Help and Information

Edited by Jenni Lynn Colson. 388 pages. 2002. 978-0-7808-0332-9.

"Particularly useful is the information about professional lactation services and chapters on breastfeeding when returning to work. . . . **Breastfeeding Sourcebook** will be useful for public libraries, consumer health libraries, and technical schools offering nurse assistant training, especially in areas where Internet access is problematic."
— American Reference Books Annual, 2003

SEE ALSO *Pregnancy & Birth Sourcebook*

■

Burns Sourcebook

Basic Consumer Health Information about Various Types of Burns and Scalds, Including Flame, Heat, Cold, Electrical, Chemical, and Sun Burns

Along with Information on Short-Term and Long-Term Treatments, Tissue Reconstruction, Plastic Surgery, Prevention Suggestions, and First Aid

Edited by Allan R. Cook. 604 pages. 1999. 978-0-7808-0204-9.

"This is an exceptional addition to the series and is highly recommended for all consumer health collections, hospital libraries, and academic medical centers."
— E-Streams, Mar '00

"This key reference guide is an invaluable addition to all health care and public libraries in confronting this ongoing health issue."
— American Reference Books Annual, 2000

"Recommended reference source."
— Booklist, American Library Association, Dec '99

SEE ALSO *Dermatological Disorders Sourcebook*

Cancer Sourcebook, 5th Edition

Basic Consumer Health Information about Major Forms and Stages of Cancer, Featuring Facts about Head and Neck Cancers, Lung Cancers, Gastrointestinal Cancers, Genitourinary Cancers, Lymphomas, Blood Cell Cancers, Endocrine Cancers, Skin Cancers, Bone Cancers, Metastatic Cancers, and More

Along with Facts about Cancer Treatments, Cancer Risks and Prevention, a Glossary of Related Terms, Statistical Data, and a Directory of Resources for Additional Information

Edited by Karen Bellenir. 1,133 pages. 2007. 978-0-7808-0947-5.

"With cancer being the second leading cause of death for Americans, a prodigious work such as this one, which locates centrally so much cancer-related information, is clearly an asset to this nation's citizens and others."
— Journal of the National Medical Association, 2004

"This title is recommended for health sciences and public libraries with consumer health collections."
— E-Streams, Feb '01

". . . can be effectively used by cancer patients and their families who are looking for answers in a language they can understand. Public and hospital libraries should have it on their shelves."
— American Reference Books Annual, 2001

"Recommended reference source."
— Booklist, American Library Association, Dec '00

SEE ALSO *Breast Cancer Sourcebook, Cancer Sourcebook for Women, Pediatric Cancer Sourcebook, Prostate Cancer Sourcebook*

■

Cancer Sourcebook for Women, 3rd Edition

Basic Consumer Health Information about Leading Causes of Cancer in Women, Featuring Facts about Gynecologic Cancers and Related Concerns, Such as Breast Cancer, Cervical Cancer, Endometrial Cancer, Uterine Sarcoma, Vaginal Cancer, Vulvar Cancer, and Common Non-Cancerous Gynecologic Conditions, in Addition to Facts about Lung Cancer, Colorectal Cancer, and Thyroid Cancer in Women

Along with Information about Cancer Risk Factors, Screening and Prevention, Treatment Options, and Tips on Coping with Life after Cancer Treatment, a Glossary of Cancer Terms, and a Directory of Resources for Additional Help and Information

Edited by Amy L. Sutton. 715 pages. 2006. 978-0-7808-0867-6.

"An excellent addition to collections in public, consumer health, and women's health libraries."
— American Reference Books Annual, 2003

"Overall, the information is excellent, and complex topics are clearly explained. As a reference book for the consumer it is a valuable resource to assist them to make informed decisions about cancer and its treatments." *— Cancer Forum, Nov '02*

"Highly recommended for academic and medical reference collections." —*Library Bookwatch, Sep '02*

"This is a highly recommended book for any public or consumer library, being reader friendly and containing accurate and helpful information."
—*E-Streams, Aug '02*

"Recommended reference source."
—*Booklist, American Library Association, Jul '02*

SEE ALSO *Breast Cancer Sourcebook, Women's Health Concerns Sourcebook*

■

Cancer Survivorship Sourcebook

Basic Consumer Health Information about the Physical, Educational, Emotional, Social, and Financial Needs of Cancer Patients from Diagnosis, through Cancer Treatment, and Beyond, Including Facts about Researching Specific Types of Cancer and Learning about Clinical Trials and Treatment Options, and Featuring Tips for Coping with the Side Effects of Cancer Treatments and Adjusting to Life after Cancer Treatment Concludes

Along with Suggestions for Caregivers, Friends, and Family Members of Cancer Patients, a Glossary of Cancer Care Terms, and Directories of Related Resources

Edited by Karen Bellenir. 6561 pages. 2007. 978-0-7808-0985-7.

■

Cardiovascular Diseases & Disorders Sourcebook, 3rd Edition

Basic Consumer Health Information about Heart and Vascular Diseases and Disorders, Such as Angina, Heart Attacks, Arrhythmias, Cardiomyopathy, Valve Disease, Atherosclerosis, and Aneurysms, with Information about Managing Cardiovascular Risk Factors and Maintaining Heart Health, Medications and Procedures Used to Treat Cardiovascular Disorders, and Concerns of Special Significance to Women

Along with Reports on Current Research Initiatives, a Glossary of Related Medical Terms, and a Directory of Sources for Further Help and Information

Edited by Sandra J. Judd. 713 pages. 2005. 978-0-7808-0739-6.

"This updated sourcebook is still the best first stop for comprehensive introductory information on cardiovascular diseases."
—*American Reference Books Annual, 2006*

"Recommended for public libraries and libraries supporting health care professionals."
—*E-Streams, Sep '05*

"This should be a standard health library reference."
—*The Bookwatch, Jun '05*

"Recommended reference source."
—*Booklist, American Library Association, Dec '00*

"... comprehensive format provides an extensive overview on this subject."
—*Choice, Association of College & Research Libraries*

■

Caregiving Sourcebook

Basic Consumer Health Information for Caregivers, Including a Profile of Caregivers, Caregiving Responsibilities and Concerns, Tips for Specific Conditions, Care Environments, and the Effects of Caregiving

Along with Facts about Legal Issues, Financial Information, and Future Planning, a Glossary, and a Listing of Additional Resources

Edited by Joyce Brennfleck Shannon. 600 pages. 2001. 978-0-7808-0331-2.

"Essential for most collections."
—*Library Journal, Apr 1, 2002*

"An ideal addition to the reference collection of any public library. Health sciences information professionals may also want to acquire the *Caregiving Sourcebook* for their hospital or academic library for use as a ready reference tool by health care workers interested in aging and caregiving." —*E-Streams, Jan '02*

"Recommended reference source."
—*Booklist, American Library Association, Oct '01*

■

Child Abuse Sourcebook

Basic Consumer Health Information about the Physical, Sexual, and Emotional Abuse of Children, with Additional Facts about Neglect, Munchausen Syndrome by Proxy (MSBP), Shaken Baby Syndrome, and Controversial Issues Related to Child Abuse, Such as Withholding Medical Care, Corporal Punishment, and Child Maltreatment in Youth Sports, and Featuring Facts about Child Protective Services, Foster Care, Adoption, Parenting Challenges, and Other Abuse Prevention Efforts

Along with a Glossary of Related Terms and Resources for Additional Help and Information

Edited by Dawn D. Matthews. 620 pages. 2004. 978-0-7808-0705-1.

"A valuable and highly recommended resource for school, academic and public libraries whether used on its own or as a starting point for more in-depth research." —*E-Streams, Apr '05*

"Every week the news brings cases of child abuse or neglect, so it is useful to have a source that supplies so much helpful information. . . . Recommended. Public and academic libraries, and child welfare offices."
—*Choice, Association of College & Research Libraries, Mar '05*

"Packed with insights on all kinds of issues, from foster care and adoption to parenting and abuse prevention."
—*The Bookwatch, Nov '04*

SEE ALSO: *Domestic Violence Sourcebook*

Childhood Diseases & Disorders Sourcebook

Basic Consumer Health Information about Medical Problems Often Encountered in Pre-Adolescent Children, Including Respiratory Tract Ailments, Ear Infections, Sore Throats, Disorders of the Skin and Scalp, Digestive and Genitourinary Diseases, Infectious Diseases, Inflammatory Disorders, Chronic Physical and Developmental Disorders, Allergies, and More

Along with Information about Diagnostic Tests, Common Childhood Surgeries, and Frequently Used Medications, with a Glossary of Important Terms and Resource Directory

Edited by Chad T. Kimball. 662 pages. 2003. 978-0-7808-0458-6.

"This is an excellent book for new parents and should be included in all health care and public libraries."
—*American Reference Books Annual, 2004*

SEE ALSO: Healthy Children Sourcebook

Colds, Flu & Other Common Ailments Sourcebook

Basic Consumer Health Information about Common Ailments and Injuries, Including Colds, Coughs, the Flu, Sinus Problems, Headaches, Fever, Nausea and Vomiting, Menstrual Cramps, Diarrhea, Constipation, Hemorrhoids, Back Pain, Dandruff, Dry and Itchy Skin, Cuts, Scrapes, Sprains, Bruises, and More

Along with Information about Prevention, Self-Care, Choosing a Doctor, Over-the-Counter Medications, Folk Remedies, and Alternative Therapies, and Including a Glossary of Important Terms and a Directory of Resources for Further Help and Information

Edited by Chad T. Kimball. 638 pages. 2001. 978-0-7808-0435-7.

"A good starting point for research on common illnesses. It will be a useful addition to public and consumer health library collections."
—*American Reference Books Annual, 2002*

"Will prove valuable to any library seeking to maintain a current, comprehensive reference collection of health resources. . . . Excellent reference."
—*The Bookwatch, Aug '01*

"Recommended reference source."
—*Booklist, American Library Association, Jul '01*

Communication Disorders Sourcebook

Basic Information about Deafness and Hearing Loss, Speech and Language Disorders, Voice Disorders, Balance and Vestibular Disorders, and Disorders of Smell, Taste, and Touch

Edited by Linda M. Ross. 533 pages. 1996. 978-0-7808-0077-9.

"This is skillfully edited and is a welcome resource for the layperson. It should be found in every public and medical library."
—*Booklist Health Sciences Supplement, American Library Association, Oct '97*

Complementary & Alternative Medicine Sourcebook, 3rd Edition

Basic Consumer Health Information about Complementary and Alternative Medical Therapies, Including Acupuncture, Ayurveda, Traditional Chinese Medicine, Herbal Medicine, Homeopathy, Naturopathy, Biofeedback, Hypnotherapy, Yoga, Art Therapy, Aromatherapy, Clinical Nutrition, Vitamin and Mineral Supplements, Chiropractic, Massage, Reflexology, Crystal Therapy, Therapeutic Touch, and More

Along with Facts about Alternative and Complementary Treatments for Specific Conditions Such as Cancer, Diabetes, Osteoarthritis, Chronic Pain, Menopause, Gastrointestinal Disorders, Headaches, and Mental Illness, a Glossary, and a Resource List for Additional Help and Information

Edited by Sandra J. Judd. 657 pages. 2006. 978-0-7808-0864-5.

"Recommended for public, high school, and academic libraries that have consumer health collections. Hospital libraries that also serve the public will find this to be a useful resource."
—*E-Streams, Feb '03*

"Recommended reference source."
—*Booklist, American Library Association, Jan '03*

"An important alternate health reference."
—*MBR Bookwatch, Oct '02*

"A great addition to the reference collection of every type of library."
—*American Reference Books Annual, 2000*

Congenital Disorders Sourcebook, 2nd Edition

Basic Consumer Health Information about Nonhereditary Birth Defects and Disorders Related to Prematurity, Gestational Injuries, Congenital Infections, and Birth Complications, Including Heart Defects, Hydrocephalus, Spina Bifida, Cleft Lip and Palate, Cerebral Palsy, and More

Along with Facts about the Prevention of Birth Defects, Fetal Surgery and Other Treatment Options, Research Initiatives, a Glossary of Related Terms, and Resources for Additional Information and Support

Edited by Sandra J. Judd. 647 pages. 2006. 978-0-7808-0945-1.

"Recommended reference source."
—*Booklist, American Library Association, Oct '97*

SEE ALSO Pregnancy & Birth Sourcebook

Contagious Diseases Sourcebook

Basic Consumer Health Information about Infectious Diseases Spread by Person-to-Person Contact through

Direct Touch, Airborne Transmission, Sexual Contact, or Contact with Blood or Other Body Fluids, Including Hepatitis, Herpes, Influenza, Lice, Measles, Mumps, Pinworm, Ringworm, Severe Acute Respiratory Syndrome (SARS), Streptococcal Infections, Tuberculosis, and Others

Along with Facts about Disease Transmission, Antimicrobial Resistance, and Vaccines, with a Glossary and Directories of Resources for More Information

Edited by Karen Bellenir. 643 pages. 2004. 978-0-7808-0736-5.

"This easy-to-read volume is recommended for consumer health collections within public or academic libraries." — E-Streams, May '05

"This informative book is highly recommended for public libraries, consumer health collections, and secondary schools and undergraduate libraries."
— American Reference Books Annual, 2005

"Excellent reference." — The Bookwatch, Jan '05

Death & Dying Sourcebook, 2nd Edition

Basic Consumer Health Information about End-of-Life Care and Related Perspectives and Ethical Issues, Including End-of-Life Symptoms and Treatments, Pain Management, Quality-of-Life Concerns, the Use of Life Support, Patients' Rights and Privacy Issues, Advance Directives, Physician-Assisted Suicide, Caregiving, Organ and Tissue Donation, Autopsies, Funeral Arrangements, and Grief

Along with Statistical Data, Information about the Leading Causes of Death, a Glossary, and Directories of Support Groups and Other Resources

Edited by Joyce Brennfleck Shannon. 653 pages. 2006. 978-0-7808-0871-3.

"Public libraries, medical libraries, and academic libraries will all find this sourcebook a useful addition to their collections."
— American Reference Books Annual, 2001

"An extremely useful resource for those concerned with death and dying in the United States."
— Respiratory Care, Nov '00

"Recommended reference source."
—Booklist, American Library Association, Aug '00

"This book is a definite must for all those involved in end-of-life care." — Doody's Review Service, 2000

Dental Care & Oral Health Sourcebook, 2nd Edition

Basic Consumer Health Information about Dental Care, Including Oral Hygiene, Dental Visits, Pain Management, Cavities, Crowns, Bridges, Dental Implants, and Fillings, and Other Oral Health Concerns, Such as Gum Disease, Bad Breath, Dry Mouth, Genetic and Developmental Abnormalities, Oral Cancers, Orthodontics, and Temporomandibular Disorders

Along with Updates on Current Research in Oral Health, a Glossary, a Directory of Dental and Oral Health Organizations, and Resources for People with Dental and Oral Health Disorders

Edited by Amy L. Sutton. 609 pages. 2003. 978-0-7808-0634-4.

"This book could serve as a turning point in the battle to educate consumers in issues concerning oral health."
— American Reference Books Annual, 2004

"Unique source which will fill a gap in dental sources for patients and the lay public. A valuable reference tool even in a library with thousands of books on dentistry. Comprehensive, clear, inexpensive, and easy to read and use. It fills an enormous gap in the health care literature." — Reference & User Services Quarterly, American Library Association, Summer '98

"Recommended reference source."
—Booklist, American Library Association, Dec '97

Depression Sourcebook

Basic Consumer Health Information about Unipolar Depression, Bipolar Disorder, Postpartum Depression, Seasonal Affective Disorder, and Other Types of Depression in Children, Adolescents, Women, Men, the Elderly, and Other Selected Populations

Along with Facts about Causes, Risk Factors, Diagnostic Criteria, Treatment Options, Coping Strategies, Suicide Prevention, a Glossary, and a Directory of Sources for Additional Help and Information

Edited by Karen Bellenir. 602 pages. 2002. 978-0-7808-0611-5.

"Depression Sourcebook is of a very high standard. Its purpose, which is to serve as a reference source to the lay reader, is very well served."
— Journal of the National Medical Association, 2004

"Invaluable reference for public and school library collections alike." — Library Bookwatch, Apr '03

"Recommended for purchase."
— American Reference Books Annual, 2003

Dermatological Disorders Sourcebook, 2nd Edition

Basic Consumer Health Information about Conditions and Disorders Affecting the Skin, Hair, and Nails, Such as Acne, Rosacea, Rashes, Dermatitis, Pigmentation Disorders, Birthmarks, Skin Cancer, Skin Injuries, Psoriasis, Scleroderma, and Hair Loss, Including Facts about Medications and Treatments for Dermatological Disorders and Tips for Maintaining Healthy Skin, Hair, and Nails

Along with Information about How Aging Affects the Skin, a Glossary of Related Terms, and a Directory of Resources for Additional Help and Information

Edited by Amy L. Sutton. 645 pages. 2005. 978-0-7808-0795-2.

"... comprehensive, easily read reference book."
—*Doody's Health Sciences Book Reviews*, Oct '97

SEE ALSO *Burns Sourcebook*

■

Diabetes Sourcebook, 3rd Edition

Basic Consumer Health Information about Type 1 Diabetes (Insulin-Dependent or Juvenile-Onset Diabetes), Type 2 Diabetes (Noninsulin-Dependent or Adult-Onset Diabetes), Gestational Diabetes, Impaired Glucose Tolerance (IGT), and Related Complications, Such as Amputation, Eye Disease, Gum Disease, Nerve Damage, and End-Stage Renal Disease, Including Facts about Insulin, Oral Diabetes Medications, Blood Sugar Testing, and the Role of Exercise and Nutrition in the Control of Diabetes

Along with a Glossary and Resources for Further Help and Information

Edited by Dawn D. Matthews. 622 pages. 2003. 978-0-7808-0629-0.

"This edition is even more helpful than earlier versions. . . . It is a truly valuable tool for anyone seeking readable and authoritative information on diabetes."
— *American Reference Books Annual*, 2004

"An invaluable reference." — *Library Journal*, May '00

Selected as one of the 250 "Best Health Sciences Books of 1999." — *Doody's Rating Service*, Mar-Apr '00

"Provides useful information for the general public."
— *Healthlines, University of Michigan Health Management Research Center*, Sep/Oct '99

". . . provides reliable mainstream medical information . . . belongs on the shelves of any library with a consumer health collection." — *E-Streams*, Sep '99

"Recommended reference source."
— *Booklist, American Library Association*, Feb '99

■

Diet & Nutrition Sourcebook, 3rd Edition

Basic Consumer Health Information about Dietary Guidelines and the Food Guidance System, Recommended Daily Nutrient Intakes, Serving Proportions, Weight Control, Vitamins and Supplements, Nutrition Issues for Different Life Stages and Lifestyles, and the Needs of People with Specific Medical Concerns, Including Cancer, Celiac Disease, Diabetes, Eating Disorders, Food Allergies, and Cardiovascular Disease

Along with Facts about Federal Nutrition Support Programs, a Glossary of Nutrition and Dietary Terms, and Directories of Additional Resources for More Information about Nutrition

Edited by Joyce Brennfleck Shannon. 633 pages. 2006. 978-0-7808-0800-3.

"This book is an excellent source of basic diet and nutrition information." — *Booklist Health Sciences Supplement, American Library Association*, Dec '00

"This reference document should be in any public library, but it would be a very good guide for beginning students in the health sciences. If the other books in this publisher's series are as good as this, they should all be in the health sciences collections."
— *American Reference Books Annual*, 2000

"This book is an excellent general nutrition reference for consumers who desire to take an active role in their health care for prevention. Consumers of all ages who select this book can feel confident they are receiving current and accurate information." — *Journal of Nutrition for the Elderly, Vol. 19, No. 4*, 2000

SEE ALSO *Digestive Diseases & Disorders Sourcebook, Eating Disorders Sourcebook, Gastrointestinal Diseases & Disorders Sourcebook, Vegetarian Sourcebook*

■

Digestive Diseases & Disorders Sourcebook

Basic Consumer Health Information about Diseases and Disorders that Impact the Upper and Lower Digestive System, Including Celiac Disease, Constipation, Crohn's Disease, Cyclic Vomiting Syndrome, Diarrhea, Diverticulosis and Diverticulitis, Gallstones, Heartburn, Hemorrhoids, Hernias, Indigestion (Dyspepsia), Irritable Bowel Syndrome, Lactose Intolerance, Ulcers, and More

Along with Information about Medications and Other Treatments, Tips for Maintaining a Healthy Digestive Tract, a Glossary, and Directory of Digestive Diseases Organizations

Edited by Karen Bellenir. 335 pages. 2000. 978-0-7808-0327-5.

"This title would be an excellent addition to all public or patient-research libraries."
— *American Reference Books Annual*, 2001

"This title is recommended for public, hospital, and health sciences libraries with consumer health collections." — *E-Streams*, Jul-Aug '00

"Recommended reference source."
— *Booklist, American Library Association*, May '00

SEE ALSO *Eating Disorders Sourcebook, Gastrointestinal Diseases & Disorders Sourcebook*

■

Disabilities Sourcebook

Basic Consumer Health Information about Physical and Psychiatric Disabilities, Including Descriptions of Major Causes of Disability, Assistive and Adaptive Aids, Workplace Issues, and Accessibility Concerns

Along with Information about the Americans with Disabilities Act, a Glossary, and Resources for Additional Help and Information

Edited by Dawn D. Matthews. 616 pages. 2000. 978-0-7808-0389-3.

"It is a must for libraries with a consumer health section." — *American Reference Books Annual*, 2002

"A much needed addition to the Omnigraphics *Health Reference Series*. A current reference work to provide people with disabilities, their families, caregivers or those who work with them, a broad range of information in one volume, has not been available until now. . . . It is recommended for all public and academic library reference collections." — *E-Streams, May '01*

"An excellent source book in easy-to-read format covering many current topics; highly recommended for all libraries." — *Choice, Association of College & Research Libraries, Jan '01*

"Recommended reference source."
— *Booklist, American Library Association, Jul '00*

Domestic Violence Sourcebook, 2nd Edition

Basic Consumer Health Information about the Causes and Consequences of Abusive Relationships, Including Physical Violence, Sexual Assault, Battery, Stalking, and Emotional Abuse, and Facts about the Effects of Violence on Women, Men, Young Adults, and the Elderly, with Reports about Domestic Violence in Selected Populations, and Featuring Facts about Medical Care, Victim Assistance and Protection, Prevention Strategies, Mental Health Services, and Legal Issues

Along with a Glossary of Related Terms and Resources for Additional Help and Information

Edited by Dawn D. Matthews. 628 pages. 2004. 978-0-7808-0669-6.

"Educators, clergy, medical professionals, police, and victims and their families will benefit from this realistic and easy-to-understand resource."
— *American Reference Books Annual, 2005*

"Recommended for all collections supporting consumer health information. It should also be considered for any collection needing general, readable information on domestic violence." — *E-Streams, Jan '05*

"This sourcebook complements other books in its field, providing a one-stop resource . . . Recommended."
— *Choice, Association of College & Research Libraries, Jan '05*

"Interested lay persons should find the book extremely beneficial. . . . A copy of *Domestic Violence and Child Abuse Sourcebook* should be in every public library in the United States."
— *Social Science & Medicine, No. 56, 2003*

"This is important information. The Web has many resources but this sourcebook fills an important societal need. I am not aware of any other resources of this type." — *Doody's Review Service, Sep '01*

"Recommended reference source."
— *Booklist, American Library Association, Apr '01*

"Important pick for college-level health reference libraries." — *The Bookwatch, Mar '01*

"Because this problem is so widespread and because this book includes a lot of issues within one volume, this work is recommended for all public libraries."
— *American Reference Books Annual, 2001*

SEE ALSO *Child Abuse Sourcebook*

Drug Abuse Sourcebook, 2nd Edition

Basic Consumer Health Information about Illicit Substances of Abuse and the Misuse of Prescription and Over-the-Counter Medications, Including Depressants, Hallucinogens, Inhalants, Marijuana, Stimulants, and Anabolic Steroids

Along with Facts about Related Health Risks, Treatment Programs, Prevention Programs, a Glossary of Abuse and Addiction Terms, a Glossary of Drug-Related Street Terms, and a Directory of Resources for More Information

Edited by Catherine Ginther. 607 pages. 2004. 978-0-7808-0740-2.

"Commendable for organizing useful, normally scattered government and association-produced data into a logical sequence."
— *American Reference Books Annual, 2006*

"This easy-to-read volume is recommended for consumer health collections within public or academic libraries." — *E-Streams, Sep '05*

"An excellent library reference."
— *The Bookwatch, May '05*

"Containing a wealth of information, this book will be useful to the college student just beginning to explore the topic of substance abuse. This resource belongs in libraries that serve a lower-division undergraduate or community college clientele as well as the general public." — *Choice, Association of College & Research Libraries, Jun '01*

"Recommended reference source."
— *Booklist, American Library Association, Feb '01*

SEE ALSO *Alcoholism Sourcebook*

Ear, Nose & Throat Disorders Sourcebook, 2nd Edition

Basic Consumer Health Information about Disorders of the Ears, Hearing Loss, Vestibular Disorders, Nasal and Sinus Problems, Throat and Vocal Cord Disorders, and Otolaryngologic Cancers, Including Facts about Ear Infections and Injuries, Genetic and Congenital Deafness, Sensorineural Hearing Disorders, Tinnitus, Vertigo, Ménière Disease, Rhinitis, Sinusitis, Snoring, Sore Throats, Hoarseness, and More

Along with Reports on Current Research Initiatives, a Glossary of Related Medical Terms, and a Directory of Sources for Further Help and Information

Edited by Sandra J. Judd. 659 pages. 2006. 978-0-7808-0872-0.

"Overall, this sourcebook is helpful for the consumer seeking information on ENT issues. It is recommended for public libraries."

—American Reference Books Annual, 1999

"Recommended reference source."

—Booklist, American Library Association, Dec '98

Eating Disorders Sourcebook, 2nd Edition

Basic Consumer Health Information about Anorexia Nervosa, Bulimia Nervosa, Binge Eating, Compulsive Exercise, Female Athlete Triad, and Other Eating Disorders, Including Facts about Body Image and Other Cultural and Age-Related Risk Factors, Prevention Efforts, Adverse Health Effects, Treatment Options, and the Recovery Process

Along with Guidelines for Healthy Weight Control, a Glossary, and Directories of Additional Resources

Edited by Joyce Brennfleck Shannon. 585 pages. 2007. 978-0-7808-0948-2.

"Recommended for health science libraries that are open to the public, as well as hospital libraries. This book is a good resource for the consumer who is concerned about eating disorders." *— E-Streams, Mar '02*

"This volume is another convenient collection of excerpted articles. Recommended for school and public library patrons; lower-division undergraduates; and two-year technical program students."

—Choice, Association of College & Research Libraries, Jan '02

"Recommended reference source."

— Booklist, American Library Association, Oct '01

SEE ALSO *Diet & Nutrition Sourcebook, Digestive Diseases & Disorders Sourcebook, Gastrointestinal Diseases & Disorders Sourcebook*

Emergency Medical Services Sourcebook

Basic Consumer Health Information about Preventing, Preparing for, and Managing Emergency Situations, When and Who to Call for Help, What to Expect in the Emergency Room, the Emergency Medical Team, Patient Issues, and Current Topics in Emergency Medicine

Along with Statistical Data, a Glossary, and Sources of Additional Help and Information

Edited by Jenni Lynn Colson. 494 pages. 2002. 978-0-7808-0420-3.

"Handy and convenient for home, public, school, and college libraries. Recommended."

— Choice, Association of College & Research Libraries, Apr '03

"This reference can provide the consumer with answers to most questions about emergency care in the United States, or it will direct them to a resource where the answer can be found."

—American Reference Books Annual, 2003

"Recommended reference source."

— Booklist, American Library Association, Feb '03

Endocrine & Metabolic Disorders Sourcebook

Basic Information for the Layperson about Pancreatic and Insulin-Related Disorders Such as Pancreatitis, Diabetes, and Hypoglycemia; Adrenal Gland Disorders Such as Cushing's Syndrome, Addison's Disease, and Congenital Adrenal Hyperplasia; Pituitary Gland Disorders Such as Growth Hormone Deficiency, Acromegaly, and Pituitary Tumors; Thyroid Disorders Such as Hypothyroidism, Graves' Disease, Hashimoto's Disease, and Goiter; Hyperparathyroidism; and Other Diseases and Syndromes of Hormone Imbalance or Metabolic Dysfunction

Along with Reports on Current Research Initiatives

Edited by Linda M. Shin. 574 pages. 1998. 978-0-7808-0207-0.

"Omnigraphics has produced another needed resource for health information consumers."

—American Reference Books Annual, 2000

"Recommended reference source."

— Booklist, American Library Association, Dec '98

Environmental Health Sourcebook, 2nd Edition

Basic Consumer Health Information about the Environment and Its Effect on Human Health, Including the Effects of Air Pollution, Water Pollution, Hazardous Chemicals, Food Hazards, Radiation Hazards, Biological Agents, Household Hazards, Such as Radon, Asbestos, Carbon Monoxide, and Mold, and Information about Associated Diseases and Disorders, Including Cancer, Allergies, Respiratory Problems, and Skin Disorders

Along with Information about Environmental Concerns for Specific Populations, a Glossary of Related Terms, and Resources for Further Help and Information

Edited by Dawn D. Matthews. 673 pages. 2003. 978-0-7808-0632-0.

"This recently updated edition continues the level of quality and the reputation of the numerous other volumes in Omnigraphics' *Health Reference Series.*"

— American Reference Books Annual, 2004

"An excellent updated edition."

— The Bookwatch, Oct '03

"Recommended reference source."

— Booklist, American Library Association, Sep '98

"This book will be a useful addition to anyone's library." *— Choice Health Sciences Supplement, Association of College & Research Libraries, May '98*

". . . a good survey of numerous environmentally induced physical disorders . . . a useful addition to anyone's library."

— Doody's Health Sciences Book Reviews, Jan '98

Ethnic Diseases Sourcebook

Basic Consumer Health Information for Ethnic and Racial Minority Groups in the United States, Including General Health Indicators and Behaviors, Ethnic Diseases, Genetic Testing, the Impact of Chronic Diseases, Women's Health, Mental Health Issues, and Preventive Health Care Services

Along with a Glossary and a Listing of Additional Resources

Edited by Joyce Brennfleck Shannon. 664 pages. 2001. 978-0-7808-0336-7.

"Recommended for health sciences libraries where public health programs are a priority."
—*E-Streams, Jan '02*

"Not many books have been written on this topic to date, and the *Ethnic Diseases Sourcebook* is a strong addition to the list. It will be an important introductory resource for health consumers, students, health care personnel, and social scientists. It is recommended for public, academic, and large hospital libraries."
—*American Reference Books Annual, 2002*

"Recommended reference source."
—*Booklist, American Library Association, Oct '01*

"Will prove valuable to any library seeking to maintain a current, comprehensive reference collection of health resources. . . . An excellent source of health information about genetic disorders which affect particular ethnic and racial minorities in the U.S."
—*The Bookwatch, Aug '01*

Eye Care Sourcebook, 2nd Edition

Basic Consumer Health Information about Eye Care and Eye Disorders, Including Facts about the Diagnosis, Prevention, and Treatment of Common Refractive Problems Such as Myopia, Hyperopia, Astigmatism, and Presbyopia, and Eye Diseases, Including Glaucoma, Cataract, Age-Related Macular Degeneration, and Diabetic Retinopathy

Along with a Section on Vision Correction and Refractive Surgeries, Including LASIK and LASEK, a Glossary, and Directories of Resources for Additional Help and Information

Edited by Amy L. Sutton. 543 pages. 2003. 978-0-7808-0635-1.

". . . a solid reference tool for eye care and a valuable addition to a collection."
—*American Reference Books Annual, 2004*

Family Planning Sourcebook

Basic Consumer Health Information about Planning for Pregnancy and Contraception, Including Traditional Methods, Barrier Methods, Hormonal Methods, Permanent Methods, Future Methods, Emergency Contraception, and Birth Control Choices for Women at Each Stage of Life

Along with Statistics, a Glossary, and Sources of Additional Information

Edited by Amy Marcaccio Keyzer. 520 pages. 2001. 978-0-7808-0379-4.

"Recommended for public, health, and undergraduate libraries as part of the circulating collection."
—*E-Streams, Mar '02*

"Information is presented in an unbiased, readable manner, and the sourcebook will certainly be a necessary addition to those public and high school libraries where Internet access is restricted or otherwise problematic." —*American Reference Books Annual, 2002*

"Recommended reference source."
—*Booklist, American Library Association, Oct '01*

"Will prove valuable to any library seeking to maintain a current, comprehensive reference collection of health resources. . . . Excellent reference."
—*The Bookwatch, Aug '01*

SEE ALSO Pregnancy & Birth Sourcebook

Fitness & Exercise Sourcebook, 3rd Edition

Basic Consumer Health Information about the Physical and Mental Benefits of Fitness, Including Cardiorespiratory Endurance, Muscular Strength, Muscular Endurance, and Flexibility, with Facts about Sports Nutrition and Exercise-Related Injuries and Tips about Physical Activity and Exercises for People of All Ages and for People with Health Concerns

Along with Advice on Selecting and Using Exercise Equipment, Maintaining Exercise Motivation, a Glossary of Related Terms, and a Directory of Resources for More Help and Information

Edited by Amy L. Sutton. 663 pages. 2007. 978-0-7808-0946-8.

"This work is recommended for all general reference collections."
—*American Reference Books Annual, 2002*

"Highly recommended for public, consumer, and school grades fourth through college." —*E-Streams, Nov '01*

"Recommended reference source."
—*Booklist, American Library Association, Oct '01*

"The information appears quite comprehensive and is considered reliable. . . . This second edition is a welcomed addition to the series."
—*Doody's Review Service, Sep '01*

Food Safety Sourcebook

Basic Consumer Health Information about the Safe Handling of Meat, Poultry, Seafood, Eggs, Fruit Juices, and Other Food Items, and Facts about Pesticides, Drinking Water, Food Safety Overseas, and the Onset, Duration, and Symptoms of Foodborne Illnesses, Including Types of Pathogenic Bacteria, Parasitic Protozoa, Worms, Viruses, and Natural Toxins

Along with the Role of the Consumer, the Food Handler, and the Government in Food Safety; a Glossary, and Resources for Additional Help and Information

Edited by Dawn D. Matthews. 339 pages. 1999. 978-0-7808-0326-8.

"This book is recommended for public libraries and universities with home economic and food science programs." — *E-Streams, Nov '00*

"Recommended reference source."
— *Booklist, American Library Association, May '00*

"This book takes the complex issues of food safety and foodborne pathogens and presents them in an easily understood manner. [It does] an excellent job of covering a large and often confusing topic."
— *American Reference Books Annual, 2000*

∎

Forensic Medicine Sourcebook

Basic Consumer Information for the Layperson about Forensic Medicine, Including Crime Scene Investigation, Evidence Collection and Analysis, Expert Testimony, Computer-Aided Criminal Identification, Digital Imaging in the Courtroom, DNA Profiling, Accident Reconstruction, Autopsies, Ballistics, Drugs and Explosives Detection, Latent Fingerprints, Product Tampering, and Questioned Document Examination

Along with Statistical Data, a Glossary of Forensics Terminology, and Listings of Sources for Further Help and Information

Edited by Annemarie S. Muth. 574 pages. 1999. 978-0-7808-0232-2.

"Given the expected widespread interest in its content and its easy to read style, this book is recommended for most public and all college and university libraries."
— *E-Streams, Feb '01*

"Recommended for public libraries."
— *Reference & User Services Quarterly, American Library Association, Spring 2000*

"Recommended reference source."
— *Booklist, American Library Association, Feb '00*

"A wealth of information, useful statistics, references are up-to-date and extremely complete. This wonderful collection of data will help students who are interested in a career in any type of forensic field. It is a great resource for attorneys who need information about types of expert witnesses needed in a particular case. It also offers useful information for fiction and nonfiction writers whose work involves a crime. A fascinating compilation. All levels."
— *Choice, Association of College & Research Libraries, Jan '00*

"There are several items that make this book attractive to consumers who are seeking certain forensic data. . . . This is a useful current source for those seeking general forensic medical answers."
— *American Reference Books Annual, 2000*

Gastrointestinal Diseases & Disorders Sourcebook, 2nd Edition

Basic Consumer Health Information about the Upper and Lower Gastrointestinal (GI) Tract, Including the Esophagus, Stomach, Intestines, Rectum, Liver, and Pancreas, with Facts about Gastroesophageal Reflux Disease, Gastritis, Hernias, Ulcers, Celiac Disease, Diverticulitis, Irritable Bowel Syndrome, Hemorrhoids, Gastrointestinal Cancers, and Other Diseases and Disorders Related to the Digestive Process

Along with Information about Commonly Used Diagnostic and Surgical Procedures, Statistics, Reports on Current Research Initiatives and Clinical Trials, a Glossary, and Resources for Additional Help and Information

Edited by Sandra J. Judd. 681 pages. 2006. 978-0-7808-0798-3.

". . . very readable form. The successful editorial work that brought this material together into a useful and understandable reference makes accessible to all readers information that can help them more effectively understand and obtain help for digestive tract problems."
— *Choice, Association of College & Research Libraries, Feb '97*

SEE ALSO *Diet & Nutrition Sourcebook, Digestive Diseases & Disorders Sourcebook, Eating Disorders Sourcebook*

∎

Genetic Disorders Sourcebook, 3rd Edition

Basic Consumer Health Information about Hereditary Diseases and Disorders, Including Facts about the Human Genome, Genetic Inheritance Patterns, Disorders Associated with Specific Genes, Such as Sickle Cell Disease, Hemophilia, and Cystic Fibrosis, Chromosome Disorders, Such as Down Syndrome, Fragile X Syndrome, and Turner Syndrome, and Complex Diseases and Disorders Resulting from the Interaction of Environmental and Genetic Factors, Such as Allergies, Cancer, and Obesity

Along with Facts about Genetic Testing, Suggestions for Parents of Children with Special Needs, Reports on Current Research Initiatives, a Glossary of Genetic Terminology, and Resources for Additional Help and Information

Edited by Karen Bellenir. 777 pages. 2004. 978-0-7808-0742-6.

"This text is recommended for any library with an interest in providing consumer health resources."
— *E-Streams, Aug '05*

"This is a valuable resource for anyone wishing to have an understandable description of any of the topics or disorders included. The editor succeeds in making complex genetic issues understandable."
— *Doody's Book Review Service, May '05*

"A good acquisition for public libraries."
— *American Reference Books Annual, 2005*

■

Head Trauma Sourcebook

Basic Information for the Layperson about Open-Head and Closed-Head Injuries, Treatment Advances, Recovery, and Rehabilitation

Along with Reports on Current Research Initiatives

Edited by Karen Bellenir. 414 pages. 1997. 978-0-7808-0208-7.

Headache Sourcebook

Basic Consumer Health Information about Migraine, Tension, Cluster, Rebound and Other Types of Headaches, with Facts about the Cause and Prevention of Headaches, the Effects of Stress and the Environment, Headaches during Pregnancy and Menopause, and Childhood Headaches

Along with a Glossary and Other Resources for Additional Help and Information

Edited by Dawn D. Matthews. 362 pages. 2002. 978-0-7808-0337-4.

■

Healthy Aging Sourcebook

Basic Consumer Health Information about Maintaining Health through the Aging Process, Including Advice on Nutrition, Exercise, and Sleep, Help in Making Decisions about Midlife Issues and Retirement, and Guidance Concerning Practical and Informed Choices in Health Consumerism

Along with Data Concerning the Theories of Aging, Different Experiences in Aging by Minority Groups, and Facts about Aging Now and Aging in the Future; and Featuring a Glossary, a Guide to Consumer Help, Additional Suggested Reading, and Practical Resource Directory

Edited by Jenifer Swanson. 536 pages. 1999. 978-0-7808-0390-9.

SEE ALSO *Physical & Mental Issues in Aging Sourcebook*

■

Healthy Children Sourcebook

Basic Consumer Health Information about the Physical and Mental Development of Children between the Ages of 3 and 12, Including Routine Health Care, Preventative Health Services, Safety and First Aid,

Healthy Sleep, Dental Care, Nutrition, and Fitness, and Featuring Parenting Tips on Such Topics as Bedwetting, Choosing Day Care, Monitoring TV and Other Media, and Establishing a Foundation for Substance Abuse Prevention

Along with a Glossary of Commonly Used Pediatric Terms and Resources for Additional Help and Information.

Edited by Chad T. Kimball. 647 pages. 2003. 978-0-7808-0247-6.

SEE ALSO *Childhood Diseases & Disorders Sourcebook*

■

Healthy Heart Sourcebook for Women

Basic Consumer Health Information about Cardiac Issues Specific to Women, Including Facts about Major Risk Factors and Prevention, Treatment and Control Strategies, and Important Dietary Issues

Along with a Special Section Regarding the Pros and Cons of Hormone Replacement Therapy and Its Impact on Heart Health, and Additional Help, Including Recipes, a Glossary, and a Directory of Resources

Edited by Dawn D. Matthews. 336 pages. 2000. 978-0-7808-0329-9.

SEE ALSO *Cardiovascular Diseases & Disorders Sourcebook, Women's Health Concerns Sourcebook*

■

Hepatitis Sourcebook

Basic Consumer Health Information about Hepatitis A, Hepatitis B, Hepatitis C, and Other Forms of Hepatitis, Including Autoimmune Hepatitis, Alcoholic Hepatitis, Nonalcoholic Steatohepatitis, and Toxic Hepatitis, with

Facts about Risk Factors, Screening Methods, Diagnostic Tests, and Treatment Options

Along with Information on Liver Health, Tips for People Living with Chronic Hepatitis, Reports on Current Research Initiatives, a Glossary of Terms Related to Hepatitis, and a Directory of Sources for Further Help and Information

Edited by Sandra J. Judd. 597 pages. 2005. 978-0-7808-0749-5.

"Highly recommended."
— *American Reference Books Annual, 2006*

∎

Household Safety Sourcebook

Basic Consumer Health Information about Household Safety, Including Information about Poisons, Chemicals, Fire, and Water Hazards in the Home

Along with Advice about the Safe Use of Home Maintenance Equipment, Choosing Toys and Nursery Furniture, Holiday and Recreation Safety, a Glossary, and Resources for Further Help and Information

Edited by Dawn D. Matthews. 606 pages. 2002. 978-0-7808-0338-1.

"This work will be useful in public libraries with large consumer health and wellness departments."
— *American Reference Books Annual, 2003*

"As a sourcebook on household safety this book meets its mark. It is encyclopedic in scope and covers a wide range of safety issues that are commonly seen in the home." — *E-Streams, Jul '02*

∎

Hypertension Sourcebook

Basic Consumer Health Information about the Causes, Diagnosis, and Treatment of High Blood Pressure, with Facts about Consequences, Complications, and Co-Occurring Disorders, Such as Coronary Heart Disease, Diabetes, Stroke, Kidney Disease, and Hypertensive Retinopathy, and Issues in Blood Pressure Control, Including Dietary Choices, Stress Management, and Medications

Along with Reports on Current Research Initiatives and Clinical Trials, a Glossary, and Resources for Additional Help and Information

Edited by Dawn D. Matthews and Karen Bellenir. 613 pages. 2004. 978-0-7808-0674-0.

"Academic, public, and medical libraries will want to add the *Hypertension Sourcebook* to their collections."
— *E-Streams, Aug '05*

"The strength of this source is the wide range of information given about hypertension."
— *American Reference Books Annual, 2005*

∎

Immune System Disorders Sourcebook, 2nd Edition

Basic Consumer Health Information about Disorders of the Immune System, Including Immune System Function and Response, Diagnosis of Immune Disorders, Information about Inherited Immune Disease, Acquired Immune Disease, and Autoimmune Diseases, Including Primary Immune Deficiency, Acquired Immunodeficiency Syndrome (AIDS), Lupus, Multiple Sclerosis, Type 1 Diabetes, Rheumatoid Arthritis, and Graves' Disease

Along with Treatments, Tips for Coping with Immune Disorders, a Glossary, and a Directory of Additional Resources.

Edited by Joyce Brennfleck Shannon. 671 pages. 2005. 978-0-7808-0748-8.

"Highly recommended for academic and public libraries." — *American Reference Books Annual, 2006*

"The updated second edition is a 'must' for any consumer health library seeking a solid resource covering the treatments, symptoms, and options for immune disorder sufferers. . . . An excellent guide."
— *MBR Bookwatch, Jan '06*

∎

Infant & Toddler Health Sourcebook

Basic Consumer Health Information about the Physical and Mental Development of Newborns, Infants, and Toddlers, Including Neonatal Concerns, Nutrition Recommendations, Immunization Schedules, Common Pediatric Disorders, Assessments and Milestones, Safety Tips, and Advice for Parents and Other Caregivers

Along with a Glossary of Terms and Resource Listings for Additional Help

Edited by Jenifer Swanson. 585 pages. 2000. 978-0-7808-0246-9.

"As a reference for the general public, this would be useful in any library." — *E-Streams, May '01*

"Recommended reference source."
— *Booklist, American Library Association, Feb '01*

"This is a good source for general use."
— *American Reference Books Annual, 2001*

∎

Infectious Diseases Sourcebook

Basic Consumer Health Information about Non-Contagious Bacterial, Viral, Prion, Fungal, and Parasitic Diseases Spread by Food and Water, Insects and Animals, or Environmental Contact, Including Botulism, E. Coli, Encephalitis, Legionnaires' Disease, Lyme Disease, Malaria, Plague, Rabies, Salmonella, Tetanus, and Others, and Facts about Newly Emerging Diseases, Such as Hantavirus, Mad Cow Disease, Monkeypox, and West Nile Virus

Along with Information about Preventing Disease Transmission, the Threat of Bioterrorism, and Current Research Initiatives, with a Glossary and Directory of Resources for More Information

Edited by Karen Bellenir. 634 pages. 2004. 978-0-7808-0675-7.

"This reference continues the excellent tradition of the *Health Reference Series* in consolidating a wealth of information on a selected topic into a format that is easy to use and accessible to the general public."
— *American Reference Books Annual, 2005*

"Recommended for public and academic libraries."
— *E-Streams, Jan '05*

■

Injury & Trauma Sourcebook

Basic Consumer Health Information about the Impact of Injury, the Diagnosis and Treatment of Common and Traumatic Injuries, Emergency Care, and Specific Injuries Related to Home, Community, Workplace, Transportation, and Recreation

Along with Guidelines for Injury Prevention, a Glossary, and a Directory of Additional Resources

Edited by Joyce Brennfleck Shannon. 696 pages. 2002. 978-0-7808-0421-0.

"This publication is the most comprehensive work of its kind about injury and trauma."
— *American Reference Books Annual, 2003*

"This sourcebook provides concise, easily readable, basic health information about injuries. . . . This book is well organized and an easy to use reference resource suitable for hospital, health sciences and public libraries with consumer health collections."
— *E-Streams, Nov '02*

"Practitioners should be aware of guides such as this in order to facilitate their use by patients and their families."
— *Doody's Health Sciences Book Review Journal, Sep-Oct '02*

"Recommended reference source."
— *Booklist, American Library Association, Sep '02*

"Highly recommended for academic and medical reference collections."
— *Library Bookwatch, Sep '02*

■

Kidney & Urinary Tract Diseases & Disorders Sourcebook

SEE *Urinary Tract & Kidney Diseases & Disorders Sourcebook*

■

Learning Disabilities Sourcebook, 2nd Edition

Basic Consumer Health Information about Learning Disabilities, Including Dyslexia, Developmental Speech and Language Disabilities, Non-Verbal Learning Disorders, Developmental Arithmetic Disorder, Developmental Writing Disorder, and Other Conditions That Impede Learning Such as Attention Deficit/Hyperactivity Disorder, Brain Injury, Hearing Impairment, Klinefelter Syndrome, Dyspraxia, and Tourette's Syndrome

Along with Facts about Educational Issues and Assistive Technology, Coping Strategies, a Glossary of Re-lated Terms, and Resources for Further Help and Information

Edited by Dawn D. Matthews. 621 pages. 2003. 978-0-7808-0626-9.

"The second edition of Learning Disabilities Sourcebook far surpasses the earlier edition in that it is more focused on information that will be useful as a consumer health resource."
— *American Reference Books Annual, 2004*

"Teachers as well as consumers will find this an essential guide to understanding various syndromes and their latest treatments. [An] invaluable reference for public and school library collections alike."
— *Library Bookwatch, Apr '03*

Named "Outstanding Reference Book of 1999."
— *New York Public Library, Feb '00*

"An excellent candidate for inclusion in a public library reference section. It's a great source of information. Teachers will also find the book useful. Definitely worth reading."
— *Journal of Adolescent & Adult Literacy, Feb 2000*

"Readable . . . provides a solid base of information regarding successful techniques used with individuals who have learning disabilities, as well as practical suggestions for educators and family members. Clear language, concise descriptions, and pertinent information for contacting multiple resources add to the strength of this book as a useful tool."
— *Choice, Association of College & Research Libraries, Feb '99*

"Recommended reference source."
— *Booklist, American Library Association, Sep '98*

"A useful resource for libraries and for those who don't have the time to identify and locate the individual publications."
— *Disability Resources Monthly, Sep '98*

■

Leukemia Sourcebook

Basic Consumer Health Information about Adult and Childhood Leukemias, Including Acute Lymphocytic Leukemia (ALL), Chronic Lymphocytic Leukemia (CLL), Acute Myelogenous Leukemia (AML), Chronic Myelogenous Leukemia (CML), and Hairy Cell Leukemia, and Treatments Such as Chemotherapy, Radiation Therapy, Peripheral Blood Stem Cell and Marrow Transplantation, and Immunotherapy

Along with Tips for Life During and After Treatment, a Glossary, and Directories of Additional Resources

Edited by Joyce Brennfleck Shannon. 587 pages. 2003. 978-0-7808-0627-6.

"Unlike other medical books for the layperson, . . . the language does not talk down to the reader. . . . This volume is highly recommended for all libraries."
— *American Reference Books Annual, 2004*

". . . a fine title which ranges from diagnosis to alternative treatments, staging, and tips for life during and after diagnosis."
— *The Bookwatch, Dec '03*

Liver Disorders Sourcebook

Basic Consumer Health Information about the Liver and How It Works; Liver Diseases, Including Cancer, Cirrhosis, Hepatitis, and Toxic and Drug Related Diseases; Tips for Maintaining a Healthy Liver; Laboratory Tests, Radiology Tests, and Facts about Liver Transplantation

Along with a Section on Support Groups, a Glossary, and Resource Listings

Edited by Joyce Brennfleck Shannon. 591 pages. 2000. 978-0-7808-0383-1.

"A valuable resource."
— *American Reference Books Annual, 2001*

"This title is recommended for health sciences and public libraries with consumer health collections."
— *E-Streams, Oct '00*

"Recommended reference source."
— *Booklist, American Library Association, Jun '00*

■

Lung Disorders Sourcebook

Basic Consumer Health Information about Emphysema, Pneumonia, Tuberculosis, Asthma, Cystic Fibrosis, and Other Lung Disorders, Including Facts about Diagnostic Procedures, Treatment Strategies, Disease Prevention Efforts, and Such Risk Factors as Smoking, Air Pollution, and Exposure to Asbestos, Radon, and Other Agents

Along with a Glossary and Resources for Additional Help and Information

Edited by Dawn D. Matthews. 678 pages. 2002. 978-0-7808-0339-8.

"This title is a great addition for public and school libraries because it provides concise health information on the lungs."
— *American Reference Books Annual, 2003*

"Highly recommended for academic and medical reference collections." — *Library Bookwatch, Sep '02*

SEE ALSO *Respiratory Diseases & Disorders Sourcebook*

■

Medical Tests Sourcebook, 2nd Edition

Basic Consumer Health Information about Medical Tests, Including Age-Specific Health Tests, Important Health Screenings and Exams, Home-Use Tests, Blood and Specimen Tests, Electrical Tests, Scope Tests, Genetic Testing, and Imaging Tests, Such as X-Rays, Ultrasound, Computed Tomography, Magnetic Resonance Imaging, Angiography, and Nuclear Medicine

Along with a Glossary and Directory of Additional Resources

Edited by Joyce Brennfleck Shannon. 654 pages. 2004. 978-0-7808-0670-2.

"Recommended for hospital and health sciences libraries with consumer health collections."
— *E-Streams, Mar '00*

"This is an overall excellent reference with a wealth of general knowledge that may aid those who are reluctant to get vital tests performed."
— *Today's Librarian, Jan '00*

"A valuable reference guide."
— *American Reference Books Annual, 2000*

■

Men's Health Concerns Sourcebook, 2nd Edition

Basic Consumer Health Information about the Medical and Mental Concerns of Men, Including Theories about the Shorter Male Lifespan, the Leading Causes of Death and Disability, Physical Concerns of Special Significance to Men, Reproductive and Sexual Concerns, Sexually Transmitted Diseases, Men's Mental and Emotional Health, and Lifestyle Choices That Affect Wellness, Such as Nutrition, Fitness, and Substance Use

Along with a Glossary of Related Terms and a Directory of Organizational Resources in Men's Health

Edited by Robert Aquinas McNally. 644 pages. 2004. 978-0-7808-0671-9.

"A very accessible reference for non-specialist general readers and consumers." — *The Bookwatch, Jun '04*

"This comprehensive resource and the series are highly recommended."
— *American Reference Books Annual, 2000*

"Recommended reference source."
— *Booklist, American Library Association, Dec '98*

■

Mental Health Disorders Sourcebook, 3rd Edition

Basic Consumer Health Information about Mental and Emotional Health and Mental Illness, Including Facts about Depression, Bipolar Disorder, and Other Mood Disorders, Phobias, Post-Traumatic Stress Disorder (PTSD), Obsessive-Compulsive Disorder, and Other Anxiety Disorders, Impulse Control Disorders, Eating Disorders, Personality Disorders, and Psychotic Disorders, Including Schizophrenia and Dissociative Disorders

Along with Statistical Information, a Special Section Concerning Mental Health Issues in Children and Adolescents, a Glossary, and Directories of Resources for Additional Help and Information

Edited by Karen Bellenir. 661 pages. 2005. 978-0-7808-0747-1.

"Recommended for public libraries and academic libraries with an undergraduate program in psychology."
— *American Reference Books Annual, 2006*

"Recommended reference source."
— *Booklist, American Library Association, Jun '00*

Mental Retardation Sourcebook

Basic Consumer Health Information about Mental Retardation and Its Causes, Including Down Syndrome, Fetal Alcohol Syndrome, Fragile X Syndrome, Genetic Conditions, Injury, and Environmental Sources

Along with Preventive Strategies, Parenting Issues, Educational Implications, Health Care Needs, Employment and Economic Matters, Legal Issues, a Glossary, and a Resource Listing for Additional Help and Information

Edited by Joyce Brennfleck Shannon. 642 pages. 2000. 978-0-7808-0377-0.

"Public libraries will find the book useful for reference and as a beginning research point for students, parents, and caregivers."
— American Reference Books Annual, 2001

"The strength of this work is that it compiles many basic fact sheets and addresses for further information in one volume. It is intended and suitable for the general public. This sourcebook is relevant to any collection providing health information to the general public."
— E-Streams, Nov '00

"From preventing retardation to parenting and family challenges, this covers health, social and legal issues and will prove an invaluable overview."
— Reviewer's Bookwatch, Jul '00

Movement Disorders Sourcebook

Basic Consumer Health Information about Neurological Movement Disorders, Including Essential Tremor, Parkinson's Disease, Dystonia, Cerebral Palsy, Huntington's Disease, Myasthenia Gravis, Multiple Sclerosis, and Other Early-Onset and Adult-Onset Movement Disorders, Their Symptoms and Causes, Diagnostic Tests, and Treatments

Along with Mobility and Assistive Technology Information, a Glossary, and a Directory of Additional Resources

Edited by Joyce Brennfleck Shannon. 655 pages. 2003. 978-0-7808-0628-3.

". . . a good resource for consumers and recommended for public, community college and undergraduate libraries." *— American Reference Books Annual, 2004*

Muscular Dystrophy Sourcebook

Basic Consumer Health Information about Congenital, Childhood-Onset, and Adult-Onset Forms of Muscular Dystrophy, Such as Duchenne, Becker, Emery-Dreifuss, Distal, Limb-Girdle, Facioscapulohumeral (FSHD), Myotonic, and Ophthalmoplegic Muscular Dystrophies, Including Facts about Diagnostic Tests, Medical and Physical Therapies, Management of Co-Occurring Conditions, and Parenting Guidelines

Along with Practical Tips for Home Care, a Glossary, and Directories of Additional Resources

Edited by Joyce Brennfleck Shannon. 577 pages. 2004. 978-0-7808-0676-4.

"This book is highly recommended for public and academic libraries as well as health care offices that support the information needs of patients and their families."
— E-Streams, Apr '05

"Excellent reference." *— The Bookwatch, Jan '05*

Obesity Sourcebook

Basic Consumer Health Information about Diseases and Other Problems Associated with Obesity, and Including Facts about Risk Factors, Prevention Issues, and Management Approaches

Along with Statistical and Demographic Data, Information about Special Populations, Research Updates, a Glossary, and Source Listings for Further Help and Information

Edited by Wilma Caldwell and Chad T. Kimball. 376 pages. 2001. 978-0-7808-0333-6.

"The book synthesizes the reliable medical literature on obesity into one easy-to-read and useful resource for the general public."
— American Reference Books Annual, 2002

"This is a very useful resource book for the lay public."
— Doody's Review Service, Nov '01

"Well suited for the health reference collection of a public library or an academic health science library that serves the general population." *— E-Streams, Sep '01*

"Recommended reference source."
— Booklist, American Library Association, Apr '01

"Recommended pick both for specialty health library collections and any general consumer health reference collection." *— The Bookwatch, Apr '01*

Oral Health Sourcebook

SEE *Dental Care & Oral Health Sourcebook*

Osteoporosis Sourcebook

Basic Consumer Health Information about Primary and Secondary Osteoporosis and Juvenile Osteoporosis and Related Conditions, Including Fibrous Dysplasia, Gaucher Disease, Hyperthyroidism, Hypophosphatasia, Myeloma, Osteopetrosis, Osteogenesis Imperfecta, and Paget's Disease

Along with Information about Risk Factors, Treatments, Traditional and Non-Traditional Pain Management, a Glossary of Related Terms, and a Directory of Resources

Edited by Allan R. Cook. 584 pages. 2001. 978-0-7808-0239-1.

"This would be a book to be kept in a staff or patient library. The targeted audience is the layperson, but the therapist who needs a quick bit of information on a particular topic will also find the book useful."
— Physical Therapy, Jan '02

"This resource is recommended as a great reference source for public, health, and academic libraries, and is another triumph for the editors of Omnigraphics."
— *American Reference Books Annual, 2002*

"Recommended for all public libraries and general health collections, especially those supporting patient education or consumer health programs."
— *E-Streams, Nov '01*

"Will prove valuable to any library seeking to maintain a current, comprehensive reference collection of health resources. . . . From prevention to treatment and associated conditions, this provides an excellent survey."
— *The Bookwatch, Aug '01*

"Recommended reference source."
— *Booklist, American Library Association, Jul '01*

SEE ALSO *Healthy Aging Sourcebook, Physical & Mental Issues in Aging Sourcebook, Women's Health Concerns Sourcebook*

■

Pain Sourcebook, 2nd Edition

Basic Consumer Health Information about Specific Forms of Acute and Chronic Pain, Including Muscle and Skeletal Pain, Nerve Pain, Cancer Pain, and Disorders Characterized by Pain, Such as Fibromyalgia, Shingles, Angina, Arthritis, and Headaches

Along with Information about Pain Medications and Management Techniques, Complementary and Alternative Pain Relief Options, Tips for People Living with Chronic Pain, a Glossary, and a Directory of Sources for Further Information

Edited by Karen Bellenir. 670 pages. 2002. 978-0-7808-0612-2.

"A source of valuable information. . . . This book offers help to nonmedical people who need information about pain and pain management. It is also an excellent reference for those who participate in patient education."
— *Doody's Review Service, Sep '02*

"Highly recommended for academic and medical reference collections." — *Library Bookwatch, Sep '02*

"The text is readable, easily understood, and well indexed. This excellent volume belongs in all patient education libraries, consumer health sections of public libraries, and many personal collections."
— *American Reference Books Annual, 1999*

"The information is basic in terms of scholarship and is appropriate for general readers. Written in journalistic style . . . intended for non-professionals. Quite thorough in its coverage of different pain conditions and summarizes the latest clinical information regarding pain treatment." — *Choice, Association of College and Research Libraries, Jun '98*

"Recommended reference source."
— *Booklist, American Library Association, Mar '98*

■

Pediatric Cancer Sourcebook

Basic Consumer Health Information about Leukemias, Brain Tumors, Sarcomas, Lymphomas, and Other Cancers in Infants, Children, and Adolescents, Including Descriptions of Cancers, Treatments, and Coping Strategies

Along with Suggestions for Parents, Caregivers, and Concerned Relatives, a Glossary of Cancer Terms, and Resource Listings

Edited by Edward J. Prucha. 587 pages. 1999. 978-0-7808-0245-2.

"An excellent source of information. Recommended for public, hospital, and health science libraries with consumer health collections." — *E-Streams, Jun '00*

"Recommended reference source."
— *Booklist, American Library Association, Feb '00*

"A valuable addition to all libraries specializing in health services and many public libraries."
— *American Reference Books Annual, 2000*

SEE ALSO *Childhood Diseases & Disorders Sourcebook, Healthy Children Sourcebook*

■

Physical & Mental Issues in Aging Sourcebook

Basic Consumer Health Information on Physical and Mental Disorders Associated with the Aging Process, Including Concerns about Cardiovascular Disease, Pulmonary Disease, Oral Health, Digestive Disorders, Musculoskeletal and Skin Disorders, Metabolic Changes, Sexual and Reproductive Issues, and Changes in Vision, Hearing, and Other Senses

Along with Data about Longevity and Causes of Death, Information on Acute and Chronic Pain, Descriptions of Mental Concerns, a Glossary of Terms, and Resource Listings for Additional Help

Edited by Jenifer Swanson. 660 pages. 1999. 978-0-7808-0233-9.

"This is a treasure of health information for the layperson." — *Choice Health Sciences Supplement, Association of College & Research Libraries, May '00*

"Recommended for public libraries."
— *American Reference Books Annual, 2000*

"Recommended reference source."
— *Booklist, American Library Association, Oct '99*

SEE ALSO *Healthy Aging Sourcebook*

■

Podiatry Sourcebook, 2nd Edition

Basic Consumer Health Information about Disorders, Diseases, Deformities, and Injuries that Affect the Foot and Ankle, Including Sprains, Corns, Calluses, Bunions, Plantar Warts, Plantar Fasciitis, Neuromas, Clubfoot, Flat Feet, Achilles Tendonitis, and Much More

Along with Information about Selecting a Foot Care Specialist, Foot Fitness, Shoes and Socks, Diagnostic Tests and Corrective Procedures, Financial Assistance for Corrective Devices, a Glossary of Related Terms, and a Directory of Resources for Additional Help and Information

Edited by Ivy L. Alexander. 543 pages. 2007. 978-0-7808-0944-4.

"Recommended reference source."
— Booklist, American Library Association, Feb '02

"There is a lot of information presented here on a topic that is usually only covered sparingly in most larger comprehensive medical encyclopedias."
— American Reference Books Annual, 2002

■

Pregnancy & Birth Sourcebook, 2nd Edition

Basic Consumer Health Information about Conception and Pregnancy, Including Facts about Fertility, Infertility, Pregnancy Symptoms and Complications, Fetal Growth and Development, Labor, Delivery, and the Postpartum Period, as Well as Information about Maintaining Health and Wellness during Pregnancy and Caring for a Newborn

Along with Information about Public Health Assistance for Low-Income Pregnant Women, a Glossary, and Directories of Agencies and Organizations Providing Help and Support

Edited by Amy L. Sutton. 626 pages. 2004. 978-0-7808-0672-6.

"Will appeal to public and school reference collections strong in medicine and women's health. . . . Deserves a spot on any medical reference shelf."
— The Bookwatch, Jul '04

"A well-organized handbook. Recommended."
— Choice, Association of College & Research Libraries, Apr '98

"Recommended reference source."
— Booklist, American Library Association, Mar '98

"Recommended for public libraries."
— American Reference Books Annual, 1998

SEE ALSO Breastfeeding Sourcebook, Congenital Disorders Sourcebook, Family Planning Sourcebook

■

Prostate & Urological Disorders Sourcebook

Basic Consumer Health Information about Urogenital and Sexual Disorders in Men, Including Prostate and Other Andrological Cancers, Prostatitis, Benign Prostatic Hyperplasia, Testicular and Penile Trauma, Cryptorchidism, Peyronie Disease, Erectile Dysfunction, and Male Factor Infertility, and Facts about Commonly Used Tests and Procedures, Such as Prostatectomy, Vasectomy, Vasectomy Reversal, Penile Implants, and Semen Analysis

Along with a Glossary of Andrological Terms and a Directory of Resources for Additional Information

Edited by Karen Bellenir. 631 pages. 2005. 978-0-7808-0797-6.

Prostate Cancer Sourcebook

Basic Consumer Health Information about Prostate Cancer, Including Information about the Associated Risk Factors, Detection, Diagnosis, and Treatment of Prostate Cancer

Along with Information on Non-Malignant Prostate Conditions, and Featuring a Section Listing Support and Treatment Centers and a Glossary of Related Terms

Edited by Dawn D. Matthews. 358 pages. 2001. 978-0-7808-0324-4.

"Recommended reference source."
— Booklist, American Library Association, Jan '02

"A valuable resource for health care consumers seeking information on the subject. . . . All text is written in a clear, easy-to-understand language that avoids technical jargon. Any library that collects consumer health resources would strengthen their collection with the addition of the Prostate Cancer Sourcebook."
— American Reference Books Annual, 2002

SEE ALSO Men's Health Concerns Sourcebook

■

Reconstructive & Cosmetic Surgery Sourcebook

Basic Consumer Health Information on Cosmetic and Reconstructive Plastic Surgery, Including Statistical Information about Different Surgical Procedures, Things to Consider Prior to Surgery, Plastic Surgery Techniques and Tools, Emotional and Psychological Considerations, and Procedure-Specific Information

Along with a Glossary of Terms and a Listing of Resources for Additional Help and Information

Edited by M. Lisa Weatherford. 374 pages. 2001. 978-0-7808-0214-8.

"An excellent reference that addresses cosmetic and medically necessary reconstructive surgeries. . . . The style of the prose is calm and reassuring, discussing the many positive outcomes now available due to advances in surgical techniques."
— American Reference Books Annual, 2002

"Recommended for health science libraries that are open to the public, as well as hospital libraries that are open to the patients. This book is a good resource for the consumer interested in plastic surgery."
— E-Streams, Dec '01

"Recommended reference source."
— Booklist, American Library Association, Jul '01

■

Rehabilitation Sourcebook

Basic Consumer Health Information about Rehabilitation for People Recovering from Heart Surgery, Spinal Cord Injury, Stroke, Orthopedic Impairments, Amputation, Pulmonary Impairments, Traumatic Injury, and More, Including Physical Therapy, Occupational Therapy, Speech/Language Therapy, Massage Therapy, Dance Therapy, Art Therapy, and Recreational Therapy

Along with Information on Assistive and Adaptive Devices, a Glossary, and Resources for Additional Help and Information

Edited by Dawn D. Matthews. 531 pages. 1999. 978-0-7808-0236-0.

"This is an excellent resource for public library reference and health collections."
— American Reference Books Annual, 2001

"Recommended reference source."
— Booklist, American Library Association, May '00

■

Respiratory Diseases & Disorders Sourcebook

Basic Information about Respiratory Diseases and Disorders, Including Asthma, Cystic Fibrosis, Pneumonia, the Common Cold, Influenza, and Others, Featuring Facts about the Respiratory System, Statistical and Demographic Data, Treatments, Self-Help Management Suggestions, and Current Research Initiatives

Edited by Allan R. Cook and Peter D. Dresser. 771 pages. 1995. 978-0-7808-0037-3.

"Designed for the layperson and for patients and their families coping with respiratory illness. . . . an extensive array of information on diagnosis, treatment, management, and prevention of respiratory illnesses for the general reader." — Choice, Association of College & Research Libraries, Jun '96

"A highly recommended text for all collections. It is a comforting reminder of the power of knowledge that good books carry between their covers."
— Academic Library Book Review, Spring '96

"A comprehensive collection of authoritative information presented in a nontechnical, humanitarian style for patients, families, and caregivers."
— Association of Operating Room Nurses, Sep/Oct '95

SEE ALSO Lung Disorders Sourcebook

■

Sexually Transmitted Diseases Sourcebook, 3rd Edition

Basic Consumer Health Information about Chlamydial Infections, Gonorrhea, Hepatitis, Herpes, HIV/AIDS, Human Papillomavirus, Pubic Lice, Scabies, Syphilis, Trichomoniasis, Vaginal Infections, and Other Sexually Transmitted Diseases, Including Facts about Risk Factors, Symptoms, Diagnosis, Treatment, and the Prevention of Sexually Transmitted Infections

Along with Updates on Current Research Initiatives, a Glossary of Related Terms, and Resources for Additional Help and Information

Edited by Amy L. Sutton. 629 pages. 2006. 978-0-7808-0824-9.

"Recommended for consumer health collections in public libraries, and secondary school and community college libraries."
— American Reference Books Annual, 2002

"Every school and public library should have a copy of this comprehensive and user-friendly reference book."
— Choice, Association of College & Research Libraries, Sep '01

"This is a highly recommended book. This is an especially important book for all school and public libraries."
— AIDS Book Review Journal, Jul-Aug '01

"Recommended reference source."
— Booklist, American Library Association, Apr '01

■

Sleep Disorders Sourcebook, 2nd Edition

Basic Consumer Health Information about Sleep and Sleep Disorders, Including Insomnia, Sleep Apnea, Restless Legs Syndrome, Narcolepsy, Parasomnias, and Other Health Problems That Affect Sleep, Plus Facts about Diagnostic Procedures, Treatment Strategies, Sleep Medications, and Tips for Improving Sleep Quality

Along with a Glossary of Related Terms and Resources for Additional Help and Information

Edited by Amy L. Sutton. 567 pages. 2005. 978-0-7808-0743-3.

"This book will be useful for just about everybody, especially the 40 million Americans with sleep disorders."
— American Reference Books Annual, 2006

"Recommended for public libraries and libraries supporting health care professionals." — E-Streams, Sep '05

". . . key medical library acquisition."
— The Bookwatch, Jun '05

■

Smoking Concerns Sourcebook

Basic Consumer Health Information about Nicotine Addiction and Smoking Cessation, Featuring Facts about the Health Effects of Tobacco Use, Including Lung and Other Cancers, Heart Disease, Stroke, and Respiratory Disorders, Such as Emphysema and Chronic Bronchitis

Along with Information about Smoking Prevention Programs, Suggestions for Achieving and Maintaining a Smoke-Free Lifestyle, Statistics about Tobacco Use, Reports on Current Research Initiatives, a Glossary of Related Terms, and Directories of Resources for Additional Help and Information

Edited by Karen Bellenir. 621 pages. 2004. 978-0-7808-0323-7.

"Provides everything needed for the student or general reader seeking practical details on the effects of tobacco use." — The Bookwatch, Mar '05

"Public libraries and consumer health care libraries will find this work useful."
— American Reference Books Annual, 2005

Sports Injuries Sourcebook, 3rd Edition

Basic Consumer Health Information about Sprains and Strains, Fractures, Growth Plate Injuries, Overtraining Injuries, and Injuries to the Head, Face, Shoulders, Elbows, Hands, Spinal Column, Knees, Ankles, and Feet, and with Facts about Heat-Related Illness, Steroids and Sport Supplements, Protective Equipment, Diagnostic Procedures, Treatment Options, and Rehabilitation

Along with a Glossary of Related Terms and a Directory of Resources for Additional Help and Information

Edited by Sandra J. Judd. 651 pages. 2007. 978-0-7808-0949-9.

"This is an excellent reference for consumers and it is recommended for public, community college, and undergraduate libraries."
— *American Reference Books Annual, 2003*

"Recommended reference source."
— *Booklist, American Library Association, Feb '03*

■

Stress-Related Disorders Sourcebook

Basic Consumer Health Information about Stress and Stress-Related Disorders, Including Stress Origins and Signals, Environmental Stress at Work and Home, Mental and Emotional Stress Associated with Depression, Post-Traumatic Stress Disorder, Panic Disorder, Suicide, and the Physical Effects of Stress on the Cardiovascular, Immune, and Nervous Systems

Along with Stress Management Techniques, a Glossary, and a Listing of Additional Resources

Edited by Joyce Brennfleck Shannon. 610 pages. 2002. 978-0-7808-0560-6.

"Well written for a general readership, the *Stress-Related Disorders Sourcebook* is a useful addition to the health reference literature."
— *American Reference Books Annual, 2003*

"I am impressed by the amount of information. It offers a thorough overview of the causes and consequences of stress for the layperson. . . . A well-done and thorough reference guide for professionals and nonprofessionals alike." — *Doody's Review Service, Dec '02*

■

Stroke Sourcebook

Basic Consumer Health Information about Stroke, Including Ischemic, Hemorrhagic, Transient Ischemic Attack (TIA), and Pediatric Stroke, Stroke Triggers and Risks, Diagnostic Tests, Treatments, and Rehabilitation Information

Along with Stroke Prevention Guidelines, Legal and Financial Information, a Glossary, and a Directory of Additional Resources

Edited by Joyce Brennfleck Shannon. 606 pages. 2003. 978-0-7808-0630-6.

"This volume is highly recommended and should be in every medical, hospital, and public library."
— *American Reference Books Annual, 2004*

"Highly recommended for the amount and variety of topics and information covered." — *Choice, Nov '03*

■

Surgery Sourcebook

Basic Consumer Health Information about Inpatient and Outpatient Surgeries, Including Cardiac, Vascular, Orthopedic, Ocular, Reconstructive, Cosmetic, Gynecologic, and Ear, Nose, and Throat Procedures and More

Along with Information about Operating Room Policies and Instruments, Laser Surgery Techniques, Hospital Errors, Statistical Data, a Glossary, and Listings of Sources for Further Help and Information

Edited by Annemarie S. Muth and Karen Bellenir. 596 pages. 2002. 978-0-7808-0380-0.

"Large public libraries and medical libraries would benefit from this material in their reference collections."
— *American Reference Books Annual, 2004*

"Invaluable reference for public and school library collections alike." — *Library Bookwatch, Apr '03*

■

Thyroid Disorders Sourcebook

Basic Consumer Health Information about Disorders of the Thyroid and Parathyroid Glands, Including Hypothyroidism, Hyperthyroidism, Graves Disease, Hashimoto Thyroiditis, Thyroid Cancer, and Parathyroid Disorders, Featuring Facts about Symptoms, Risk Factors, Tests, and Treatments

Along with Information about the Effects of Thyroid Imbalance on Other Body Systems, Environmental Factors That Affect the Thyroid Gland, a Glossary, and a Directory of Additional Resources

Edited by Joyce Brennfleck Shannon. 599 pages. 2005. 978-0-7808-0745-7.

"Recommended for consumer health collections."
— *American Reference Books Annual, 2006*

"Highly recommended pick for basic consumer health reference holdings at all levels."
— *The Bookwatch, Aug '05*

■

Transplantation Sourcebook

Basic Consumer Health Information about Organ and Tissue Transplantation, Including Physical and Financial Preparations, Procedures and Issues Relating to Specific Solid Organ and Tissue Transplants, Rehabilitation, Pediatric Transplant Information, the Future of Transplantation, and Organ and Tissue Donation

Along with a Glossary and Listings of Additional Resources

Edited by Joyce Brennfleck Shannon. 628 pages. 2002. 978-0-7808-0322-0.

"Along with these advances [in transplantation technology] have come a number of daunting questions for potential transplant patients, their families, and their health care providers. This reference text is the best single tool to address many of these questions. . . . It will be a much-needed addition to the reference collections in health care, academic, and large public libraries."
— *American Reference Books Annual, 2003*

"Recommended for libraries with an interest in offering consumer health information." — *E-Streams, Jul '02*

"This is a unique and valuable resource for patients facing transplantation and their families."
— *Doody's Review Service, Jun '02*

■

Traveler's Health Sourcebook

Basic Consumer Health Information for Travelers, Including Physical and Medical Preparations, Transportation Health and Safety, Essential Information about Food and Water, Sun Exposure, Insect and Snake Bites, Camping and Wilderness Medicine, and Travel with Physical or Medical Disabilities

Along with International Travel Tips, Vaccination Recommendations, Geographical Health Issues, Disease Risks, a Glossary, and a Listing of Additional Resources

Edited by Joyce Brennfleck Shannon. 613 pages. 2000. 978-0-7808-0384-8.

"Recommended reference source."
— *Booklist, American Library Association, Feb '01*

"This book is recommended for any public library, any travel collection, and especially any collection for the physically disabled."
— *American Reference Books Annual, 2001*

SEE ALSO *Worldwide Health Sourcebook*

■

Urinary Tract & Kidney Diseases & Disorders Sourcebook, 2nd Edition

Basic Consumer Health Information about the Urinary System, Including the Bladder, Urethra, Ureters, and Kidneys, with Facts about Urinary Tract Infections, Incontinence, Congenital Disorders, Kidney Stones, Cancers of the Urinary Tract and Kidneys, Kidney Failure, Dialysis, and Kidney Transplantation

Along with Statistical and Demographic Information, Reports on Current Research in Kidney and Urologic Health, a Summary of Commonly Used Diagnostic Tests, a Glossary of Related Terms, and a Directory of Resources for Additional Help and Information

Edited by Ivy L. Alexander. 649 pages. 2005. 978-0-7808-0750-1.

"A good choice for a consumer health information library or for a medical library needing information to refer to their patients."
— *American Reference Books Annual, 2006*

Vegetarian Sourcebook

Basic Consumer Health Information about Vegetarian Diets, Lifestyle, and Philosophy, Including Definitions of Vegetarianism and Veganism, Tips about Adopting Vegetarianism, Creating a Vegetarian Pantry, and Meeting Nutritional Needs of Vegetarians, with Facts Regarding Vegetarianism's Effect on Pregnant and Lactating Women, Children, Athletes, and Senior Citizens

Along with a Glossary of Commonly Used Vegetarian Terms and Resources for Additional Help and Information

Edited by Chad T. Kimball. 360 pages. 2002. 978-0-7808-0439-5.

"Organizes into one concise volume the answers to the most common questions concerning vegetarian diets and lifestyles. This title is recommended for public and secondary school libraries." — *E-Streams, Apr '03*

"Invaluable reference for public and school library collections alike." — *Library Bookwatch, Apr '03*

"The articles in this volume are easy to read and come from authoritative sources. The book does not necessarily support the vegetarian diet but instead provides the pros and cons of this important decision. The Vegetarian Sourcebook is recommended for public libraries and consumer health libraries."
— *American Reference Books Annual, 2003*

SEE ALSO *Diet & Nutrition Sourcebook*

■

Women's Health Concerns Sourcebook, 2nd Edition

Basic Consumer Health Information about the Medical and Mental Concerns of Women, Including Maintaining Health and Wellness, Gynecological Concerns, Breast Health, Sexuality and Reproductive Issues, Menopause, Cancer in Women, Leading Causes of Death and Disability among Women, Physical Concerns of Special Significance to Women, and Women's Mental and Emotional Health

Along with a Glossary of Related Terms and Directories of Resources for Additional Help and Information

Edited by Amy L. Sutton. 746 pages. 2004. 978-0-7808-0673-3.

"This is a useful reference book, which makes the reader knowledgeable about several issues that concern women's health. It is recommended for public libraries and home library collections." — *E-Streams, May '05*

"A useful addition to public and consumer health library collections."
— *American Reference Books Annual, 2005*

"A highly recommended title."
— *The Bookwatch, May '04*

"Handy compilation. There is an impressive range of diseases, devices, disorders, procedures, and other physical and emotional issues covered . . . well organized, illustrated, and indexed." — *Choice, Association of College & Research Libraries, Jan '98*

SEE ALSO *Breast Cancer Sourcebook, Cancer Sourcebook for Women, Healthy Heart Sourcebook for Women, Osteoporosis Sourcebook*

Workplace Health & Safety Sourcebook

Basic Consumer Health Information about Workplace Health and Safety, Including the Effect of Workplace Hazards on the Lungs, Skin, Heart, Ears, Eyes, Brain, Reproductive Organs, Musculoskeletal System, and Other Organs and Body Parts

Along with Information about Occupational Cancer, Personal Protective Equipment, Toxic and Hazardous Chemicals, Child Labor, Stress, and Workplace Violence

Edited by Chad T. Kimball. 626 pages. 2000. 978-0-7808-0231-5.

"As a reference for the general public, this would be useful in any library." —*E-Streams, Jun '01*

"Provides helpful information for primary care physicians and other caregivers interested in occupational medicine. . . . General readers; professionals." —*Choice, Association of College & Research Libraries, May '01*

"Recommended reference source." —*Booklist, American Library Association, Feb '01*

"Highly recommended." —*The Bookwatch, Jan '01*

Worldwide Health Sourcebook

Basic Information about Global Health Issues, Including Malnutrition, Reproductive Health, Disease Dispersion and Prevention, Emerging Diseases, Risky Health Behaviors, and the Leading Causes of Death

Along with Global Health Concerns for Children, Women, and the Elderly, Mental Health Issues, Research and Technology Advancements, and Economic, Environmental, and Political Health Implications, a Glossary, and a Resource Listing for Additional Help and Information

Edited by Joyce Brennfleck Shannon. 614 pages. 2001. 978-0-7808-0330-5.

"Named an Outstanding Academic Title." —*Choice, Association of College & Research Libraries, Jan '02*

"Yet another handy but also unique compilation in the extensive *Health Reference Series*, this is a useful work because many of the international publications reprinted or excerpted are not readily available. Highly recommended." —*Choice, Association of College & Research Libraries, Nov '01*

"Recommended reference source." —*Booklist, American Library Association, Oct '01*

SEE ALSO *Traveler's Health Sourcebook*

Teen Health Series
Helping Young Adults Understand, Manage, and Avoid Serious Illness

List price $65 per volume. **School and library price $58 per volume.**

Alcohol Information for Teens
Health Tips about Alcohol and Alcoholism

Including Facts about Underage Drinking, Preventing Teen Alcohol Use, Alcohol's Effects on the Brain and the Body, Alcohol Abuse Treatment, Help for Children of Alcoholics, and More

Edited by Joyce Brennfleck Shannon. 370 pages. 2005. 978-0-7808-0741-9.

"Boxed facts and tips add visual interest to the well-researched and clearly written text."
— *Curriculum Connection, Apr '06*

Allergy Information for Teens
Health Tips about Allergic Reactions Such as Anaphylaxis, Respiratory Problems, and Rashes

Including Facts about Identifying and Managing Allergies to Food, Pollen, Mold, Animals, Chemicals, Drugs, and Other Substances

Edited by Karen Bellenir. 410 pages. 2006. 978-0-7808-0799-0.

Asthma Information for Teens
Health Tips about Managing Asthma and Related Concerns

Including Facts about Asthma Causes, Triggers, Symptoms, Diagnosis, and Treatment

Edited by Karen Bellenir. 386 pages. 2005. 978-0-7808-0770-9.

"Highly recommended for medical libraries, public school libraries, and public libraries."
— *American Reference Books Annual, 2006*

"It is so clearly written and well organized that even hesitant readers will be able to find the facts they need, whether for reports or personal information. . . . A succinct but complete resource."
— *School Library Journal, Sep '05*

Body Information for Teens
Health Tips about Maintaining Well-Being for a Lifetime

Including Facts about the Development and Functioning of the Body's Systems, Organs, and Structures and the Health Impact of Lifestyle Choices

Edited by Sandra Augustyn Lawton. 458 pages. 2007. 978-0-7808-0443-2.

Cancer Information for Teens
Health Tips about Cancer Awareness, Prevention, Diagnosis, and Treatment

Including Facts about Frequently Occurring Cancers, Cancer Risk Factors, and Coping Strategies for Teens Fighting Cancer or Dealing with Cancer in Friends or Family Members

Edited by Wilma R. Caldwell. 428 pages. 2004. 978-0-7808-0678-8.

"Recommended for school libraries, or consumer libraries that see a lot of use by teens."
— *E-Streams, May '05*

"A valuable educational tool."
— *American Reference Books Annual, 2005*

"Young adults and their parents alike will find this new addition to the *Teen Health Series* an important reference to cancer in teens."
— *Children's Bookwatch, Feb '05*

Complementary and Alternative Medicine Information for Teens
Health Tips about Non-Traditional and Non-Western Medical Practices

Including Information about Acupuncture, Chiropractic Medicine, Dietary and Herbal Supplements, Hypnosis, Massage Therapy, Prayer and Spirituality, Reflexology, Yoga, and More

Edited by Sandra Augustyn Lawton. 405 pages. 2006. 978-0-7808-0966-6.

Diabetes Information for Teens
Health Tips about Managing Diabetes and Preventing Related Complications

Including Information about Insulin, Glucose Control, Healthy Eating, Physical Activity, and Learning to Live with Diabetes

Edited by Sandra Augustyn Lawton. 410 pages. 2006. 978-0-7808-0811-9.

Diet Information for Teens, 2nd Edition

Health Tips about Diet and Nutrition

Including Facts about Dietary Guidelines, Food Groups, Nutrients, Healthy Meals, Snacks, Weight Control, Medical Concerns Related to Diet, and More

Edited by Karen Bellenir. 432 pages. 2006. 978-0-7808-0820-1.

"Full of helpful insights and facts throughout the book. . . . An excellent resource to be placed in public libraries or even in personal collections."
— *American Reference Books Annual, 2002*

"Recommended for middle and high school libraries and media centers as well as academic libraries that educate future teachers of teenagers. It is also a suitable addition to health science libraries that serve patrons who are interested in teen health promotion and education." — *E-Streams, Oct '01*

"This comprehensive book would be beneficial to collections that need information about nutrition, dietary guidelines, meal planning, and weight control. . . . This reference is so easy to use that its purchase is recommended." — *The Book Report, Sep-Oct '01*

"This book is written in an easy to understand format describing issues that many teens face every day, and then provides thoughtful explanations so that teens can make informed decisions. This is an interesting book that provides important facts and information for today's teens." — *Doody's Health Sciences Book Review Journal, Jul-Aug '01*

"A comprehensive compendium of diet and nutrition. The information is presented in a straightforward, plain-spoken manner. This title will be useful to those working on reports on a variety of topics, as well as to general readers concerned about their dietary health."
— *School Library Journal, Jun '01*

Drug Information for Teens, 2nd Edition

Health Tips about the Physical and Mental Effects of Substance Abuse

Including Information about Marijuana, Inhalants, Club Drugs, Stimulants, Hallucinogens, Opiates, Prescription and Over-the-Counter Drugs, Herbal Products, Tobacco, Alcohol, and More

Edited by Sandra Augustyn Lawton. 468 pages. 2006. 978-0-7808-0862-1.

"A clearly written resource for general readers and researchers alike." — *School Library Journal*

"This book is well-balanced. . . . a must for public and school libraries."
— *VOYA: Voice of Youth Advocates, Dec '03*

"The chapters are quick to make a connection to their teenage reading audience. The prose is straightforward and the book lends itself to spot reading. It should be useful both for practical information and for research, and it is suitable for public and school libraries."
— *American Reference Books Annual, 2003*

"Recommended reference source."
— *Booklist, American Library Association, Feb '03*

"This is an excellent resource for teens and their parents. Education about drugs and substances is key to discouraging teen drug abuse and this book provides this much needed information in a way that is interesting and factual." — *Doody's Review Service, Dec '02*

Eating Disorders Information for Teens

Health Tips about Anorexia, Bulimia, Binge Eating, and Other Eating Disorders

Including Information on the Causes, Prevention, and Treatment of Eating Disorders, and Such Other Issues as Maintaining Healthy Eating and Exercise Habits

Edited by Sandra Augustyn Lawton. 337 pages. 2005. 978-0-7808-0783-9.

"An excellent resource for teens and those who work with them."
— *VOYA: Voice of Youth Advocates, Apr '06*

"A welcome addition to high school and undergraduate libraries." — *American Reference Books Annual, 2006*

"This book covers the topic in a lucid manner but delves deeper into every aspect of an eating disorder. A solid addition for any nonfiction or reference collection." — *School Library Journal, Dec '05*

Fitness Information for Teens

Health Tips about Exercise, Physical Well-Being, and Health Maintenance

Including Facts about Aerobic and Anaerobic Conditioning, Stretching, Body Shape and Body Image, Sports Training, Nutrition, and Activities for Non-Athletes

Edited by Karen Bellenir. 425 pages. 2004. 978-0-7808-0679-5.

"Another excellent offering from Omnigraphics in their *Teen Health Series*. . . . This book will be a great addition to any public, junior high, senior high, or secondary school library."
— *American Reference Books Annual, 2005*

Learning Disabilities Information for Teens

Health Tips about Academic Skills Disorders and Other Disabilities That Affect Learning

Including Information about Common Signs of Learning Disabilities, School Issues, Learning to Live with a Learning Disability, and Other Related Issues

Edited by Sandra Augustyn Lawton. 337 pages. 2005. 978-0-7808-0796-9.

"This book provides a wealth of information for any reader interested in the signs, causes, and consequences

of learning disabilities, as well as related legal rights and educational interventions. . . . Public and academic libraries should want this title for both students and general readers."
— *American Reference Books Annual, 2006*

Mental Health Information for Teens, 2nd Edition
Health Tips about Mental Wellness and Mental Illness

Including Facts about Mental and Emotional Health, Depression and Other Mood Disorders, Anxiety Disorders, Behavior Disorders, Self-Injury, Psychosis, Schizophrenia, and More

Edited by Karen Bellenir. 400 pages. 2006. 978-0-7808-0863-8.

"In both language and approach, this user-friendly entry in the *Teen Health Series* is on target for teens needing information on mental health concerns."
— *Booklist, American Library Association, Jan '02*

"Readers will find the material accessible and informative, with the shaded notes, facts, and embedded glossary insets adding appropriately to the already interesting and succinct presentation."
— *School Library Journal, Jan '02*

"This title is highly recommended for any library that serves adolescents and parents/caregivers of adolescents."
— *E-Streams, Jan '02*

"Recommended for high school libraries and young adult collections in public libraries. Both health professionals and teenagers will find this book useful."
— *American Reference Books Annual, 2002*

"This is a nice book written to enlighten the society, primarily teenagers, about common teen mental health issues. It is highly recommended to teachers and parents as well as adolescents."
— *Doody's Review Service, Dec '01*

Sexual Health Information for Teens
Health Tips about Sexual Development, Human Reproduction, and Sexually Transmitted Diseases

Including Facts about Puberty, Reproductive Health, Chlamydia, Human Papillomavirus, Pelvic Inflammatory Disease, Herpes, AIDS, Contraception, Pregnancy, and More

Edited by Deborah A. Stanley. 391 pages. 2003. 978-0-7808-0445-6.

"This work should be included in all high school libraries and many larger public libraries. . . . highly recommended."
— *American Reference Books Annual, 2004*

"*Sexual Health* approaches its subject with appropriate seriousness and offers easily accessible advice and information."
— *School Library Journal, Feb '04*

Skin Health Information for Teens
Health Tips about Dermatological Concerns and Skin Cancer Risks

Including Facts about Acne, Warts, Hives, and Other Conditions and Lifestyle Choices, Such as Tanning, Tattooing, and Piercing, That Affect the Skin, Nails, Scalp, and Hair

Edited by Robert Aquinas McNally. 429 pages. 2003. 978-0-7808-0446-3.

"This volume, as with others in the series, will be a useful addition to school and public library collections."
— *American Reference Books Annual, 2004*

"There is no doubt that this reference tool is valuable."
— *VOYA: Voice of Youth Advocates, Feb '04*

"This volume serves as a one-stop source and should be a necessity for any health collection."
— *Library Media Connection*

Sports Injuries Information for Teens
Health Tips about Sports Injuries and Injury Protection

Including Facts about Specific Injuries, Emergency Treatment, Rehabilitation, Sports Safety, Competition Stress, Fitness, Sports Nutrition, Steroid Risks, and More

Edited by Joyce Brennfleck Shannon. 405 pages. 2003. 978-0-7808-0447-0.

"This work will be useful in the young adult collections of public libraries as well as high school libraries."
— *American Reference Books Annual, 2004*

Suicide Information for Teens
Health Tips about Suicide Causes and Prevention

Including Facts about Depression, Risk Factors, Getting Help, Survivor Support, and More

Edited by Joyce Brennfleck Shannon. 368 pages. 2005. 978-0-7808-0737-2.

Tobacco Information for Teens
Health Tips about the Hazards of Using Cigarettes, Smokeless Tobacco, and Other Nicotine Products

Including Facts about Nicotine Addiction, Immediate and Long-Term Health Effects of Tobacco Use, Related Cancers, Smoking Cessation, Tobacco Use Prevention, and Tobacco Use Statistics

Edited by Karen Bellenir. 440 pages. 2007. 978-0-7808-0976-5.

Health Reference Series